Y0-BXH-077

Red Cell Metabolism and Function

ADVANCES IN EXPERIMENTAL MEDICINE AND BIOLOGY

Editorial Board:

Nathan Back *Chairman, Department of Biochemical Pharmacology, School of Pharmacy, State University of New York, Buffalo, New York*

N. R. Di Luzio *Chairman, Department of Physiology, Tulane University School of Medicine, New Orleans, Louisiana*

Alfred Gellhorn *University of Pennsylvania Medical School, Philadelphia, Pennsylvania*

Bernard Halpern *Director of the Institute of Immuno-Biology, Paris, France*

Ephraim Katchalski *Department of Biophysics, The Weizmann Institute of Science, Rehovoth, Israel*

David Kritchevsky *Wistar Institute, Philadelphia, Pennsylvania*

Abel Lajtha *New York State Research Institute for Neurochemistry and Drug Addiction, Ward's Island, New York*

Rodolfo Paoletti *Institute of Pharmacology, University of Milan, Milan, Italy, and Institute of Pharmacology, University of Cagliari, Cagliari, Italy*

[International Conference on Red Cell Metabolism
and Function, 1st, University of Michigan, 1969.

Red Cell Metabolism and Function

Proceedings of the First International Conference on Red Cell
Metabolism and Function, held at the University of Michigan,
Ann Arbor, October 1-3, 1969

Edited by

George J. Brewer

Departments of Human Genetics and Medicine
(Simpson Memorial Institute)
University of Michigan
Ann Arbor, Michigan

QP96
A1
I 612r
1969
(1970)

 PLENUM PRESS • NEW YORK–LONDON • 1970

249541

Library of Congress Catalog Card Number 77-110798

SBN 306-39006-X

© 1970 Plenum Press, New York
A Division of Plenum Publishing Corporation
227 West 17th Street, New York, N.Y. 10011

United Kingdom edition published by Plenum Press, London
A Division of Plenum Publishing Corporation, Ltd.
Donington House, 30 Norfolk Street, London W.C.2, England

All rights reserved

No part of this publication may be reproduced in any form
without written permission from the publisher

Printed in the United States of America

PREFACE

In the last six years, a remarkable series of studies have demonstrated an intimate relationship between red cell metabolism and the function of the cell as an organ of gas transport. First came the demonstration of binding of organic phosphocompounds of the red cell to hemoglobin; this was followed by studies that demonstrated modification of hemoglobin oxygen affinity by such binding. At present we are in an exhilirating phase of accrual of data showing that the levels of these phosphorylated intermediates can be rapidly altered in the red cell to modulate hemoglobin function. At one time it was said that the red cell was an inert bag full of hemoglobin. Now we know not only that the cell has an active metabolism crucial to its viability, but that this metabolism is just as crucial to the whole organism in the proper adjustment of oxygen transport.

On October first, second and third, 1969, red cell biochemists, general biochemists, geneticists, cardio-pulmonary physiologists, exercise physiologists, experts in blood storage, and representatives from many other disciplines met in the Towsley Center for Continuing Medical Education at the University of Michigan, Ann Arbor, to present recent findings and discuss developments in this new interdisciplinary field. The meeting was dedicated to Dr. Alfred Chanutin, Professor Emeritus of the University of Virginia, to honor his retirement in 1967 and in recognition of his great contributions to the studies outlined in the first paragraph of this preface.

The program dealt with our present understanding of binding of organic phosphocompounds, and certain other substances, to hemoglobin, and how the binding affects oxygen dissociation properties. Interaction with the acid-base status of the blood was emphasized, as was interaction with carboxyhemoglobin, particularly in smokers. Changes in levels of phosphorylated intermediates in several hypoxic conditions, and the resulting effect on oxygen dissociation, were reported. Metabolic control mechanisms in the red cell and mechanisms of pulmonary and systemic gas transport were discussed at length. The effect of exercise on gas transport and red cell intermediates, and comparative aspects of gas transport were considered. An entire session was devoted to the serious problem of the capability of stored blood to transport oxygen after transfusion, particularly after the first 1-2 weeks of storage, in view of the marked decline of organic phosphocompounds during storage.

This volume, the Proceedings of the above Conference, represents a comprehensive coverage of these new and important developments. The major part of the volume is comprised of the formal manuscripts, which present a rich bounty of new data and formulations. At the end is appended the recorded discussions of the papers, in sequence according to the order of the presentations. In toto, the volume displays the interchange of current thinking on the problems of oxygen transport in health and disease.

The Editor would like to acknowledge the invaluable assistance of Mrs. Lynne Bowbeer in the organization of the Conference, assistance with the Conference, and in compilation of this volume. I am very grateful to Dr. John W. Eaton for generously given advice and assistance. I also thank Colonel Lawrence Rose, Dr. and Mrs. John Faulkner, Miss Lucia Feitler, Mr. David Bowbeer, Mr. Conrad Knutsen, Mr. Dinu Patel, Miss Kathleen Hilden, Mrs. Eleanor Miller, Dr. C.J.D. Zarafonetis, Dr. James Neel, Mr. Robert Richards, Mrs. Katherine French, and Dean William Hubbard, Jr. for their help and support. Financial support from the US Army Medical Research and Development Command and Abbott Laboratories made the Conference possible. The staff of Plenum Press has been most patient and helpful.

THE EDITOR

October 17, 1969

TABLE OF CONTENTS

IV. ERYTHROCYTE FUNCTION AFTER BLOOD STORAGE

Session 5 - G. Bartlett, Chairman

PARTICIPANTS

Poul Astrup, Dept. of Clinical Chemistry, Rigshospitalet, Copenhagen, Denmark

Grant Bartlett, Laboratory of Comparative Biochemistry, San Diego, California

George J. Brewer, Departments of Human Genetics and Medicine, (Simpson Memorial Institute), University of Michigan, Ann Arbor, Michigan

Alfred Chanutin, Department of Biochemistry, University of Virginia, Charlottesville, Virginia

R. Ben Dawson, US Army Medical Research Laboratory, Fort Knox, Kentucky

Carl-Henric deVerdier, Department of Clinical Chemistry, Akademiska Sjukhuset, Uppsala, Sweden

Raymond Dern, Department of Medicine, Loyola University, Chicago, Illinois

John W. Eaton, Department of Human Genetics, University of Michigan, Ann Arbor, Michigan

John Faulkner, Department of Physiology, University of Michigan, Ann Arbor, Michigan

✓ Giles Filley, Department of Physiology, University of Colorado, Denver, Colorado

Lars Garby, Department of Clinical Physiology, Akademiska Sjukhuset, Uppsala, Sweden

Eckehart Gerlach, Department of Physiology, University of Freiburg, Freiburg, Germany

Santiago Grisolia, Department of Biochemistry, University of Kansas, Kansas City, Kansas

✓ Robert Grover, Department of Medicine, University of Colorado, Denver, Colorado

Magnus Hjelm, Department of Clinical Chemistry, University Hospital, Uppsala, Sweden

J. Horejsi, Institute of Hematology and Blood Transfusion, Prague, Czechoslovakia

Claude Lenfant, Department of Medicine, University of Washington, Seattle, Washington

J.A. Loos, Central Laboratory for Blood Transfusion, Amsterdam, The Netherlands

James Metcalfe, Department of Medicine, University of Oregon, Portland, Oregon

Mikael Rørth, Department of Clinical Chemistry, Rigshospitalet,
    Copenhagen, Denmark

Zelda Rose, The Institute for Cancer Research, Philadelphia,
    Pennsylvania

Charles E. Shields, US Army Medical Research Laboratory, Fort
    Knox, Kentucky

Robert Valeri, US Naval Hospital, Chelsea, Massachusetts

John Williamson, Department of Biophysics and Biochemistry,
    University of Pennsylvania, Philadelphia, Pennsylvania

Jose Carreras Barnes, Dept. of Biochemistry, University of Kansas, Kansas City, Kansas

✓Heinz Bartels, Hannover, Germany

Albert Bernadini, Brooks Air Force Base, San Antonio, Texas

Robert H. Bigley, University of Oregon, Portland, Oregon

H. Franklin Bunn, Thorndike Memorial Laboratory, Boston City Hospital, Boston, Massachusetts.

Samuel Charache, Johns Hopkins Hospital, Baltimore, Maryland

Ching Jer Chern, Dept. of Biochemistry, Michigan State University, East Lansing, Michigan

H.B. Collier, Dept. of Clinical Pathology, University of Alberta, Edmonton, Alberta, Canada

Jane DesForges, Hematology Laboratory, Boston City Hospital, Boston, Massachusetts

Alice Diederich, Dept. of Biochemistry, University of Kansas, Kansas City, Kansas

Dennis Diederich, Dept. of Biochemistry, University of Kansas, Kansas City, Kansas

Kenneth R. Dirks, US Army Medical Research and Development Command, Washington, D.C.

Gabriel Duc, Babies Hospital, New York, New York

Knud Engel, Babies Hospital, New York, New York

Sidney E. Epstein, Abbott Laboratories, North Chicago, Illinois

Albert J. Eusebi, The Bryn Mawr Hospital, Bryn Mawr, Pennsylvania

Normand L. Fortier, Naval Blood Research Laboratory, Chelsea, Massachusetts

Bertil Glader, Dept. of the Army, Walter Reed Army Institute of Research, Washington, D.C.

Tibor J. Greenwalt, American National Red Cross, Washington, D.C.

Donald R. Harkness, Hematology Dept., Miami Veteran's Hospital, Miami, Florida

Ralph Henderson, Dept. of Biochemistry, University of Texas, Galveston, Texas

H. Clark Hoagland, Mayo Clinic, Rochester, Minnesota

Alan S. Keitt, University of Florida College of Medicine, Gainesville, Florida

Stephen Kimzey, NASA Manned Spacecraft Center, Houston, Texas

Fabian J. Lionetti, Blood Research Institute, Brookline, Massachusetts

Leonard Miller, The Children's Hospital of Philadelphia, Philadelphia, Pennsylvania

Allan J. Morris, Dept. of Biochemistry, Michigan State University, East Lansing, Michigan

William Munson, US Army Medical Research and Development Command, Washington, D.C.

Thomas F. Necheles, Boston City Hospital, Boston, Massachusetts

John C. Nixon, Dept. of Hematology, St. Joseph Mercy Hospital, Ann Arbor, Michigan

Armando R. Orlina, Michael Reese Research Foundation and Blood
    Center, Chicago, Illinois
Frank Oski, The Children's Hospital of Philadelphia, Philadelphia,
    Pennsylvania
Robert Petitt, Mayo Clinic, Rochester, Minnesota
L.F. Plzak, US Army Medical Research and Development Command,
    Washington, D.C.
Lawrence R. Rose, US Army Medical Research and Development
    Command, Washington D.C.
Robert E. Sage, Boston City Hospital, Boston, Massachusetts
J. Gerald Scott, Toronto General Hospital, Toronto, Ontario,
    Canada
A. William Shafer, University of Oklahoma, Oklahoma City,
    Oklahoma
Ernest R. Simon, Dept. of Medicine, University of New Mexico,
    Albuquerque, New Mexico
Robert F. Skora, Research and Engineering Dept., Kimberly-Clark
    Corporation, Neenah, Wisconsin
Philip Slawsky, Hematology Laboratory, Boston City Hospital,
    Boston, Massachusetts
L. Michael Snyder, Department of Hematology, Saint Vincent Hospital,
    Worcester, Massachusetts
Martin Steinberg, New England Medical Center Hospitals, Boston,
    Massachusetts
Thomas D. Stevenson, Department of Pathology, The Ohio State
    University Hospital, Columbus, Ohio
Paul Strumia, The Bryn Mawr Hospital, Bryn Mawr, Pennsylvania
Scott N. Swisher, Olin Health Center, Michigan State University,
    East Lansing, Michigan
Kouichi R. Tanaka, Department of Medicine, Harbor General Hospital,
    Torrance, California
Catherine Tanser, The Royal Victoria Hospital, Montreal, Quebec,
    Canada
John D. Torrance, Division of Hematology, University of Washington
    Hospital, Seattle, Washington
John H. Triebwasser, Brooks Air Force Base, San Antonio, Texas
W.L. Warner, Travenol Laboratories, Inc., Morton Grove, Illinois
Robert I. Weed, Dept. of Medicine, University of Rochester,
    Rochester, New York
Martin H. Welch, Veterans Administration Hospital, Oklahoma City,
    Oklahoma

DEDICATION

OF THE FIRST INTERNATIONAL CONFERENCE ON RED CELL METABOLISM
AND FUNCTION TO
DR. ALFRED CHANUTIN
UNIVERSITY OF VIRGINIA

It's a great pleasure for me to dedicate this meeting and
the Proceedings which will subsequently be published to Dr.
Alfred Chanutin, Professor Emeritus of Biochemistry, University of
Virginia.

Dr. Chanutin was born June 3, 1897 in New Haven, Connecticut.
He received his Ph.B. from Sheffield Scientific School, Yale
University in 1917. He was an Assistant in the Dept. of Medicine
at the University of Pennsylvania in 1919, an Assistant in the
Dept. of Physiology at Cornell Medical School in 1920, and
obtained his Ph.D. from Yale in 1923. He was an Instructor in
Physiology at the University of Illinois for a year and then
accepted a position as Associate Professor of Biochemistry at the
University of Virginia in 1924. He has been at Virginia since
that time. Dr. Chanutin was promoted to Professor of Biochemistry,
and became the first Chairman of the Department of Biochemistry
at Virginia, in 1929. He retired in 1967 after serving a record
term at Virginia of 38 years as a full professor.

Dr. Chanutin is a member of the Society for Experimental
Biology and Medicine, the Southern Society of Clinical Investi-
gation, the Radiation Research Society, the American Society of
Biological Chemistry, the American Chemistry Society, Alpha
Omega Alpha, and Sigma Xi. He has been a member of the Hematology
Study Section of the National Institutes of Health, and the
Subcommittee on Sterilization of Blood and Plasma of the National
Research Council. He has served as a Consultant to the Research
and Development Command, Office of the Surgeon General, to the
Medical Division of the Chemical Corps and to other groups too
numerous to mention.

Aside from his work on red cell biochemistry to which we will
turn in a moment, he is widely known for studies on creatine
metabolism, the biochemistry of renal insufficiency produced by
partial nephrectomy, the biochemical effects of chemical warfare
agents, trauma, thermal injury and Xray-irradiation, studies on
fractionation and electrophoresis of plasma proteins, and studies
on protein-calcium interaction.

But it is for his work in the field of red cell biochemistry
that we particularly wish to honor him here today. Glancing over
Dr. Chanutin's bibliography, there are some 2 dozen publications
on the red cell, mostly in the last dozen years. His interests
in the red cell, like his interests in general, are wide ranging.

His papers include work on preservation of human red cells,
metabolism of human red cells in health and disease, and electrophoresis of hemolysates of fresh and stored cells. In a series of
papers beginning in 1957, Dr. Chanutin and his co-workers began to
note differences in hemoglobin electrophoretic patterns according
to the condition of the blood e.g. the patterns were different
after the blood had been stored for long periods. In 1963
Sugita and Chanutin suggested that the alterations in electrophoretic patterns could be explained by the formation of a complex
between hemoglobin and phosphoric acid esters, such as 2,3-
diphosphoglycerate (DPG) and adenosine triphosphate (ATP), the
two phosphorylated intermediates present in largest amounts in
the human red cell. They demonstrated that incubation of stored
hemolysates with DPG and ATP would regenerate the original
electrophoretic patterns. These effects were further elucidated
and expanded in papers in 1964 and 1965. This series of
observations led Dr. Chanutin to study the effects of these same
phosphorylated intermediates on the oxygen dissociation properties
of hemoglobin, with the results published in a landmark paper in
1967 (Chanutin and Curnish, 1967) entitled "Effect of Organic
and Inorganic Phosphates on the Oxygen Equilibrium of Human
Erythrocytes." Of course, we all know the significance of these
observations. It is possibly an acceptable view that publications
beginning in 1967 from other laboratories featuring the effects of
phosphorylated intermediates on hemoglobin oxygen dissociation
properties were also stimulated by the early Chanutin papers on
the binding effects between phosphorylated intermediates and
hemoglobin.

        The papers submitted to this conference stand in testimony
to the importance of this area of study initiated in large part
by Dr. Chanutin. The story has unfolded in truly dramatic fashion
as we find that changes in levels of intermediates such as DPG
can explain long-puzzling and important phenomena such as the
differences in the oxygen dissociation curve between hemoglobin
and intact cells, and the right-shifted oxygen dissociation curve
of high altitude anemia, pulmonary disease, and of exercise.
The interdisciplinary nature of this conference demonstrates how
widespread the ramifications of this area have become. It is
obvious that the pulmonary physiologist, the exercise physiologist,
the hematologist, those interested in biochemical control
mechanisms, and those interested in blood storage, as well as
other disciplines, must take note of the red cell findings if they
are to understand oxygen transport.

        Now if I may interject a personal note. In organizing this
conference, Dr. Chanutin's advice and help have been invaluable.
And as I talked to people around the country, I became aware that
he had been just as helpful over the years to other people. This
man is beloved at his home University of Virginia and by colleagues
across this country, as well as overseas.

Dr. Chanutin, it is our pleasure to honor you with this meeting, with these contributions, and with the published volume which will result from this conference.

George J. Brewer, M.D.
Conference Chairman

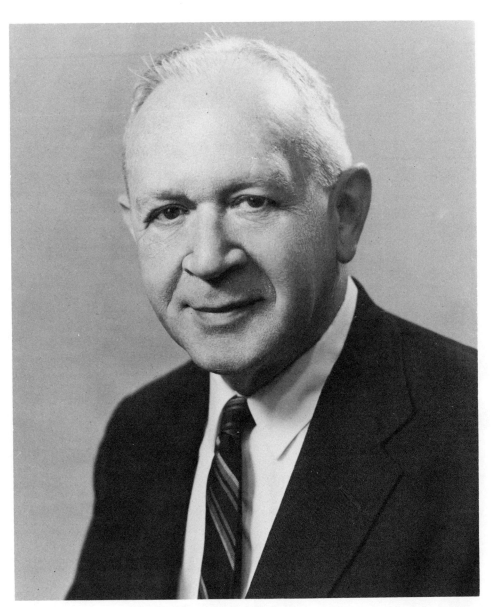

DR. ALFRED CHANUTIN

I

RELATIONSHIP BETWEEN RED CELL METABOLISM AND FUNCTION

SESSION 1 - A. Chanutin, Chairman

SESSION 2 - C.-H. deVerdier, Chairman

BINDING OF ORGANIC PHOSPHATES TO HEMOGLOBIN A AND HEMOGLOBIN F

Lars Garby and Carl-Henric de Verdier

Department of Clinical Physiology and Department of

Clinical Chemistry, University Hospital, Uppsala, Sweden

A new physiological system for the regulation of the oxygen affinity to hemoglobin has been discovered during the last two years. Addition of 2,3-diphosphoglycerate (DPG) and adenosine triphosphate (ATP) to dilute hemoglobin solutions dramatically decreased the affinity of the hemoglobin for oxygen (Benesch & Benesch, 1967; Chanutin and Curnish, 1967) and a close inverse relation was found (Akerblom et al., 1968; Engel & Duc, 1968; Lenfant et al., 1968) between the oxygen affinity and the concentration of these phosphocompounds in intact human erythrocytes.

The effect of these phosphocompounds on the oxygen affinity of the hemoglobin is most probably due to direct binding. The details of the binding are not yet clear. The data available at the present time have been obtained by using different methods as well as different solvent conditions. The present paper is an attempt to summarize the available data and to comment upon the different results.

There are three aspects of the binding that appears to be of primary interest in the present context. First, there is the question of the site(s) of binding. Second, we would like to know just how the binding is related to the conformational changes of the subunits and the tetramer that take place during loading and unloading of the oxygen. Third, in attempts to evaluate the importance of the binding for the glycolytic processes and their regulation in the intact cell it is necessary to know the numerical values of the association constants under conditions prevailing in the intact cells.

We can discuss the site(s) of binding on the basis of indirect data only. There is first the observation (Benesch & Benesch, 1969) that β chains but not α chains bind DPG. There is further the agreement that deoxygenated hemoglobin has a higher affinity to-

3

wards DPG (and ATP) (Benesch et al., 1968; Chanutin and Curnish, 1969; Garby et al., 1969) and this fact, together with the observation(Muirhead et al., 1967) that the β chains move apart by some 6 A during deoxygenation makes binding to the inside of the β chains highly attractive. The pH dependence of the binding (Garby et al., 1968; Benesch et al., 1969; Garby et al., 1969) shows increased affinity with increasing hydrogen ion concentration with an inflexion point between pH 7 and pH 8. This behaviour makes a histidine residue the most likely candidate for binding but the interpretation is complicated because of the dissociation of DPG which has two groups with an average pK of about 7. One of the histidine residues on the inside of the β chains, His β-H21, has been suggested (Garby et al., 1969; deVerdier & Garby, 1969) because of its favorable position and orientation to binding within the cavity, because both hemoglobin F (γ-H21 Ser) and hemoglobin Hiroshima (β-H21 $\rightarrow$ Asp) have a high oxygen affinity and because the affinity of DPG to hemoglobin F is markedly lower than that to hemoglobin A (deVerdier & Garby, 1969). It would be of considerable interest to find out about the DPG binding to Hb Hiroshima as well as to Hb Rainier (β-H23 Tyr $\rightarrow$ His), Hb Yakima (β-G1 Asp $\rightarrow$ His), Hb Kempsey (β-G1 Asp $\rightarrow$ Asn) which all show a high oxygen affinity.

The submolecular mechanisms by which binding of DPG might influence the conformation of the hemoglobin molecule have been discussed in some detail recently (Hamilton et al., 1969) but so far the available data do not permit any firm conclusions.

Although there is agreement that DPG binds more avidly to deoxygenated hemoglobin than to oxygenated hemoglobin (cp. above), the problem of the numerical values for the affinity of DPG to these two forms of hemoglobin has not yet been settled. Benesch, Benesch & Yu (1968) studied the binding in very dilute (about 0.5 g%) solutions of hemoglobin in 0.1 M NaCl at pH 7.3 and found no binding to oxygenated hemoglobin. Under these conditions, deoxygenated hemoglobin bound maximally 1 mole of DPG per mole of hemoglobin tetramer with an association constant of about 5×10^{-4} litres/mole at room temperature. Benesch, Benesch & Yu (1969) estimated indirectly the temperature dependence of the binding and found that the reaction was strongly exothermic: 13 kcal of heat are liberated when one mole of DPG combines with one mole of deoxyhemoglobin. Under these same conditions and at room temperature, the association constant increases to about 13×10^4 litres/ mole when the pH is lowered to 7.0 and decreases to about 1×10^4 litres/mole at pH 7.8. Chanutin & Hermann (1969) also worked with very dilute hemoglobin solutions. They used a cacodylate buffer of low ionic strength (Γ /2 0.033) and a pH of 6.5. They performed the experiments in the cold room. Under these conditions, both oxygenated and deoxygenated hemoglobin bound DPG and ATP, the affinities being higher for the deoxygenated form. Both forms showed evidence of three binding sites with one of the sites having a much larger affinity than the other two. The association constants of the "high-affinity" sites were 14×10^4 and 7×10^4 litres/mole for the deoxygenated and oxygenated forms respectively. When the differences in pH, temperature and ionic strength are taken into account it appears that the association constant for the deoxygenated form is considerably lower than that obtained by Benesch and coworkers (1968). This difference is difficult to explain. The discrepancy between the authors with respect to the binding to oxygenated hemoglobin may be due to the differences in temperature, pH and ionic strength since low values of these sol- vent parameters tend to increase the binding affinity.

Garby, Gerber, and deVerdier (1968; 1969) performed binding studies at $+4^{\circ}C$ in concentrated (about 20 g%) hemoglobin solutions in a salt medium closely approximating that in the intact erythro- cyte. Under these conditions both hemoglobin forms bound DPG with an affinity to oxygenated hemoglobin several times less than that to deoxygenated hemoglobin. Furthermore, they found evidence for (at least) three binding sites. There was a strong cooperation between the first two sites whereas the affinity for the third site was quite small. The pH dependence was rather similar to that found by Benesch et al. (1969). When the difference in temperature is taken into account, it appears that the overall affinity of deoxy- genated hemoglobin to DPG under these conditions is considerably smaller than that found by Benesch et al. (1969) and rather more similar to that found by Chanutin and Hermann (1969). The difference is difficult to explain. However, the temperature and pH dependence and also the affinity proper may be different in different hemoglo- bin concentrations.

The uncertainties involved in the comparisons between the different studies with respect to temperature, pH, ionic strength and composition makes it extremely difficult to extrapolate the data to the conditions prevailing in the intact cell with a hemo- globin concentration of about 30 g%. If such an extrapolation is nevertheless made with respect to temperature and pH, we get the following values (Table 1) for the concentration of free DPG in cells with a hemoglobin concentration of 5 mM, a temperature of $37^{\circ}C$, a pH of 7.3 and with 4, 5 and 6 mM, respectively of total DPG concentration.

Table 1. Estimates of the concentration (mM) of free 2,3-DPG in human erythrocytes in vivo

	Concentration of total DPG					
Data from	4 mM		5 mM		6 mM	
	Deox	Ox	Deox	Ox	Deox	Ox
Benesch et al. (1969)	0.2	4.0	0.5	5.0	1.2	6.0
Chanutin et al. (1969)	1.0	1.5	1.5	2.0	2.2	2.7
Garby et al. (1969)	2.0	3.0	2.5	4.0	3.0	5.0

The data have been corrected to $37^{\circ}C$ and a pH of 7.3 using the data for temperature and pH dependence given by Benesch et al.(1969).

The binding of ATP to deoxygenated and oxygenated hemoglobin has been studied by Chanutin and Hermann (1969) and by Garby, Gerber and deVerdier (1969). Chanutin and Hermann performed their studies in very dilute hemoglobin solutions at pH 6.5 in a cacodylate buffer of low ionic strength whereas Garby et al studied the binding in 20 g% hemoglobin solutions with a salt composition closely corresponding to that in intact cells. Both groups found evidence of several binding sites and also that the affinity for ATP washigher with the deoxygenated form than with the oxygenated form. Garby et al. also found a rather strong pH dependence, quite similar to that found for DPG. Both groups studied the binding at +4°C and, in view of the marked temperature dependence of the DPG binding reported by Benesch et al. (1969), extrapolation to 37°C would be very uncertain.

Although the available data do not give a firm basis for speculations concerning the influence of binding of these two organic phosphates on the glycolytic rate and its regulation in intact erythrocytes, the following points may be worth mentioning (cp. also Benesch & Benesch, 1969; Garby, Gerber & deVerdier, 1969; deVerdier, Garby & Hjelm, 1969): 1) A time-average increase in the relative concentration of deoxygenated hemoglobin in the circulation would tend to decrease the concentration of free DPG in the cells and, through a release of the product inhibition of DPG at the level of the DPG mutase reaction, increase the concentration of total (bound and free) DPG. This mechanism would be highly suitable for regulation of the erythrocyte oxygen release capacity. 2) A decrease in the blood pH would tend to decrease the total concentration of erythrocyte DPG through inhibition of the DPG mutase reaction and stimulation of the DPG phosphatase reaction. This decrease might be partly or fully compensated by the higher affinity of both hemoglobin forms for DPG at a lower pH. 3) The low pH of erythrocytes in the spleen together with the low oxygen tension in that organ would tend to increase the binding of ATP. This mechanism has been suggested (Garby et al., 1969) to be responsible for the ATP-dependent transformation of the splenic cells into rigid spheres as described by Weed and collaborators (1969). 4) The binding to hemoglobin of most other phosphocompounds in the erythrocyte is unknown. It seems to be an important task clarify this matter in the near future. The effect on oxygen binding of these compounds is probably of minor importance because of their small amounts in comparison to DPG and ATP. However, for the understanding of regulating mechanisms within the glycolytic system it is necessary to establish the free concentration of these intermediates. The problem is complicated because it is entirely possible that different compounds may compete for the same binding sites. For example, it is quite possible that the inhibitory effect of DPG on the hexokinase activity in a hemolysate (Dische, 1941) could be due to a release of glucose-6-phosphate from hemoglobin. This hypothesis is strongly supported by the lack of effect of DPG in experiments with a hemoglobin-free hexokinase preparation (deVerdier & Garby, 1965).

REFERENCES

Akerblom, O., deVerdier, C.-H., Garby, L. and Hogman, C. (1968).
    Scand. J. Clin. Lab. Invest. 21:245.
Benesch, R., Benesch, R.E. and Yu, C.I. (1968). Proc. Nat. Acad.
    Sci. 59:526.
Benesch, R. and Benesch, R.E. (1969). Nature 221:618.
Benesch, R.E., and Benesch, R., and Yu, C.I. (1969). Biochemistry
    8:2567
Benesch,R. and Benesch, R.E. (1967). Biochem. Biophys. Res. Comm.
    26:162.
Chanutin, A. and Curnish, R.R. (1967). Arch. Biochem. Biophys.
    121:96.
Chanutin, A. and Hermann, E. (1969). Arch. Biochem. Biophys. 131:180.
deVerdier, C.-H. and Garby, L. (1969). Scand. J. Clin. Lab. Invest.
    23:149.
deVerdier, C.-H., Garby, L. and Hjelm, M. (1969). Acta Soc. Med.
    Upsal. In press
Engel, K. and Duc, G. (1968). Nature 219:936.
Garby, L., Gerber, G. and deVerdier, C-H. (1968). In Stoffwechsel
    und Membranpermeabilitaet von Erytrhocyten und Thrombocyten.
    G. Thieme, Stuttgart, 1968.
Garby, L., Gerber, G. and deVerdier, C.-H. (1969). Europ. J. Biochem.
    10:110.
Hamilton, H.B., Iuchi, I., Miyaji, T. and Shibata, S. (1969). J.
    Clin. Invest. 48:525.
Lenfant, C., Torrance, J., English, G., Finch, C.A., Reynfarje, C.,
    Ramos, J. and Faura, J. (1968)., J. Clin. Invest. 47:2652.
Muirhead, H., Cox, J.M., Mazzarella, L. and Perutz, M. (1967).
    J. Mol. Biol. 28:117.
Weed, R.I., LaCelle, P.L. and Merrill, E.W. (1969). J. Clin.
    Invest. 48:795.

EFFECT OF GLUTATHIONE AND SOME OTHER SUBSTANCES ON THE OXYGEN

DISSOCIATION CURVE OF HEMOGLOBIN AND EXPERIMENTAL THERAPY OF

HEMORRHAGIC SHOCK WITH SOLUTIONS ENRICHED WITH GLUTATHIONE

J. Horejsi , M.D. D.Sc.

Medical Faculty of the Charles University, Institute
of Haematology, Prague, Czechoslovakia

I. Effect of Glutathione and Some Other Substances on the
    Oxygen Dissociation Curve of Hemoglobin

In recent years some very significant studies have been
published demonstrating the important role of reduced glutathione
(GSH) in the metabolism of the red blood cell and also its
function in protecting hemoglobin from irreversible oxidation to
methemoglobin. Glutathione also appears to play an important
role in the specific function of hemoglobin, i.e. the mediation
of oxygen transport from the atmospheric air to the tissues.
Many years ago our attention was drawn to the mechanism of
oxygen transport in different anemias, especially in pernicious
anemia. The dissociation curve of oxyhemoglobin was determined -
using classical laboratory procedures - by equilibrating blood
samples with gas mixtures of definite partial pressures of oxygen and 40 mm Hg of CO_2. The shape and position of the curve
were characterized by the so called Hill's constant, which
determines the relationship between x - partial pressure of
oxygen and y - the percentage of oxy-hemoglobin formed under
given experimental conditions.

$$K = \frac{y}{x^n\ (100-y)} \qquad\qquad n=2.5$$

Our normal values for this constant are within the range
18.10^{-4} to 39.10^{-4}. In pernicious anemia we found significantly
lower values, between 47.10^{-5} and 79.10^{-5}. This means that the
curves corresponding to these values of Hill's constant are
shifted to the right. Similar changes of the position of the
dissociation curve in anemias were described at that time also by
others (e.g. Litarczek, 1930). When trying to find an inter-

9

pretation of this phenomenon we turned our attention to the level
of GSH in erythrocytes. Preliminary experiments in which red
cells separated from the blood of patients with pernicious
anemia were suspended in normal plasma indicated that the change
of the dissociation curve was linked with the red cell and not
with the plasma. This was confirmed in studies in which normal
red cells were suspended in plasma from pernicious anemia
patients. It is very well known that GSH is present in the cell
and not in the plasma and this drew our attention to the content
of GSH in erythrocytes. In our first experiments, GSH was
determined by iodometric titration. Later we used a colorimetric
reaction with alloxan which is more specific because the UV
absorption of the alloxan-GSH complex is different from alloxan-
cysteine. The content of GSH was expressed by the so called
Index of Gabbe

$$I = \frac{GSH\ mg\ \%}{erythrocytes\ in\ millions}$$

We have found an indirect correlation, between Hill's constant and the Index of Gabbe, which is not linear, but has
approximately hyperbolic shape (Figure 1). Subsequently, we
investigated the influence of glutathione upon the dissociation
curve by experiments in vitro. After the addition of GSH to the
blood we found a distinct decrease of Hill's constant, indicating
a shift of the dissociation curve to the right. An analogous
effect is also observed when cysteine is used instead of glutathione. Both experiments are demonstrated in Figure 2.

The blocking of SH groups by heavy metals (e.g. organic
compounds of mercury such as phenylmercuric borate) has the
opposite effect. In this case, Hill's constant increases and the
dissociation curve shifts to the left. This effect of mercuric
compounds was also observed by Riggs and Wollbach (1956) who
assumed an influence of GSH upon the interaction of heme units.
The effect of mercuric compounds can be suppressed by the addition
of either GSH or cysteine. The results of one such experiment
are presented in Figure 3.

In another series of experiments we used crystalline human
hemoglobin which was prepared by Drabkin's method from hemolyzed
blood. The results of these experiments are rather peculiar. The
solutions of pure crystalline hemoglobin, free from stroma, did
not exhibit any effect of GSH on the dissociation curve. However,
when stroma previously separated from the hemolysate were added to
the solution of purified hemoglobin, the effect of GSH on the
dissociation curve reappeared. We assumed therefore that the
effect of GSH on the dissociation curve of hemoglobin was influenced
by some component present in the membrane of the erythrocyte.

It is well known that the membrane of the erythrocyte contains significant carbonic anhydrase activity. The role of this
enzyme in the transportation of CO_2 by the red cell is well known.

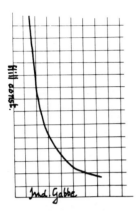

1. The relation of
   Hill's constant
   and index of Gabbe

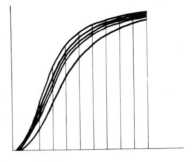

2. Right-side shift of
   the dissoc. curve
   caused by rising conc.
   of GSH (5-10-15-20 mg%)

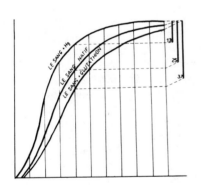

3. Shifts of the dissoc.
   curve caused by GSH
   and Hg salt

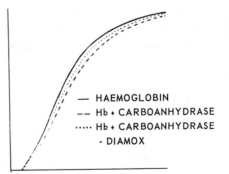

4. Shift of the dissoc.
   curve caused by
   carbonanhydrase

We wondered if carbonic anhydrase might also influence the oxygen dissociation curve of hemoglobin. We have purified carbonic anhydrase according to the technique of Keilin and Mann, and added it to whole blood and hemolysates. The results (see Figure 4) indicate that increasing concentrations of carbonic anhydrase are accompanied by progressive shifts of the dissociation curve to the right, and that the addition of GSH further increases this phenomenon. Further, blocking of the carbonic anhydrase activity by either cyanate or by Diamox has an opposite effect, shifting the dissociation curve to the left.

The Bohr effect, in the opinion of some authors is due to the influence of SH groups, decreasing attractive forces between proton and sulphur. This is caused by the shift of an electron in the supposed coupling which occurs in the course of oxygenation. The linkage between vinyl and sulfhydryl radicals increases the stability of the bivalent iron by oxidation or by activation of pi electrons.

SH compounds belong to a group of agents with oxidoreducing power. Therefore, in our experiments we tried to find out if any other oxidoreducing substance would prove to have an effect similar to that of GSH. For these experiments we have used ascorbic acid in concentrations from 0.3 to 1.0 mg in 10 ml of blood. The pH of the solution of ascorbic acid was adjusted to pH 7.0 immediately before use. Our results indicate that with higher concentrations of ascorbic acid in the blood or hemolysates there is a distinct shift of the dissociation curve to the right (Figure 5). The relation of Hill's constant and concentration of ascorbic acid is a linear and negative (Figure 6). The influence of ascorbic acid may be diminished or abolished through addition of the salts of Cu $(CuCl_2)$.

The present experimental results do not give us a satisfactory explanation of the mechanism of action of ascorbic acid. We have observed that ascorbic acid increases the effect of carbonic anhydrase. On the other hand (in contrast with the influence of GSH on the dissociation curve) ascorbic acid is active also in solutions of pure crystalline hemoglobin, in the absence of erythrocytic stroma.

Another significant difference between GSH, cysteine, and ascorbic acid was observed in biological experiments in which reduced GSH was used for treatment of severe experimental hemorrhagic shock in dogs. I shall speak about these experiments in more detail later in this paper. Here I should like to say only that GSH, added either to the blood or blood-expanders, increases the survival of experimental animals whereas cysteine and ascorbic acid are absolutely ineffective.

I should like to report now on another series of experiments in which we have studied some problems of synthesis of GSH in the red cell. The synthesis of GSH from its constituent

amino acids (glycine, cysteine, and glutamic acid) proceeds very
quickly. Detectable incorporation of C^{14} glycine and of S^{35}
cysteine occurs in 4 1/2 hours. It is interesting that the
incorporation of C^{14} glutamic acid has not been fully proved. In
our experiments we were able to prove - using chromatography of
extracellular medium and of the hemolysate - that glutamic acid
almost did not penetrate into the red cell. On the other hand
glutamine penetrates easily and is being incorporated into GSH.

Our attention has been directed to two questions:

1) Can the synthesis of GSH be accomplished also with
precursors other than the three constituent aminoacids? Speaking
more concretely: Can methionine provide sulphur for the formation
of cysteine in the presence of serine?

2) Can GSH be synthetised only by the intact red cell or
also by its stroma?

In our experiments we used the colorimetric method with
alloxan for the determination of GSH. In another series of
experiments we used labeled amino acids - S^{35} methionine and
cysteine and measured the activity of GSH, isolated by precipi-
tation with cadmium salt.

A. Erythrocytes from fresh ACD blood were used. The washed
cells were incubated in Ringer-phosphate buffer containing
glucose and adenine-1-phosphate and corresponding quantities of
amino acids. Time of incubation was 3 hours at 37°C in Warburg
vessels filled with nitrogen.

When erythrocytes were incubated in the glutamic acid-
glycine-cysteine mixture in the presence of adenylate, the increments of GSH in 3 hours were about 200 uM (209-579 uM, the
average being 297 uM). Erythrocytes incubated in Ringer phosphate
buffer only, with no amino acids added, served as controls.
Increments of GSH in this case varied from 5.5 - 68 uM (average
29.1).

On incubating red cells in mixtures of amino acids where
methionine and serine were added instead of cysteine, the increase
of GSH reached the same values as were found in previous
experiments with added cysteine (164 - 328 uM, average 220 uM).

B. Stroma was prepared from erythrocytes isolated from
fresh ACD blood by hemolysis with distilled water and ether.

Suspensions of stroma in Ringer-phosphate buffer were
incubated with glycine, glutamic acid, cysteine, and adenylate.
In one series of experiments ATP was added, in another, ommitted.
In another series of experiments methionine was substituted for
cysteine, alpha-oxoglutaric acid for serine and glutamic acid.
In experiments where stroma was suspended in the incubation
mixture containing glycine, glutamic acid and cysteine, the
average increment of GSH was about 210 uM (112-297 uM). But in
the mixtures containing methionine and serine instead of cysteine
no GSH formation was observed. The results of all mentioned

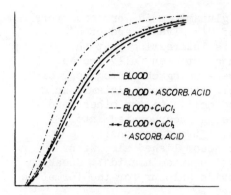

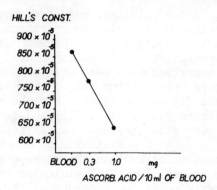

5. Shift of the dissoc. curve caused by as-corbic acid

6. The relation of Hill´s const. and conc. of ascorbic acid

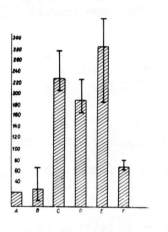
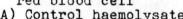

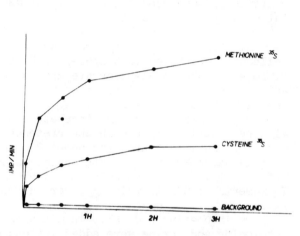

7. Synthesis of GSH in red blood cell
A) Control haemolysate
B) Red cell suspension incub. 3 hrs.
C) Red cell suspension incub. with glu-gly-meth.-ser.
D) Stroma incub. with glu-gly-cys.
E) Red cell suspension incub. with glu-gly-cys.
F) Stroma incub. with glu-gly-meth.-ser.

8. Incorpor. of cysteine ^{35}S and methionine ^{35}S into GSH of the red cell

experiments are summarized in Figure 7.

     C. In the last series of experiments, the direct incorporation of 35 cysteine and of methionine was followed. Washed red cells were incubated in Ringer-phosphate buffer solution containing adenine-l-monophosphate, glycine, glutamic acid, methionine, and serine. Labeled methionine was added in quantities corresponding to an activity of 30 uC and the rest of the total necessary amount was supplemented by non-radioactive amino acid. In another set of xperiments cysteine was used instead of methionine and serine, while other experimental conditions remained the same. The mixture was incubated for 3 hours at 37°C in a Warburg apparatus, vessels filled with nitrogen. After the incubation period, the red cells were hemolysed, the hemolysates deproteinized and GSH was isolated by precipitation with Cd^{++} salt. The precipitate was isolated by centrifugation, washed, and suspended in double-distilled water. After being dissolved in phosphoric acid, an aliquot was dried and the activity of the sample measured by GM tube. Results of measurements represented by the number of impulses per 3 min. are given in Figure 8.

     From all experiments reported here we have concluded:
     1) The human erythrocyte can synthesize GSH from its constituent amino acids under anaerobic conditions in the presence of adenylate. The erythrocyte stroma has the same capacity. Intact erythrocytes can synthesize GSH not only from glycine, cysteine and glutamic acid, but also from methionine and serine instead of cysteine, and alpha-oxoglutaric acid in place of glutamic acid or glutamine. The transsulfuration is probably the same as has been described in the liver - intermediate products being cystathionine and homocysteine. The transamination of alpha-oxoglutaric acid to glutamic acid has been described in our laboratories by Mircevova and also by Sass (1963).
     The synthesis of GSH from methionine cannot be detected with isolated stroma. The enzymes necessary for transsulfuration are probably present in the erythrocytic medium and are removed with hemolysis.
     2) GSH has a definite influence on dissociation curve of oxyhemoglobin. Its higher concentrations in blood cause the right side shift of the curve, whereas blocking of SH is characterized by left shift. Similar influences on the shape and position of the dissociation curve are displayed also by cysteine, carbonic anhydrase and ascorbic acid. However, only the addition of GSH to the blood or blood expanders will produce a therapeutic effect in severe experimental hemorrhagic shock.
     It is not yet possible to give an interpretation of the reasons for the influence of GSH on the dissociation curve of hemoglobin. It has been proved that GSH added to the medium (be it saline, ACD or plasma) in which red cells are suspended, does

not penetrate into the cell, and in spite of that it has an influence on the dissociation curve. This is perhaps due to the shift of electric charges resulting from the accumulation of a greater number of free SH reactive groups on the surface of the red cell. This charge shift could cause the changes of configuration of the hemoglobin molecule which, it is now known, take place during the oxygenation and deoxygenation of hemoglobin.

In our laboratory experiments have been proposed to resolve this question through studies of the interrelations of hemoglobin structure and function.

II. Experimental Therapy of Hemorrhagic Shock with Solutions Enriched with Glutathione

In the first half of my paper I have tried to demonstrate how the dissociation curve of hemoglobin can be influenced by reduced GSH and some other agents (carbonic anhydrase and ascorbic acid).

We have found that on increasing the content of GSH in blood or hemolysate, the dissociation curve of oxyhemoglobin shifts to the right. This change has (as is evident from Figure 2) quite significant influence upon the quantity of oxygen released from a given quantity of oxygen is, under these conditions, significantly higher. This effect seems to give at least partial explanation of the clinical observation that some anemias, in particular pernicious anemia, are not accompanied by a more serious hypoxia, even if the anemia is quite severe. This observation stimulated further studies on the possible utilization of this effect for therapeutic purposes. Our experimental studies were performed on a series of 260 dogs.

The experiments in dogs were carried out with a standard model of severe hemorrhagic shock. In dogs of the average weight 17.5 kg the arteria and vena femoralis were prepared and into the artery one side a manometer was inserted and from the artery on the other side blood was let out at a rate of 1 ml/kg/min until the blood pressure sank to 110 torr. Then the blood letting was continued so that during the following 15 min. the blood pressure dropped to 40 torr. The pressure was maintained for 60-80 min. at this level. The blood which was let out was used for preparation of blood preserves. After the expiration of the period of hypotension, the infusion of either blood or another blood expander was started at a rate of 1 ml/kg/min. The total volume of the liquid infused varied according to the previous loss of blood.

Under these experimental conditions, about 50% of the experimental animals died when treated with the transfusion of blood. Another series of animals was treated with blood to which GSH had been added. First, the dosage of GSH necessary for a manifest therapeutic effect had to be established. We used blood preserves fortified with 8, 16, and 40 mg per 100 ml of GSH. As is apparent from Figure 9, the optimal effect was obtained with the concentration of 40 mg/100 ml of blood. At this concentration more than 90% of the experimental animals survived the acute loss of blood.

This therapeutic effect is evidently produced by the increased content of GSH in the blood preserve, as follows from several circumstances:

1) There exists an apparent direct proportionality between the therapeutic effect and the dose of GSH used.

2) Other compounds containing SH groups did not exhibit any therapeutic effect. The addition of cysteine to the blood had no detectable effect.

3) The addition of amino acid constituents of GSH (glutamic acid, cysteine, and glycine) in respective molar proportions corresponding to 40 mg of GSH did not exhibit any favorable therapeutic effect.

In 18 dogs which had received blood containing 40 mg % GSH, we investigated the changes of the dissociation curve of oxy-hemoglobin. The Hill's constant values were determined before the experiment, immediately after the administration of blood with GSH, and finally 1 and 2 hrs. later. The results are presented in the table below.

	Aver. val.	Range
Hill's const. in control blood	$3,39.10^{-4}$	$1,30.10^{-4} - 8,4.10^{-4}$
Hill c. after the applic. of GSH	$1,34.10^{-4}$	$3,0.10^{-5} - 2,9.10^{-4}$
Hill c. after 1 hr.	$1,45.10^{-4}$	$7,7.10^{-5} - 1,95.10^{-4}$
Hill c. after 2 hrs.	$2,40.10^{-4}$	$1,10.10^{-4} - 7,8.10^{-4}$

The administration of blood with GSH causes a decrease of Hill's constant which means a shift of the dissociation curve to the right. The decrease remains at almost the same value during the first hour, and even after 2 hrs the values do not return to the initial level. Such a course was observed in all experimental animals with a single exception in which no change followed the administration of GSH. A subsequent analysis of GSH solution administered revealed that the greater part of GSH was present in oxidized form (our solutions of GSH are always prepared immediately before use, and are kept under nitrogen till the time of use. In the single case mentioned above, a solution which had been stored for a relatively long period was used).

In a control experiment on a group of 3 dogs, to which pre-served blood containing 50 mg% of ascorbic acid was administered, no therapeutic effect was observed, and the changes of the Hill's

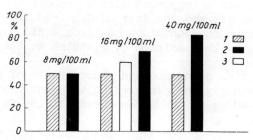

9 .   The survival of experimental animals submitted to standardized haemorrhagic shock and treated with blood, packed cells and blood fortified with GSH (blood
pressure 40 mm Hg/70 minutes)

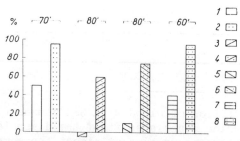

10 .   The influence of fortification with glutathione on the survival of dogs exposed
to severe haemorrhagic shock and treated with blood, dextran and modified hetero-
plasma (1 = blood; 2 = blood with GSH; 3 = mean-molecular dextran; 4 = mean-
molecular dextran with GSH; 5 = high-molecular dextran; 6 = high-molecular
dextran with GSH, 7 = modified bovine serum; 8 = modified bovine serum with GSH)

constant were insignificant.

In our further experiments we tried to prove the therapeutic effect of blood expanders used in treatment of hemorrhagic shock. We used the most important types of substitutive solutions: despecified (antigenic properties removed by processing) bovine plasma, hemoplasma, BK8 solution (a Russian plasma expander), Subtosan, Dextran (both of medium and high molecular weight), Macrodex and homologous plasma. Administration of these solutions without GSH for treatment of hemorrhagic shock (the same standard model was used as described before) give favorable therapeutic results in between 60 - 70% of the dose.

In Figure 10 the therapeutic results achieved with different preparations fortified with GSH are demonstrated. In the group treated with blood with GSH added, 95% survived (in contrast to 50% treated with blood alone). Very marked differences are apparent in both groups treated with Dextran. The group receiving Dextran of medium molecular weight had 100% mortality, while the addition of GSH raised the precentage of survival to 60%. In the group treated with high molecular weight Dextran the results were still more favorable - a survival rate of 75% (vs 15% in the controls). Fortification with GSH showed a favorable effect also in the administration of despecified bovine plasma 85% survival vs 45% in controls. All our results were statistically evaluated with the aid of X^2 test and all were highly significant.

In our experiments GSH appeared to be a substance favorably influencing the treatment of experimental hemorrhagic shock. The interpretation of this effect is not easy. The shift of the dissociation curve to the right observed at an increased concentration of GSH in the blood both in vitro and in vivo may certainly favorably influence the conditions regulating the supply of oxygen to the tissues. In our opinion, however, this is only a partial interpretation of the whole mechanism. GSH plays an important role in the metabolism not only of the red cell but also of other tissues. GSH plays an important role in the activation and preservation of activity of enzymes which are SH dependent and this might perhaps offer additional explanation of our observations. Further experiments concerning this problem are now in progress and we have completed necessary preparations for the application of GSH fortification in treatment of hemorrhagic shock in humans.

REFERENCES

Bunn, H.F., May, M.H., Kocholaty, W.F., Schields, Ch.E. (1969).
    J. Clin. Invest. 48:311.
Drabkin, D.L. (1949). Arch. Biochem. 21,1:224.
Horejsi, J. (1933). Cas. lek. ces. 72:227.
Horejsi, J. (1933). Cas. lek. ces. 72:287.
Horejsi, J. (1961). Problemi gematologii i perelivanija krovi.
    9:30.

Horejsi, J. (1968). Pokroky v biochemii (Advances in Biochemistry.
    Glutathione, Its Significance for the Function of the Red
    Blood Cell). Stat.zdrav.naklad., Praha.
Horejsi, J., and Komarkova, A. (1960). Clin. Chim. Acta 5:392.
Horejsi, J., and Sterba, O. (1966). Folia Haemat. 86:220
Horejsi, J., Lehky, T., Mircevova, L., Nikl, J., Perez, R.,
    Sterba, O., and Zmeskalova, D. (1961). Physiologia Bohemo-
    Slovenica.
Huisman, T.H.J., Dogy, A.M., Horton, B.F., and Nechtman, C.M.
    (1966). J. Lab. Clin. Med. 67:355.
Litarczek, G., Aubert, Cosmulesco, Comanesco (1930). Le Sang
    4,2:188.
Murawski, K., Zakrzewski, K. (1964). Acta Biochem. Polon. 11:379.
Riggs, A., Wolbach, R.A. (1956). J. Gener. Physiol. 39,4:585.
Sass, M.D. (1963). Nature 200:1209.
Taylor, J.F., Antonini, E., and Wyman, J. (1963). J. Biol. Chem.
    238:2660

VARIATION IN 2,3-DIPHOSPHOGLYCERATE AND ATP LEVELS IN HUMAN

ERYTHROCYTES AND EFFECTS ON OXYGEN TRANSPORT

John W. Eaton, George J. Brewer, Jerome S. Schultz, and
Charles F. Sing
University of Michigan, Depts. of Human Genetics,
Medicine (Simpson Memorial Institute), and Chemical
Engineering

INTRODUCTION

The discovery of the effects of 2,3-diphosphoglycerate (DPG) and adenosine triphosphate (ATP) on the oxygen dissociation characteristics of hemoglobin (Chanutin & Curnish, 1967; Benesch & Benesch, 1967) has greatly increased our appreciation of the association between red cell metabolism and function. Recent evidence makes it clear that, through variations in the levels of ATP and DPG, the metabolism of the human red cell may help maintain normoxia. Increases in the concentration of DPG will produce corresponding decreases in the oxygen affinity of hemoglobin. Elevation of red cell DPG content and shifting of the hemoglobin-oxygen dissociation curve to higher pO_2's have been observed in a number of conditions characterized by hypoxia, such as exposure to high altitude (Lenfant et al., 1968; Eaton et al., 1968), anemia and pulmonary disease (Brewer & Eaton, 1969). Significant adjustments in the level of DPG in the circulating red cell may occur quite rapidly, as will be discussed in the paper by Faulkner (this volume).

Other physiological variables known to have significant effects on the position of the dissociation curve, such as temperature or pH, are not usually changed enough in vivo to

This work was supported in part by NIH Grants 5-T01-GM-71-11, AM 09381, GM 15152, NIH Career Development Award AM07959 (GJB), by US AEC Contract AT (11-1)-1552 and in part by Contract DADA 17-69-C-9103 with the US Army and Navy Medical Research and Development Commands. A portion of this work was presented in preliminary form at the Central Society for Clinical Research.

modify greatly the amount of oxygen delivered by the blood. Increases in the levels of DPG within the red cell, however, require
only the gradual accumulation of a normal intermediate of red cell
metabolism. A subtle metabolic modulation of this sort has none
of the associated side effects which normally accompany, for
instance, a large change in blood pH.

In this paper, we intend to discuss the relationship of levels
of red cell DPG and ATP to the gas transport function of the red
cell. We shall consider some examples of the ways in which DPG
and, therefore, the metabolism of the red cell are used to make
both gross and fine adjustments to variations in the availability
of oxygen.

VARIATION IN LEVELS OF RED CELL DPG

The concentration of erythrocyte DPG appears to be quite
responsive to the oxygen delivery demands which are placed on the
red cell. In a sample of normal individuals, it has been found
that whole blood hemoglobin (which is presumably an approximation
of the oxygenating capacity of the blood) and red cell DPG are
negatively correlated (Eaton & Brewer, 1968a and 1968b).
Individuals who, for one reason or another, have relatively high
whole blood hemoglobin levels usually display DPG concentrations
which are lower than normal. On the other hand, those with low
hemoglobins will probably have rather high DPG levels. This
relationship in conjunction with further data to be presented
here indicate that red cell DPG concentration may be of use as a
"fine tuning" mechanism for the respiratory system, allowing a
more perfect integration of oxygen transport with level of oxygen
use.

It is now known that an increase of the red cell DPG concentration may be a significant adaptive mechanism in hypoxias of
various etiologies. Blood from residents of higher altitudes has
been found to have a right shifted oxygen dissociation curve and,
as has been recently reported, relatively high levels of red cell
DPG (Lenfant et al., 1968; Eaton et al., 1968). The excellent
work of Lenfant and co-workers has demonstrated that increased
levels of red cell DPG may be seen in individuals transferred to
higher altitudes as soon as six hours after exposure (Lenfant et
al., 1968). They report that this adjustment (and the associated
curve shift) is complete after 24 hours. It is not yet certain
how great a part in man's altitude adaptation the increase in
red cell DPG levels plays, but the shift of the oxygen dissociation
curve to the right has frequently been cited as a central part of
altitude adaptation in the human (for example, Hurtado, 1964).

Elevations in levels of red cell DPG also seem to be involved
in adaptation to the stress of prolonged exercise. In a group of
10 individuals engaged in a game of basketball, the red cell DPG
was found to be elevated 20% over the baseline values after one
hour of play. Further work employing a bicycle ergometer has

shown that the amount of change in red cell DPG levels is closely related to the physical stress as reflected in the elevation of blood lactate (r = +0.743, $p <$ 0.01) (Eaton et al., 1969). We do not yet know how great a change may be produced in DPG during exercise, but the increases we have noted during only one hour of exercise are probably of significance in increasing the delivery of oxygen to the active muscle beds.

The mechanism usually advanced to explain the DPG rise during hypoxia has been that of the increasingly desaturated hemoglobin binding more DPG, and the enzymes of glycolysis replacing the newly bound DPG with enough free DPG to restore the previous free levels (Eaton & Brewer, 1968a; Benesch and Benesch, 1969). This, then, would produce an over-all increase in the level of red cell DPG. As indirect support of this theory, we have found that exposure of rats to hyperoxia will result in a decrease of the levels of both ATP and DPG within the circulating red cell (Brewer & Eaton, unpublished observations). This reduction in ATP and DPG during exposure to hyperoxia is probably brought about through the average saturation of the red cell being increased. This, in turn, should produce transiently higher levels of free ATP and free DPG which are subsequently reduced. The results of exposure to both hyperoxia and hypoxia, then, indicate that the state of oxygenation of the red cell is at least one of the factors controlling the amounts of ATP and DPG within the circulating red cell. In this way, the oxygen delivering capacity of the red cell may be governed, at least in part, by a relatively simple feed-back system, in which the functioning of the red cell is maintained at an adequate level merely by factors in the cell "sensing" the amount of oxygen which the cell is called upon to transport. Evidence for an additional possible mechanism will be presented in a subsequent paper by Brewer et al.

EFFECTS OF DPG VARIATION IN OXYGEN TRANSPORT

Introduction

Among those studying the red cell and oxygen transport, it has been the dogma for quite some time that a shift of the dissociation curve to the right will significantly increase the amount of oxygen which is delivered to the tissues. However, as far as we are aware, there has been little or no experimental evidence gathered to support this assumption. The relevance of the oxygen dissociation curve to the physiological uptake and release of oxygen is quite indirect. The curve is constructed by measuring the saturation of hemoglobin with oxygen after equilibration with gas mixtures of specific oxygen tensions. However, under physiological conditions, the red cell does not come to equilibrium with tissue oxygen tensions. Because of this, the rate of oxygen release, as well as the pO_2 at which it occurs, is vitally important. In the following section, which deals with some experimentally derived data on the rate of oxygen exchange, the variations in oxygen delivery by whole blood which may result in part from differences in the concentrations of red cell DPG are considered.

As far as we are aware, there is no satisfactory answer available as to what a given shift in the oxygen dissociation curve means as far as changes in oxygen delivery _in vivo_. Previous studies of the rate of oxygen uptake and release by single red cells and by red cells mixed with saline have shown that significant differences exist between the cells of different individuals. These differences have been ascribed by at least one author to variations in the red cells themselves (Baumberger _et al._, 1967).

Unfortunately, all previously employed techniques of measuring rates of oxygen uptake and release by red cells involve lengthy preparations, resulting in the red cell's being in an unphysiologic state by the time the measurements were made. Further, no extensive comparative work had been done on groups of more than ten or fifteen individuals. Finally, no previous work had attempted to relate variations in the rates of oxygen uptake and release to differences in the metabolic state of the red cell.

We have designed and built an apparatus called a "rogeometer" (for rate of gas exchange-ometer) which permits rapid and relatively simple measurement of the rate at which whole fresh blood will release oxygen. A description of this apparatus and of our preliminary results with it follow.

Materials and Methods

Normal subjects were laboratory personnel and staff members of the University of Michigan Medical Center. All patients were selected from the wards and outpatient clinics of the University Hospital. Patients were considered significantly anemic if their hemoglobin levels were below 12.0 grams% for males and 11.0 grams% for females. Patients with pulmonary or vascular disease producing significant hypoxia as indicated by abnormal pulmonary function and blood gas studies were also included. The specific diagnoses of the various patients are indicated in the tables.

Hemoglobin values and hematocrit levels of whole blood were determined by standard hematologic techniques. Assay of erythrocyte ATP was carried out by a previously described method (Brewer & Powell, 1966), which was adapted to smaller quantities of blood. During these studies we observed that acid-citrate-dextrose used as an anticoagulant added to the color development in the chromatropic acid method. For this reason we have employed heparin, which does not contribute color. One-half ml of blood was precipitated with 2 ml of 6.7% trichloracetic acid (TCA). After extraction of the TCA with ether, the extract was used for the measurement of both ATP and DPG. Because of the inaccuracies involved in measuring these small quantities, the final volume of

the TCA extract was assumed to be the sum of the volumes of blood
and TCA used (2.5 ml). (In the original methods for ATP and DPG,
the actual amount of TCA extract was measured.) While the con-
vention we have adopted here does not effect comparative studies,
it does result in slightly higher calculated levels of both ATP
and DPG than we have previously reported (mean level of ATP in
Caucasians is now 3.84 µmoles per gram hemoglobin, was previously
3.47; mean level of DPG in Caucasians is now 13.2 µmoles per gram
hemoglobin, was previously 11.6).

The measurement of DPG by the chromatropic acid method was
done with the technique of Bartlett (1959). However, we have
modified the procedure as follows: A ratio of 0.1 ml of TCA
extract to 4.0 ml chromatropic solution was used, and incubation
time at $100^{\circ}C$ was increased from 120 to 135 minutes to insure
complete hydrolysis. Since plasma contributes some optical density
in the chromatropic acid method, and the amount varies somewhat
from individual to individual, plasma extracts were made from each
sample. The optical density of the whole blood extract was then
corrected by subtracting the contribution of the plasma.

Oxygen exchange in gas permeable capillary tubes has been
treated experimentally and theoretically by several authors in
recent years (Buckles et al., 1968). However, these authors have
concentrated on the oxygenation of blood flowing through these
tubes, usually with the idea of designing systems for artificial
lung applications. Because of the small diameter of these tubes,
flow is usually laminar, and the oxygenation process is thought to
be controlled by the rate of gas diffusion through the permeable
tube wall and plasma to the red cell. Good correspondence between theory and experiment for oxygenation of blood flowing through
gas permeable tubes is obtained if the blood is considered to be
a homogeneous solution of hemoglobin, and if the kinetics of the
hemoglobin-oxygenation reaction are very rapid so that local
equilibrium can be assumed. Experimental studies on the deoxygenation of blood in gas permeable fiber tubes have not been
previously reported. Colton and Drake (1969) have made some computer calculations on blood desaturation in tubes, similar to
those given by Buckles et al (1968) for oxygenation. Since
desaturation of blood is much slower than saturation, we expected
that desaturation rate experiments in such tubes might be most
sensitive to differences between individuals.

As a result of the above considerations, an instrument called
a "rogeometer" (for rate of gas exchange-ometer has been devised
to measure the rate of oxygen release by whole fresh blood. The
operation of this apparatus is as follows (see Figure 1):
Heparinized blood, immediately after withdrawal from the vein is
equilibrated in a rotating tonometer with air and 5% CO_2 for 30
minutes. It is important that all procedures be done promptly,
so that the metabolic status of the red cell remains as close to
physiologic as possible. The oxygenated blood is then withdrawn
into a 10 ml multifit glass syringe which is placed on a constant

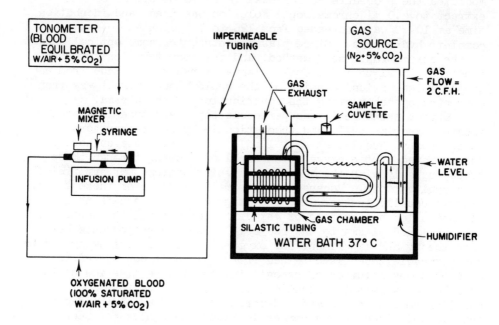

Figure 1. The rogeometer (rate of gas exchange-ometer). See text for details.

flow infusion pump adjusted to deliver 1.56 ml per 10 minutes. The syringe is attached to a length of gas impermeable tubing, such as polyethylene, which leads to a gas permeable Silastic^R tubing (approximately 150 cm long, with an inside diameter of 0.635 mm), enclosed in a small (approximately three inches on each side) gas-tight chamber. The chamber containing the Silastic tubing is immersed in a water bath maintained at 37°C. A gas mixture of 95% N_2 and 5% CO_2 is warmed to 37°C, humidified, and then allowed to flow through the box at a rate of about 2 cubic feet per hour. As the blood passes through the Silastic tubing it loses some of its oxygen. The rate of pumping has been adjusted so that the blood of normal individuals loses about 20 to 30% of its oxygen, in keeping with the average physiological level of desaturation. When the blood comes out of the box, it once again travels through gas-impermeable polyethylene tubing to be collected (after the first 0.5 ml has been discarded) under a layer of mineral oil in an oximeter cuvette. After sufficient blood has been collected (approximately 1.5 ml for a macro-oximeter cuvette and about 0.2 ml for a micro-oximeter), the oxygen saturation is measured. An additional quantity of blood is collected for ATP and DPG assays and is precipitated immediately with TCA. The time elapsed from drawing the blood from the vein until the end of the experimental procedure is about 45 minutes. Multiple determinations of the amount of desaturation on samples from single individuals indicate that the results are quite reproducible (i.e., differences between repeated samples ±3% of the amount of desaturation).

There have, however, been a few technical and theoretic problems. First, the tubing which we employ has a diameter of 0.635 mm, many times the thickness of the average capillary. Hence, a relatively large volume of blood is exchanging its oxygen through a small surface area. This difference does not, however, diminish the value of the observations made with the rogeometer, since the oxygen release is partially controlled by a pO_2 gradient extending from the red cell to the capillary wall and thence to the tissues. In the case of our device, the gradient is simply enlarged. The amount of oxygen unloaded is still dependent on the steepness of this gradient, which, in turn, depends in part on the saturation of the blood and the position of the oxygen dissociation curve.

Second, it has been found that the concentration of hemoglobin in the whole blood sample will have an effect on the rate of oxygen release. A number of experiments, employing varying hemoglobin concentrations (from 6 to 24 grams%) made up from the same samples of whole blood, have shown that increasing the hemoglobin concentration will produce a small decrease in the percent desaturation of the sample. However, the effect of hemoglobin level on desaturation is much less than expected for a diffusion limited process.*

*The regression of desaturation on hemoglobin was -0.3294 with a standard deviation of 0.086.

A simplified mathematical model based on a linearized hemoglobin saturation curve (Thews, 1959) was used to estimate the effect of operation parameters on the desaturation rate. An effective diffusivity of oxygen in whole blood, defined by $De = \dfrac{Dwb}{(1 + R)}$, where De is effective diffusivity, Dwb is diffusion of oxygen in whole blood, and R is the slope of the linear saturation curve (ml of oxygen bound to hemoglobin per ml dissolved oxygen) can be used to calculate desaturation rates (Crank, 1956). The diffusivity of oxygen in whole blood (Dwb) decreases with higher hematocrits (Hershey and Karhan, 1968), and R is directly proportional to hemoglobin concentration.

Under the laminar flow conditions in the Silastic tube and with the assumptions noted above, gas transport in this situation is formally analogous to the classical Graetz heat for which graphical solutions are available. Buckles et al. (1968) have also calculated the effect of the diffusion resistance of the permeable tubing and in our case, as in theirs, the mass resistance parameter (γ) had a value of about 0.1.

Expected desaturation rates for the operating conditions of the rogeometer based on the simplified diffusion model are given in Table 1. For the range of values considered, it is apparent that measured desaturation rates are slower than predicted, and that the experimental rates are less dependent on hemoglobin level than expected for a simple diffusional process. All of the subsequent data in this paper have been adjusted for the experimentally determined effects of variation in hemoglobin. This was done using the regression coefficient derived above.

Table 1. Expected desaturation rates at different hemoglobin levels (assuming Silastic tubing of length 150 cm and inside diameter 0.635 mm, and also assuming laminar flow).

Hemoglobin concentration	Dwb cm^2/sec	R*	Expected % desaturation
8	3.80×10^{-5}	66.5	39
16	3.45×10^{-5}	133	20
24	3.05×10^{-5}	199	15

*Values for R obtained from a linearized oxygen dissociation curve, by assuming the curve to be a straight line from 0 to 55 mm Hg PO_2. See text for further details.

Results

Our results with normal individuals indicate that there is a negative correlation between an individual's whole blood hemoglobin

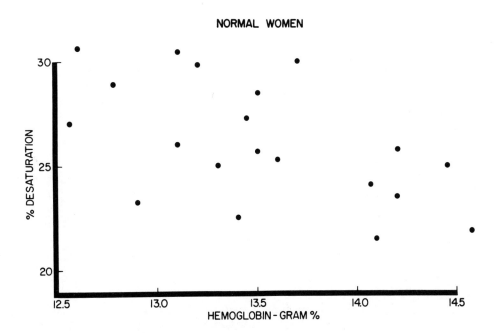

Figure 2.   The negative correlation between whole blood hemoglobin level and % desaturation in the rogeometer in a sample of 20 normal women.

level and the rate of oxygen release (see Table 2 and Figure 2).
That is, since they desaturated to a greater degree, those subjects with relatively low whole blood hemoglobin values unloaded
approximately as much oxygen as those with high whole blood hemoglobins. The existence of this negative correlation implies that
whole blood hemoglobin level may not be an adequate predictor of
the oxygenating capacity of a normal individual's blood. Indeed,
there is no significant relationship between hemoglobin concentration and the absolute amount of oxygen unloaded in our system.

Table 2. Correlation of rate of desaturation with the variables
shown, in a sample of normal men and women.

	DPG	ATP	DPG + ATP	Whole Blood Hemoglobin Levels
20 normal women	+0.456*	+0.243	+0.466*	-0.598**
20 normal men	+0.351	+0.064	+0.386	-0.300

*Significant at p 0.05
**Significant at p 0.01

There is a positive correlation between the rate of desaturation in the rogeometer and both DPG and the sum DPG+ATP (Table 2).
The correlation is significant in our sample of 20 females, but
not in our sample of males. However, in both sexes the correlation
coefficients are in agreement with the idea that variations in
levels of ATP and DPG will influence the rate of oxygen release
as well as shifting the position of the oxygen dissociation curve.

The rate of desaturation of whole blood of females is significantly greater than that of men (Table 3). Therefore,
although the absolute amount of oxygen delivered by the whole
blood of the two sexes is not detectably different, the females
in our sample unloaded significantly greater proportions of their
oxygen than the males. The negative correlations between whole
blood hemoglobin and red cell DPG content which we had previously
reported in much larger samples of males and females, were also
present (but not at significant levels in this smaller sample).

The results of studies on 10 anemic men, 10 anemic women,
and 9 men with pulmonary or pulmonary-vascular disease are shown
in Tables 4,5, and 6. The mean rate of desaturation was significantly increased in all three groups. There was considerable
variation, however, among the patients within all three groups,
with values ranging from normal to two or more times above the
normal mean.

Levels of DPG in the red cells of these three patient groups
were markedly elevated. As with rates of desaturation, there was
considerable heterogeneity among patients in the degree of elevation of the DPG levels. The levels of ATP were also significantly

Table 3. Means and standard deviations - normal subjects

	N	% Desaturation	DPG*	ATP*	DPG+ATP	Gram% Hemoglobin
Normal Women (Mean ± 1 S.D.)	20	26.42±3.00**	13.56±2.62	3.89±0.49	17.45±2.80	13.51±0.60
Normal Men (Mean ±1 S.D.)	20	23.86±2.56**	12.80±2.32	3.80±0.43	17.19±2.90	15.43±0.68
"t" values for differences of means		2.89	0.97	0.66	0.30	9.40
p Value		<0.01	NS†	NS†	NS†	<0.001

*Expressed as umoles/gram hemoglobin
**Means adjusted to common hemoglobin value
†NS = Non-significant

TABLE 4

Anemic men

Diagnosis	Hemo-globin	%Desatu-ration	DPG	ATP	DPG+ATP
Chronic granulocytic leukemia	10.25	29.50	22.60	6.89	24.58
Acute leukemia	6.89	31.21	38.03	4.13	42.16
Acute leukemia	8.01	37.44	32.71	5.07	37.78
Acute leukemia	8.65	27.33	29.57	3.46	33.03
Lymphosarcoma	11.27	26.77	23.29	3.81	27.10
Myeloid metaplasia	10.25	32.80	26.57	3.56	30.13
Uremia	5.88	30.34	25.61	4.15	29.76
Uremia	5.77	39.28	47.50	6.10	53.60
Acute leukemia	6.60	46.16	27.40	6.63	34.03
Lymphosarcoma	7.85	29.20	26.68	6.43	33.11
Mean ±1 S.D.:	8.14 (±1.94)	33.00 (±6.15)	30.00 (±7.65)	5.03 (±1.38)	35.03 (±7.86)
"t" value*	15.26	7.11	9.37	3.71	9.11
p	< 0.001	< 0.001	< 0.001	< 0.001	< 0.001

*Anemic men vs. normal men (data shown in Table 3) with contrasting means adjusted to a common hemoglobin value for comparison of the % desaturation. Adjusted mean for normal, 22.98, and for anemic, 34.20% desaturation

Table 5

Anemic Women

Diagnosis	Hemo-globin	%Desatu-ration	DPG	ATP	DPG+ATP
Subacute leukemia	8.70	24.27	28.74	3.00	31.74
Myeloid metaplasia	9.85	29.69	42.53	2.83	45.36
Anemia of chronic disease*	10.74	37.70	42.25	3.32	45.57
Chronic lymphocytic leukemia	7.85	30.95	30.47	3.67	34.14
Uremia	7.48	32.07	34.23	4.97	39.20
Chronic lymphocytic leukemia	8.28	29.41	24.17	4.41	28.58
Uremia	5.41	37.20	25.34	8.06	33.40
Immune hemolytic anemia	6.98	55.19	32.23	5.22	37.45
Iron deficiency	10.82	24.67	18.07	3.11	21.18
Acute leukemia	7.04	32.72	16.84	3.09	19.93
Mean ±1 S.D.	8.31 (±1.74)	33.39 (±8.84)	29.49 (±8.82)	4.17 (±1.61)	33.65 (±8.81)
t value*	12.12	4.21	7.55	7.13	7.59
p	< 0.001	< 0.001	< 0.001	< 0.001	< 0.001

*Anemic women vs. normal women (data shown in Table 3) with contrasting means adjusted to a common hemoglobin value for comparison of the % desaturation. Adjusted mean for normal, 25.24, and for anemic, 34.25% desaturation.

Table 6

Male patients with pulmonary or pulmonary vascular disease

Diagnosis	Hemo-globin	%Desatu-ration	DPG	ATP	DPG+ATP
Interstitial fibrosis*	13.90	26.66	16.49	4.67	21.16
Pulmonary vascular disease**	12.40	43.26	30.11	5.28	35.39
Obesity and chronic bronchitis	17.09	30.01	15.18	4.19	19.37
Emphysema	15.70	28.47	29.78	7.52	37.30
Emphysema	16.02	32.36	10.56	3.96	14.52
Emphysema	15.60	36.50	12.82	4.07	16.89
Emphysema	18.21	27.74	24.43	4.04	28.47
Emphysema	16.56	29.69	22.45	3.40	25.85
Emphysema	15.00	28.50	13.45	3.89	17.34
Mean ±1 S.D.	15.61 (±1.72)	31.47 (±5.16)	19.47 (±7.42)	4.56 (±1.23)	24.03 (±8.25)
"t" value***	0.40	4.99	3.71	2.49	3.34
p	NS	<0.001	<0.001	<0.05	<0.01

*Muscular dystrophy

**Pulmonary vascular insufficiency due to multiple pulmonary emboli

***Men with pulmonary disease vs. normal men (data shown in Table 3) with contrasting means adjusted to a common hemo-globin value for comparison of the % desaturation. Adjusted mean for normal, 24.22, and for pulmonary disease, 31.43% desaturation.

elevated in all three groups as was, of course, the total level of
DPG plus ATP.

Discussion

Our data, both from normals and from patients with fairly
severe hypoxemias, indicate that the red cell is capable of
making both fine and gross adjustments to facilitate the delivery
of oxygen in vivo. This adjustment is, in a sense, a "programming"
for a specific rate of oxygen release. Baumberger et al. (1967)
had earlier reported that significant differences seemed to exist
in rate of oxygen delivery between the red cells of different
individuals. These authors suggested that variations in the red
cells themselves were probably involved, and that "in the intact
red cell there are factors that affect oxygen exchange which are
much more decisive than the dissociation constants of the
hemoglobin-oxygen reactions."

As the red cell passes through the various parts of the
circulatory system, it rarely, if ever, reaches complete equilibrium with the oxygen pressures in its immediate environment.
Because of this, the amount of oxygen actually unloaded by the red
cell will be a function of both the oxygen affinity of the hemoglobin (as determined by the position of the oxygen dissociation
curve) and the rate at which the oxygen is loaded or unloaded as
influenced by diffusion and kinetic factors. The measurements
made with the rogeometer are influenced by much the same factors
as govern desaturation in vivo, and we therefore expect that rates
measured by this device under standard conditions will serve as
valuable clinical indicies of the in vivo blood function to
supplement other procedures.

Previous studies of the rate of oxygen transport have dealt
with numerically small samples and have largely ignored the
possibility of the existence of differences between individuals.
Our results conclusively demonstrate that there are wide variations
between individuals in the rate at which their blood will unload
oxygen. These variations seem to be partly related to differences
in the red cell content of DPG and ATP. The correlation of DPG+
ATP with the rate of oxygen release is positive (see Table 2),
in that the higher the sum DPG+ATP, the greater the rate of oxygen
release. However, a correlation such as this does not extablish
a causal relationship. In the present case, it seems most likely
that a causal connection does exist, but final proof must await
additional experimentation.

As might be expected from the negative correlation between
the level of whole blood hemoglobin and the rate of desaturation
of blood in the rogeometer, there is no consistent relationship
between the hemoglobin concentration and the amount of oxygen
which is unloaded. This lack of relationship between whole blood
hemoglobin and amount of oxygen delivered implies an adjustment of

the red cells of each individual, so that, regardless of the level of whole blood hemoglobin, approximately the same amount of oxygen may be released. The most reasonable mechanism for this adjustment of the oxygen delivering capacity of the red cell would be variations in the levels of DPG (and, perhaps, ATP) within the circulating red cell.

Our results with individuals with hypoxic diseases indicate that the red cell is capable of making a significant portion of the adjustments required to maintain normoxia during reduced availability of oxygen. Previous authors have reported a decrease in the oxygen affinity of hemoglobin (i.e. a shift of the dissociation curve to the right) in hypoxemic diseases such as anemia and cardiopulmonary disorders (Edwards et al., 1968; Morse et al., 1950; Dill et al., 1928; Kennedy & Valtis, 1954; Mulhausen et al., 1967). We now know that, at least in our experimental apparatus, there may be a tremendous increase in the amount of oxygen unloaded per unit hemoglobin. In many of the anemic patients, the decrement in amount of oxygen transported by the whole blood due to the reduction in whole blood hemoglobin level appears to be completely compensated by the increase in oxygen delivery per unit volume of blood. There is, however, considerable heterogeneity among the anemic patients in our sample, and some do not seem to be making adequate adjustments in the level of function of the red cell. This suggests that some patients with severe hypoxias may eventually be therapeutically helped by modification of the red cell to allow more rapid oxygen release.

The levels of red cell DPG and ATP are very much higher in all three patient groups. This increase in the levels of these intermediates is probably at least partly responsible for the much greater rate of oxygen release. However, there is certainly not a direct correspondence between changes in these intermediates and increases in desaturation rates, implying that additional factors also influence rate of oxygen transport by the red cell.

The shift of the oxygen dissociation curve to the right which may be produced by an increase in the concentration of red cell DPG is probably one of the most economical adjustments to hypoxia which can be made. This response to oxygen lack involves only an increase in a normal metabolite of the red cell, and the maintenance of these increased levels. Almost all the other modes of physiological adaptation to hypoxia of which we are aware require a greater total energy expenditure, especially if they are sustained over a long period of time. Work done by this laboratory and others shows that the level of red cell DPG and, therefore, the position of the oxygen dissociation curve, is extremely flexible (Eaton et al., 1969; Lenfant et al., 1968). Considering the rapidity with which this response may occur, and in view of the effects of this response, we may conclude that the increased oxygen delivery made possibly by changes in erythrocyte DPG (and

ATP) is an important physiological adjustment, allowing the maintenance of normal oxygen tensions in the stressed and unstressed human.

CONCLUSIONS

Variations in the metabolism of the human red cell seem to be very important in the maintenance of respiratory homeostasis. The normal individual appears to make some use of variations in the levels of DPG as a "fine tuning" mechanism, allowing the close adjustment of the respiratory system with the level of oxygen use. The existence of such an adjustment is apparent both from the negative correlation which has been found between whole blood hemoglobin levels and DPG and from the relationship which exists between the levels of DPG+ATP and the rate of oxygen release by the whole blood.

In the normal human subjected to hypoxic stress, the adjustment of the red cells' oxygen transport potential may be vital to complete adaptation. Significant increases in DPG levels have been reported to occur at high altitude (after both short- and long-term exposure) and during relatively short periods of moderate physical exertion. In the face of both these hypoxic stresses, the adjustment of oxygen delivery through changes in the level of DPG may significantly promote the delivery of oxygen and help maintain adequate tissue oxygen delivery.

Individuals with severe, long-standing hypoxias such as anemia and pulmonary dysfunction frequently display tremendous elevations of red cell DPG and ATP. These elevations produce large shifts of the oxygen dissociation curve and appear to raise the rate of oxygen delivery as much as two fold. An increase in oxygen delivery of this magnitude may obviously be a very important part of adaptation to the greatly reduced availability of oxygen in these pathologies.

REFERENCES

Bartlett, G.R. (1959). J. Biol. Chem. 234:469.

Baumberger, J.P., Leong, H.C., and Neville, J. R. (1967). J. Appl. Physiol. 23:40.

Benesch, R. and Benesch, R.E. (1967). Biochem. Biophys. Res. Comm. 26:162.

Benesch, R. and Benesch, R.E. (1969). Nature 221:618.

Brewer, G.J. and Powell, R.D. (1966). J. Lab. & Clin. Med. 67:726.

Brewer, G.J. and Eaton, J. W. (1969). J. Clin. Invest. 48:11a (abst).

Buckles, R.G., Merrill, E. W., Gilliland, E.R. (1968). Amer. Inst. Chem. Eng. J. 14:703.

Chanutin, A. and Curnish, R.R. (1967). Arch. Biochem. Biophys. 121:96.

Colton, C.F. and Drake, R.F. (1969). Amer. Soc. Art. Int. Organs. 15th Annual Meeting, April, 1969, Atlantic City.

Crank, J. (1956). The Mathematics of Diffusion, p. 121. Oxford
  University Press, London.
Dill, D.B., Bock, A. V., Caulaert, C.,Folling, A., Hurxthal, L.M.
  and Henderson, L.J. (1928). J. Biol. Chem. 78:191.
Eaton, J. W. and Brewer, G.J. (1968a). Proc. Nat. Acad. Sci.
  61:756.
Eaton, J.W. and Brewer, G.J. (1968b). Clin. Res. 16:454.
Eaton, J.W., Brewer, G.J. and Grover, R.F. (1969). J. Lab. & Clin.
  Med. 73:603.
Eaton, J.W., Faulkner, J.A. and Brewer, G.J. (1969). Proc. Soc.
  Exp. Biol. & Med. In press.
Edwards, M.J., Novy, M.J., Walters, C.L. and Metcalfe, J. (1968).
  J. Clin. Invest. 47:1851.
Hershey, D. and Karhan, T. (1968). Amer. Inst. Chem. Eng. J.
  14:969.
Hurtado, A. (1964). In Handbook of Physiology. Section 4.
  Adaptation to the Environment. D.B. Dill, ed. American
  Physiological Society, Washington, D.C.
Kennedy, A.C. and Valtis, D.J. (1954). J. Clin. Invest. 33:1372.
Lenfant, C., Torrance, J., English, E., Finch, C.A., Reynfarje,
  C., Ramos, J. and Faura, J. (1968). J. Clin. Invest. 47:
  2652.
Morse, M., Cassels, D.E. and Holder, M. (1950). J. Clin. Invest.
  29:1098.
Mulhausen, R., Astrup, P., and Kjeldsen, K. (1967). Scand. J.
  Clin. Lab. Invest. 19:291.
Thews, G. (1959). Pfluger. Arch. Ges. Physiol. 268:308.

BINDING OF 2,3-DIPHOSPHOGLYCERATE (DPG) TO OXYHEMOGLOBIN; LEVELS AND EFFECT OF DPG ON OXYGEN AFFINITY OF NORMAL AND ABNORMAL BLOOD.

S. Grisolia, J. Carreras, D. Diederich, and S. Charache

University of Kansas Medical Center, and Johns Hopkins

Medical Institutions

My awareness of 2,3-diphosphoglycerate (DPG) started over 20 years ago when I occupied a bench in a laboratory shared by my teacher Ochoa with Greenwald, who had some 20 years earlier discovered DPG in the red cell (1). Nevertheless, my interest in DPG came about in a round about way. In the late 40's was demonstrated for the first time the use of ATP, at the enzyme level, for synthetic reactions, i.e., urea and glutamine synthesis (2). At the suggestion of Ochoa, Ratner and then I started to use 3 PGA in a generating system for ATP; a technique which, by the way, became so popular that possibly it has been forgotten, if ever recognized, that it originated with Ochoa. The need of a glycolytic system free from interfering phosphatases led me to purify phosphoglyceromutase, which up to then had been studied only in crude preparations. Possibly a misfortune was the fact that Rodwell, then one of my students was lucky in crystallizing the enzyme for the first time; since that time I have been most reluctant to lose interest in the phosphoglycerate area. Of course today with the advances in enzymology, it is only a matter of patience to achieve enzyme crystallization as pointed out recently by Theorell (3).

Our studies led very quickly to phosphoglyceromutases which do not require DPG and to the fact that the DPG dependent phosphoglyceromutase does not need DPG as a necessary cofactor in the sense that it would be used and reformed, as postulated by Cori and coworkers, every time 3 PGA is converted into 2 PGA and vice versa. In other words, we started to suspect that the satisfying explanation of the role of DPG for mutase action alone was a red herring. Of course DPG was long suspected of being related to red cell viability since it was noted by many workers that its disappearance paralleled the decreased survival of stored human erythrocytes. On

39

THE 1,3-PHOSPHOGLYCERATE TRIDENT SHUNT

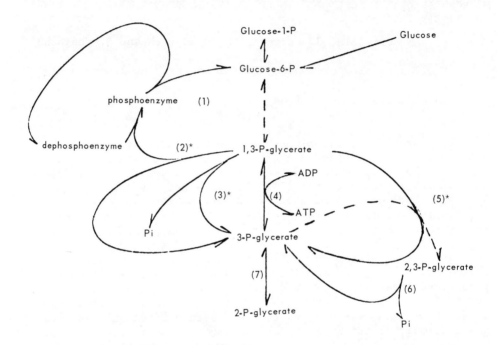

Figure 1. (1) Phosphoglucomutase; (2) Alpers' Pathway;
(3) Diederich's Acyl Phosphatase; (4) Phosphoglycerate Kinase;
(5) Diphosphoglycerate Mutase; (6) Diphosphoglycerate Phosphatase; (7) 2,3-Phosphoglycerate Dependent Phosphoglyceromutase
(also manifests 2,3-diphosphoglycerate phosphatase activity);
* Indicates the 3 steps at which 1,3 P-glycerate may shunt away
from the "normal" pathway catalyzed by phosphoglycerate kinase.

this basis and from extensive work of our coworkers and others,
it became evident to me that DPG had other roles just as important
as that for P-glyceromutase (4,5). All these points have been
extensively discussed before (6,7,8) and need not be covered here.
The exciting findings of Chanutin (9) showing binding of DPG to
hemoglobin and of Benesch et al. (10) demonstrating a shift in the
O_2 saturation curve of hemoglobin by DPG have stimulated considerable interest, as evidenced by the bringing together of such a
distinguished group for this conference under the leadership of
Dr. Brewer. This meeting should exemplify the present high level
of sophistication in biochemistry and, at the same time, the need
to closely integrate and bring about interrelationships between
metabolic pathways, mechanisms and structure at the molecular level.
These interrelations should provide the fundamental framework for
a proper understanding of regulation of enzyme activity and thus
help to clarify the hardest problem which confronts modern biology,
that is to translate the results of "in vitro" conditions to those
which occur in the living cell. This point has already been stressed in the literature by many, including myself (8,11,12,13). I
was delighted by the findings and suggestions of Benesch since for
many years, as indicated above, we have thought about and searched
for a major physiologic role for DPG. Indeed, we postulated long
ago there might be changes in conformation of hemoglobin induced by
DPG and even tried to interest crystallographers to seek evidence.
It is my purpose, since there are so many experts in the audience,
and due to time limitation, to illustrate briefly some of the
points which have interested us in the area of DPG with particular
emphasis on comparing the behavior of phosphoglyceromutase and
hemoglobin towards DPG.

Alpers has shown recently that 1,3-diphosphoglycerate can
phosphorylate phosphoglucomutase (3). Figure 1 illustrates there
is at the level of 1,3-diphosphoglycerate in the glycolytic scheme,
a multi-shunt, which, as of now, involves at least three pathways.
It is an enlarged version of the shunt part of the phosphoglycerate
cycle (8). Thus, it may be called the diphosphoglycerate trident
shunt, (or if you permit me some levity, the phosphoglycerate tri-
cycle). This triple shunt involves, in addition to the Alpers
reaction, the formation of DPG which, via phosphatase, will be
converted into Pi and return P-glycerate to the Emden-Meyerhof
scheme or, yield the same products directly, via acylphosphatase.

There are two points which I should like to stress. One is
that the trident shunt (3) could be of much interest in regulation,
since, as shown, it may operate at the 6 and 3 carbon levels in the
Emden-Meyerhof scheme and since it may be under enzymatic control,
via the acylphosphatase [the smallest enzyme thus far described
(14)]. This enzyme may prevent chemotropic effects such as brought
about by powerful chemical reagents which are made in large quantities as is the case for 1,3-diphosphoglycerate (on the order of

moles per day for man) (12,15). Second, the complex control of
these reactions "in vivo" may obscure the quantitative aspects of
synthesis and utilization of DPG in addition to the fact that P-
glyceromutase itself is a DPG phosphatase which Alpers believes is
of primary importance in the control of DPG in the red cell (per-
sonal communication).

With this scheme as the background, I will try to cover now
several points as follows: A) Outline a sensitive automatic and
specific enzymatic method for analysis of DPG. B) Binding studies
of DPG to oxyhemoglobin. C) The presence of firmly bound DPG to
hemoglobin in normal and abnormal hemoglobins and values of DPG in
blood of normal and abnormal individuals with special emphasis on
its possible relation to O_2 affinity.

A. <u>Automatic Procedure</u>. In 1957, we presented a micro-pro-
cedure (16) based on the catalytic effect of DPG on phosphoglyceromutase. Since that time, estimation of DPG based on its identification by chromatography has been described (17). We automated
recently (18) "Method 4" (16) which is based on the colorimetric
estimation of the pyruvate formed by coupling mutase to enolase
and pyruvate kinase. The method can be used to determine the
DPG in human blood at about five hundred-fold dilution. Two
reagent mixtures are prepared. Mixture A contains: ADP, 3-phospho-
glycerate, Tris-PO_4 buffer, $MgCl_2$ and EDTA. Mixture B contains:
pyruvic kinase, enolase and P-glyceromutase. Prior to use, mixture
A and B are mixed. The analysis is carried out using a Technicon
Auto-Analyzer employing Sampler Model II, Proportioning Pump Model
1 and Dialyzer. Samples and assay mixtures are pumped in at the
same ratio, passed through mixing coils, and then into the dialyzer.
The mixture is dialyzed against water, mixed with 2,4 dinitro-
phenylhydrazine in 1 N HCl, and then with 1.75 M NaOH. The mixture
passes via a flow cell through a Gilford Spectrophotometer #2000,
set to record absorbance at 540 mμ. A plot of A versus concentration yields an essentially linear curve to 10 mμmoles/ml DPG.

We have recently adapted the Technicon components to a Gilford
300-N with data lister 4006. We replaced the ordinary cell with a
10 mm flow cell; this is the most convenient size because it is
easier to keep it free from bubbles. The manual reading signal in
the 4006 <u>is activated</u> with a 306D synchronous-motor driven Duo-Set
Repeat Cycle Timer, Automatic Timing & Control, Inc. (King of
Prussia, Pennsylvania),set to 30 seconds. At about 15 minutes from
the starting of the run, i.e., when the samples are to begin to
pass through the flow cell the timer is changed to read every 2
seconds. The peaks are easily seen in the "adding machine tape".
They can also be identified by distance. While ideally it would
be best to use a peak-trough reader, the present arrangement is
most satisfactory. Indeed, with little practice it is easier, less
time consuming, more exact and certainly less expensive than the

use of the 2000 Gilford recorder, In fact, I must say that we
consider recorders somewhat obsolete.

The automated method has about one-fourth the variability of
the manual method, is essentially foolproof and permits the assay
of hundreds of samples per day with accuracy and at a moderate cost.
It seems that it may be useful in other laboratories as it has been
in ours as is further exemplified below.

B. Binding studies of DPG to oxyhemoglobin and presence of
firmly bound DPG. DPG was reported by Benesch and Benesch to bind to
oxy and deoxygenated β chains of hemoglobin (10,19). Dissociation of
the DPG was postulated to be required before oxygenation of Hb could
take place (19). Findings that agree with these are: Red cells
depleted of DPG by incubation with iodoacetate developed increased
affinity for oxygen (20). The high oxygen affinity of stored blood
could be related to its low content of DPG and ATP, and restoration
of DPG and ATP by incubation with inosine is associated with a
return of oxygen affinity to normal. Lenfant (21,22), et al.
reported a decrease in oxygen affinity in individuals who moved to
high altitude, and an increase in DPG content of red cells (23).
Eaton, et al. reported that persons living at about 11,000 feet
had higher DPG than others living at sea level (24). Association
between a decrease in oxygen affinity and elevated levels of DPG
had been documented in two moderately anemic patients with pyruvate
kinase (PK) deficiency (25), and in patients with sickle cell
anemia (26).

Behavior on Sephadex columns and of ultrafiltration through
membranes indicates that binding of DPG to oxyhemoglobin may occur
readily (27). The hemoglobin was "stripped" of DPG by gel filtra-
tion through Sephadex G-25 columns (10,19). In some 16 experiments
the hemoglobin solutions retained nearly 10% of their original DPG,
i.e., showing molar ratios of DPG/hemoglobin of 0.1 to 0.15. This
is in disagreement with the results of Benesch et al. (10,19).
The solutions were concentrated by diafiltration through a Diaflo
PM-30 membrane. Experiments were carried out using a fixed-volume
diafiltration assembly. By this technique we demonstrated extensive
binding of DPG to oxyhemoglobin at a wide range of concentrations,
even approximating those which occurred in the red cell. Again
extensive binding of DPG to oxyhemoglobin was demonstrated (27)
by the technique of Pfleiderer and Auricchio (28).

As reported above, there is a portion of DPG bound which cannot
be removed by Sephadex as described by Benesch (10). The amount of
DPG retained by hemoglobin passed through Sephadex G-25 fine
columns depended upon the column dimensions. For example, hemoglobin passed through 2.5 x 30 cm columns as described by Benesch,
et al. (10), retained 2-3 mμmoles of DPG per mg. However, using

1.2 x 100 cm columns, the molar binding ratios decreased to 0.04 to 0.06 but longer columns will not remove this DPG. Since there are strong similarities between the binding of DPG to hemoglobin and to phosphoglyceromutase (7,29), we tested whether DPG could be removed or converted to monophosphoglycerates on denaturation of the protein with acid or heat, as is the case with muscle phosphoglyceromutase (30). Neither radioactivity nor DPG are released on denaturation of the protein. To further clarify the binding, separation of tryptic peptides was carried out (31). The peptide and radioactivity elution profiles demonstrate binding of DPG to peptide(s). Aliquots of the tube containing the peak radioactivity were examined by thin layer and compared with the original digest. This peak contained two major peptides, as yet unidentified.

Recently, Benesch has illustrated the effect of environmental factors on DPG binding (32). This area has been extensively covered in our laboratory in general (13) and for DPG and P-glycerate mutase in particular (8). Figure 2 illustrates the marked influence of ionic strength on binding of DPG to Hb. As previously shown, moderate changes in ionic strength similar to those illustrated may affect the kinetic constants of P-glycerate mutase enormously (8).

C. <u>Presence of firmly bound DPG to normal and abnormal Hb and DPG values in normal and abnormal blood</u>. As we have briefly outlined (26) and as to be reported in full elsewhere (33), we attempted to answer two questions: 1) Are elevated levels of DPG present in the red cells of patients with disorders known to be associated with decreased oxygen affinity, and 2) are conditions within red cells different from those in dilute solutions of hemoglobin so that high DPG could cause decreased oxygen affinity in such patients?

Sickle cell anemia (SS) blood was studied since it shows decreased oxygen affinity (34,35), while the oxygen affinity of sickle cell hemoglobin equals that of hemoglobin A (36). The mean DPG concentration in blood from 34 healthy donors was 4.47 μmoles/ml packed red cells (S.D. 0.53 μmole/ml). The mean concentration in blood from 32 patients with sickle cell anemia was 6.25 μmoles/ml (S.D. 0.91 μmole/ml); the difference is statistically significant (p<.001).

Among patients with sickle cell anemia, DPG concentrations did not appear to be correlated with either hematocrit value or reticulocyte count. Elevated DPG was found in some patients with severe anemia associated with uremia, and in three patients with megaloblastic anemia. Five carriers of hemoglobin Chesapeake had slightly elevated levels, while DPG was increased in five patients with cyanotic heart disease. Oxygen affinity of blood from an extremely anemic SS patient was studied. While the dissociation curve was somewhat farther to the right than that of less anemic SS patients,

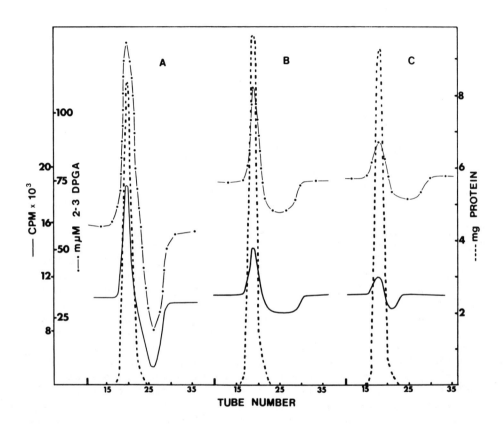

Figure 2.   The influence of ionic strength on binding of DPG to
oxyhemoglobin.   Experiment A, 0.02 M NaCl; experiment B, 0.1 M NaCl
and experiment C, 0.12 M KCl - 0.02 M NaCl.

the DPG concentration did not differ from that of the total population of SS patients.

Two SS patients were selected since they had the lowest and
highest DPG concentrations. Oxygen affinity was found to be the
same, their curves falling about 6-7 mm Hg to the right of the
curve for normal blood. Oxygen affinity of lysed normal and SS
blood was measured, with and without addition of DPG. Oxygen
affinity of both types of hemolysate was decreased by addition of
DPG.

DPG was added to hemolysates from two normal men with AA
hemoglobin. Oxygen affinity was related to DPG concentration in a
curvilinear fashion, maximum decreases in affinity were at about
10 µmoles DPG/ml. No further decrease in oxygen affinity was
found at high DPG concentrations. A hemolysate oxygen affinity
identical with that of normal whole blood was found at about 5
µmoles DPG/ml RBC. A hemolysate affinity similar to that of SS
blood was observed at about 8 µmoles DPG/ml RBC.

As illustrated above, there is binding of DPG to oxyhemoglobin
and ionic strength has a marked influence upon the binding. We
tested the binding of DPG to normal and abnormal hemoglobins.
Figure 3 illustrates binding to normal and to Kansas hemoglobin.
As shown the DPG measurements and radioactivity values agree very
well for normal but not for Hb Kansas. With Hb Kansas the trough
clearly indicates binding but there is little indication at the
peak as measured by DPG assay. Nevertheless the radioactivity
measurement clearly indicate binding. The discrepancy is due to
phosphatase activity. Indeed in this particular experiment, the
blood samples remained in the cold for several hours before assay.
It seems at first glance there is no advantage in using DPG assay
over radioactivity measurements. There is however an absolute
need, for without it splitting of DPG would remain undetected and
quantitative measurement based on radioactivity would not be reliable. I stress that for these comparative studies one needs both
types of data. Any additional precaution such as working in the
cold, using freshly prepared DPG solutions, etc., will not preclude
DPG changes and may introduce interference by other factors affecting binding. However, with resonable precautions, e.g., completing
all analysis during the day, it is possible to carry on comparative
studies as those presented in Table 1. Table 2 illustrates the
residual DPG binding to several types of hemoglobin. It is seen
that Kansas hemoglobin binds twice as much as normal hemoglobin.
Interestingly, the SS hemoglobin has very little residual binding.
Table 3 presents a comparison of phosphoglycerate mutase, DPG
phosphatase and DPG binding to normal and abnormal hemoglobins.
SS hemoglobin shows no phosphatase. Indeed, under the conditions
tested the level of DPG raises slightly. This is of particular
interest since it is not clear as yet what is the contribution of

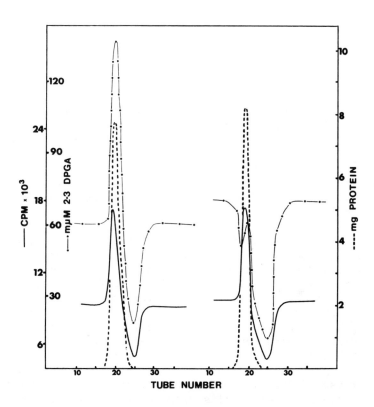

Figure 3. Binding of DPG to normal and to Kansas hemoglobin. The data for the left hand portion of the figure corresponds to normal and that of the right portion to Kansas hemoglobin.

the dual function of phosphoglyceromutase as a phosphatase (8), within the erythrocyte (37) and on the P-glycerate triple shunt (3). It seems then that binding measurements, particularly residual DPG binding, may be of much interest in understanding the behavior of both normal and abnormal hemoglobin.

General Discussion

As already discussed the oxygen affinity of blood is decreased in anemias of several etiologies (38); possibly this shift in the oxygen dissociation curve helps to maintain an adequate oxygen supply to the tissues (39). Our data, and those of Eaton and Brewer (40), indicate the DPG is increased in the red cells of some of those persons; it seems reasonable that the two findings may be related. DPG is elevated when hypoxia is caused by heart disease, as shown here and recently reported by Oski (41), and by residence at high altitude (23,24). It could be argued that in all these conditions, the average concentration of deoxyhemoglobin per cell is increased.

The proposal that deoxyhemoglobin binds DPG better, thus the unbound DPG decreases, relieving inhibition of diphosphoglyceromutase (42), and then more DPG is produced, increasing the total DPG (43), is most attractive. Some doubt as to whether elevated levels of DPG could lower oxygen affinity was raise by the original studies of Benesch and Benesch (10); maximal effects were exerted at $1-2 \times 10^{-3}$ M DPG below the concentration in normal red cells. Predictions based upon Benesch's hypothesis are: 1) Concentrations of DPG inhibiting the mutase should be within the range found in red cells of patients. 2) Increases in deoxyhemoglobin should parallel those of DPG. 3) DPG should be decreased in the red cells containing abnormal hemoglobins with increased oxygen affinity, and conversely. 4) It should be possible to lower oxygen affinity of hemoglobin in vitro, to the degree observed in blood of patients, by adding DPG.

It is then of interest that the diphosphoglyceromutase is inhibited by DPG (44,45) in the proper range. (Addition of deoxyhemoglobin to an enzyme system in vitro should relieve inhibition and increase in total DPG may be observed.) On the other hand the metabolism of DPG is slow, compared to circulation time and reoxygenation of red cells; it is unlikely that deoxygenated hemoglobin persists long in the hyperkinetic circulation of anemic persons to significantly increase DPG. If it would, increase in DPG should parallel the severity of anemia. We did not observe such correlation in SS patients. These arguments do not hold at high altitude, and there one would expect a somewhat disproportionate increase in DPG for binding leading to further increases in

TABLE 1.   RESIDUAL 2,3 DPG BINDING TO HEMOGLOBIN

Type Hb	Protein		2,3 DPG	Molar ratio
	mg/ml	µmolar	µmolar	2,3 DPG/Hb
Normal 1	9.8	152	9.7	0.0638
Normal 2	10.6	164	9.7	0.059
Kansas	10.3	159	16.8	0.106
SS	6.45	10	<1.8	0.018
Paroxysmal Noct. Hemoglobinuria	5.9	092	4.9	0.0533
Dog	5.65	087	5.1	0.0586
Sheep	10.8	167	<0.6	0.0036

TABLE 2.   2,3 DPG BINDING TO OXYHEMOGLOBIN

NaCl Molar	Type Hb	Hb Eluted mµmoles	Bound 2,3 DPG mµmoles	Molar ratio 2,3 DPG/Hb
0.1	Adult 1	145	29.0	0.20
0.1	Adult 2	155	26.8	0.17
0.1	Kansas	104	42.6	0.42
0.1	SS	153	15.0	0.10
0.02	Adult 1	116	167.0	1.43
0.02	Adult 2	137	142.0	1.03
0.02	Kansas	116	140.0	1.21
0.02	SS	95	36.8	0.41

TABLE 3. RESUMÉ OF MUTASE, DPG PHOSPHATASE, FIRMLY BOUND DPG AND DPG BINDING TO SEVERAL HEMOGLOBINS

Type Hb	Mutase Units/mg Hb	Phosphatase mμmoles/mg Hb/hr	"Residual" DPG Molar Ratio	μmoles DPG Bound in	
				01. M NaCl	0.02 M NaCl
A	0.086	1.1	0.059	0.20	1.43
K	0.091	1.86	0.106	0.417	1.21
SS	0.10	00	0.018	0.10	0.4

concentration of deoxyhemoglobin. Eaton and Brewer pointed out that increases in deoxyhemoglobin under these conditions seem insufficient to account for observed increases in DPG (24).

DPG was higher than normal in carriers of hemoglobin Chesapeake, which has high oxygen affinity (46). However, the level of hemoglobin Rainier, which has very high oxygen affinity (47) is normal, while levels in hemoglobin Kansas (48) and in hemoglobin Seattle, which have decreased oxygen affinity, are slightly elevated. These data suggest that there is no straight forward relationship between the state of oxygenation of hemoglobin within red cells and the amount of DPG they contain.

Benesch et al. estimated that the energy of binding of DPG hemoglobin is 6.4 Kc/mole (19). It should be pointed out (49) that oneml of blood consumes 2.10 mg glucose/min or ∿14 mg (∿82 μmoles) for the blood of a 70 Kg man. Reportedly 75% of the metabolism of glucose in the red cell is via glycolysis, and the rest via the pentose shunt. Thus 60 μmoles of glucose would yield 120 μmoles ATP from glycolysis plus 120 μmoles ATP via shunt. Of course if much of the ATP is used for the formation of DPG there will be little net synthesis of ATP from glycolysis! Under basal metabolic conditions a 70 Kg man uses ca 250 ml of O_2 (0.011 moles) per min (50). On the basis of Hb $(O_2)_\eta$ where η = 2 moles O_2 scission of the DPG-Hb bond would consume about 0.035 Kc/minute, this is about 50 Kc/day. In the basal state, a normal man needs some 1600 Kc/day (50), suggesting that the chemical work of oxygenating hemoglobin under those conditions consumes about 3% of total calories. Or put another way the consumption of 1 mole of oxygen yields some 46 Kc and the transport of 1 mole of oxygen will require 3.2 Kc or nearly 6%. Assuming 7 Kc per mole ATP, 15 to 50 more ATP will be needed than the red cell can produce for O_2 transport. Of course these are minimum examples since under normal living conditions and under exercise the ratio will be higher by a factor of several folds. Therefore it is apparent at first glance that ATP produced by the red cell can not contribute significantly to DPG binding. Indeed, it looks like ATP is not directly involved in oxygen transport by hemoglobin. These figures are indeed gross estimates, but their magnitude suggests that the thermodynamics of the proposed reaction between DPG and deoxyhemoglobin have not been entirely clarified. On the other hand we do not know with certainly the extent of binding nor the percentage of bound DPG in the cell.

Hemolysed blood is just a model of the internal environment of red cells. However, it is free of extraneous effects on oxygen affinity produced by addition of nucleotides or metabolic inhibitors due to prolonged dialysis. Addition of DPG to the lysates decreased oxygen affinity to that of normal blood, regardless of whether lysates were prepared from normal or SS blood.

Our data, and those of others (22,24,51), indicate that DPG
exerts effects at concentrations considerably above the 1:1 hemo-
globin:DPG mole ratio found by Benesch and Benesch. Those authors
concluded that DPG was bound to one of the basic amino acid
residues lining the central cavity of the hemoglobin molecule, so
that one molecule of DPG could be bound to both β chains simultaneously (19,37). Independent studies suggested that histidine
residues in the H helices (52), or lysine residues (53), may be the
sites involved. Histidine B H 21 has been replaced by aspartic
acid in hemoglobin Hiroshima, which has an increased affinity for
oxygen, and it has been suggested that loss of a binding site for
DPG may be responsible for the abnormal dissociation curve (54).

All data suggest that elevated levels of DPG within red cells
could be a cause of decreased oxygen affinity of blood, but that
binding of DPG to hemoglobin, and the effect of DPG on oxygen
affinity, may be more complex than originally anticipated. Organic
phosphates do exert a profound influence on the oxygen affinity of
hemoglobin; failure of attempts to crystallize deoxyhemoglobin in
the presence of DPG suggest that the metabolite may also affect
the state of aggregation of molecules within the cell. Abnormal
aggregation of molecules of hemoglobin S, independent of DPG
concentration, has been suggested as an explanation of abnormal
oxygen affinity in sickle cell anemia (55). It seems quite likely
that these factors, and others, act in concert to govern this most
important physiologic function.

As tested by both radioactivity and by enzymatic assay, the
amount of firmly bound DPG is small, ca. 5% of the total DPG which
may be bound to oxyhemoglobin. The binding may be similar to
muscle phosphoglyceromutase binding of DPG; this enzyme is not
isolated as a phosphoenzyme nor is there detectable bound DPG.
However, even if the amount of P-enzyme or bound DPG is very small,
it is sufficient to maintain catalytic activity (5). This behavior is even more extreme in the case of the yeast enzyme (56).
Nevertheless, the basic mechanism for both enzymes most likely
necessitates covalent interaction of the cofactor and the protein.
Alternatively, and since only ca 1/20 mole of DPG per mole of
hemoglobin is bound, a certain type of hemoglobin may bind the material. Possibly, either newly formed or older hemoglobin may bind
the DPG. It is of interest that red cells possess a small amount
of adenoyl DPG, (ca. 5% the amount of DPG) (57).

While sedimentation, circular dichroism, and optical rotatory
dispersion measurements have shown no distinct differences in
average molecular weight or conformation between DPG-free deoxyhemoglobin and a mixture of it with the metabolite, nor is there a
difference between mixtures of deoxy- or oxyhemoglobin and DPG,
it is of interest that crystals of horse oxy and deoxyhemoglobin,

provided by Dr. Max Perutz, were free of DPG. Attempts to crystallize human hemoglobin in the presence of DPG proved most difficult,
and the crystals obtained were quite imperfect.

We are all aware that hemoglobin in the red cell is the most
concentrated protein known and often simply by lysing the red cell,
hemoglobin may crystallize. It is my considerate opinion, as
previously suggested (8), that the main role of DPG in the red cell
is that of affecting conformation resulting in deaggregation which
in turn prevents hemoglobin from crystallizing in vivo.

Acknowledgments
        Supported by PHS, Grants AM01855, AM13119, HE 02799-13,
the American Heart Association, the Kansas Heart Association
and the Life Insurance Medical Research Fund, G-68-30. J.
Carreras (on leave of absence from the University of Barcelona)
is a Special Fellow of PHS, 1 F05 TW01388-01. I wish to thank
J. Luque, A. Diederich, K.Moore, H. Grady and S. Burke for their
contributions to the work presented here.

Bibliography

1. Greenwald, I., J. Biol. Chem., 63, 339, 1925.
2. Grisolia, S., in Phosphorus Metabolism (McElroy and Glass,
    eds.), p. 619, The Johns Hopkins Press, Baltimore, 1951.
3. FEBS Symposium, Metabolic Regulation and Enzyme Action, (Sols
    and Grisolia, eds.), Academic Press, London and New York,
    In Press, 1969.
4. Grisolia, S., in Methods in Enzymology, (Colowick and Kaplan,
    eds.), V, 236, Academic Press, New York and London, 1962.
5. Grisolia, S., and Cleland, W.W., Biochem., 7, 1115, 1968.
6. Grisolia, S., and Joyce, B., J. Biol. Chem., 234, 1335, 1959.
7. Cascales, M., and Grisolia, S., Biochem., 5, 3116, 1966.
8. Grisolia, S., in Homologous Enzymes and Biochemical Evolution,
    (Thoai and Roche, eds.), p. 167, Gordon and Breach Science
    Publishers, New York, 1968.
9. Chanutin, A., and Curnish, R.R., Arch. Biochem. Biophys., 121,
    96, 1967.
10. Benesch, R., Benesch, R.E., and Yu, C.I., Proc. U.S. Nat. Acad.
    Sci., 59, 526, 1968.
11. Warren, J.C., Carr, D.O., and Grisolia, S., Biochem. J., 93,
    409, 1964.
12. Grisolia, S., Lancet, II, 1033, 1968.
13. Grisolia, S., Physiological Rev., 44, 657, 1964.
14. Diederich, D.A., and Grisolia, S., J. Biol. Chem., 294, 2412,
    1969.
15. Grisolia, S., Biochem. Biophys. Res. Commun., 32, 56, 1968.

16. Towne, J.C., Rodwell, V.W., and Grisolia, S., J. Biol. Chem.,
    226, 777, 1957.
17. Bartlett, G.R., J. Biol. Chem., 234, 466, 1959.
18. Grisolia, S., Moore, K., Luque, J., and Grady, H., Anal.
    Biochem., In Press, 1969.
19. Benesch R., Benesch, R.E., and Enoki, Y., Proc. Nat. Acad.
    Sci. U.S., 61, 1102, 1968.
20. Engel, K., and Duc, G., Nature, 219, 936, 1968.
21. Akerblom, O., de Verdier, C.H., Garby, L., and Högman, C.,
    Scand. J. Clin. Lab. Invest., 21, 245, 1968.
22. Bunn, H.F., May, M.H., Kocholaty, W.F., and Shields, C.E.,
    J. Clin. Invest., 48, 311, 1969.
23. Lenfant, C., Torrance, J., English, E., Finch, C.A.,
    Reynafarje, C., Ramos, J., and Faura, J., J. Clin. Invest.,
    47, 2652, 1968.
24. Eaton, J.W., Brewer, G.J., and Grover, R.F., J. Lab. Clin. Med.,
    73, 603, 1969.
25. Mourjinis, A., Walters, C., Edwards, M.J., Koler, R.D.,
    Vanderheiden, B., and Metcalf, J., Clin. Res., 17, 153, 1969.
26. Charache, S., Fiedler, A.J., Grisolia, S., and Hellegers, A.E.,
    Clin. Res., 16, 301 (Abstr.), 1968.
27. Luque, J., Diederich, D., and Grisolia, S., Biochem. Biophys.
    Res. Commun., 36, 1019, 1969.
28. Pfleiderer, G., and Auricchio, F., Biochem. Biophys. Res.
    Commun., 16, 53, 1964.
29. Torralba, A., and Grisolia, S., J. Biol. Chem., 241, 1713, 1966.
30. Grisolia, S., and Jacobs, R., J. Biol. Chem., 241, 5926, 1966.
31. Diederich, A., Diederich, D., Luque, J., and Grisolia, S.,
    FEBS Letters, In Press, 1969.
32. Benesch, R.E., Benesch, R., and Yu, C.I., Biochem., 8, 2567,
    1969.
33. Charache, S., Grisolia, S., Fiedler, A., and Hellegers, A.,
    (Submitted for publication).
34. Becklake, M.R., Griffiths, S.B., McGregor, M., Goldman, H.I.,
    and Schreve, J.P., J. Clin. Invest., 34, 751, 1955.
35. Bromberg, P.A., and Jensen, W.N., J. Lab. Clin. Med., 70,
    480, 1967.
36. Allen, D.W., and Wyman, J. Jr., Rev. Hématol., 9, 155, 1954.
37. Harkness, D., Ponce, J., and Grayson, V., Comp. Biochem.
    Physiol., 28, 129, 1969.
38. Kennedy, A.C., and Valtis, D.J., J. Clin. Invest., 33, 1372,
    1954.
39. Edwards, M.J., Novy, M.J., Walters, C.L., and Metcalfe, J.,
    J. Clin. Invest., 47, 1851, 1968.
40. Eaton, J.W., Brewer, G.J., Proc. Nat. Acad. Sci., U.S., 61,
    756, 1968.
41. Oski, F., Miller, W., Delivoria-Papadopoulos, M., and Gottlieb,
    A., Society for Pediatric Research, 39th Annual Meeting, 46,
    (Abstr.) 1969.

42. Rapoport, S., and Luebering, J., J. Biol. Chem., 196, 583, 1952.
43. Benesch, R., and Benesch, R.E., Nature, 221, 618, 1969.
44. Rose, Z.B., J. Biol. Chem., 243, 4810, 1968.
45. Joyce, B.K., and Grisolia, S., J. Biol. Chem., 234, 1330, 1959.
46. Charache, S., Weatherall, D.J., and Clegg, J.B., J. Clin. Invest., 45, 813, 1966.
47. Stamatoyannopoulos, G., Yoshida, A., Adamson, J., and Heinenberg, S., Science, 159, 741, 1968.
48. Bonaventura, J., and Riggs, A., J. Biol. Chem., 243, 980, 1968.
49. Bishop, C., in The Red Blood Cell, (Bishop and Surgenor, eds.), p. 153, Academic Press, New York and London, 1964.
50. Gemmill, C.L., and Brobeck, J.R., in Medical Physiology, (Mountcastle, ed.), 1, 473, C.V. Mosby, St. Louis, 1968.
51. Rörth, M., Scand. J. Clin. Lab. Invest., 22, 208, 1968.
52. Perutz, M.F., and Lehmann, H., Nature, 219, 902, 1968.
53. Benesch, R.E., Benesch, R., and Yu, C.I., Fed. Proc., 28, 604, (Abstr.), 1969.
54. Hamilton, H.B., Iuchi, I., Miyaji, T., and Shibata, S., J. Clin. Invest., 48, 525, 1969.
55. Bromberg, P.A., and Jensen, W.N., J. Clin. Invest., 44, 1031, (Abstr.), 1965.
56. Bogart, D., and Grisolia, S., (unpublished observations).
57. Hashimoto, T., Tatibana, M., and Yoshikawa, H., J. Biochem., 50, 471, 1961.

DEPENDENCE OF OXYHEMOGLOBIN DISSOCIATION AND INTRA-ERYTHROCYTIC 2.3-DPG ON ACID-BASE STATUS OF BLOOD. I.IN VITRO STUDIES ON REDUCED AND OXYGENATED BLOOD

Mikael Rørth

Department of Clinical Chemistry A,

Rigshospitalet,Copenhagen,Denmark

INTRODUCTION

According to the conception of the regulation of the intraerythrocytic 2.3-DPG concentration,introduced recently,the most important regulatory factor should be the level of reduced hemoglobin in the erythrocytes (i.e.either the "average" level in the circulatory system or the maximal level attained on the venous side) (GARBY AND DE VERDIER,1969,BENESCH AND BENESCH,1969). The main support for this hypothesis comes from the well-known increase in 2.3-DPG concentration seen under several hypoxic conditions (LENFANT ET AL.,1968).The adaptional nature of this regulatory mechanism should be imitable in vitro under proper incubation conditions. This paper describes the results of some in vitro experiments,where we have studied the effect of pH,deoxygenation and addition of different substances to human blood.

The aim of this study was to provide information, that ultimatively could help us to evaluate some of the physiological and pathological problems in this field.

As well our in vitro studies as our in vivo studies have concentrated on the effect of pH on the 2.3-DPG concentration and on the oxyhemoglobin dissociation curve (characterized by the T50 value).It seems to be generally accepted,that 2.3-DPG is the most important regulator of oxyhemoglobin dissociation at constant pH and temperature.

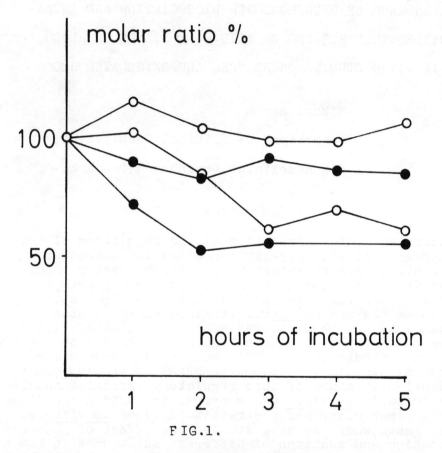

FIG.1.

Variation in 2.3-DPG concentration during incubation
at constant pH.Concentrations are given as per cent
of start value.
     2 upper curves : pH 7.55
     2 lower curves : pH 7.05.
● : 18.5% oxygen ,   ○ : 0% oxygen.

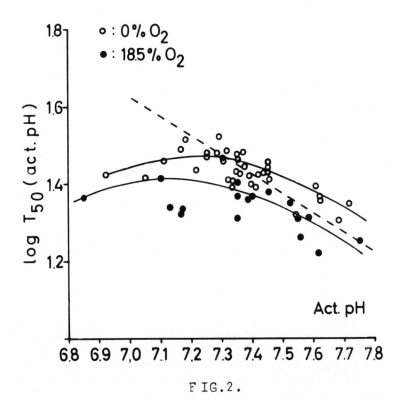

F IG.2.

Effect of pH on T50 at actual pH. The dotted line
indicates the T50 variation according to the Bohr
effect ($\Delta \log Po_2$ = - 0.50 Δ pH).

MATERIALS AND METHODS

Throughout the study freshly drawn heparinized blood
from young healthy subjects was used.Immediately after
the blood was drawn,it was poured into Visking bags,
1 ml in each.The bags were mounted in 1.5 l dialysis
chambers,3 bags in each.The dialysis chambers contained
Krebs-Ringer solution with glucose (3 g/l),the bicarbonate concentration was varied.The dialysis system was
equilibrated with humidified gas mixtures containing
18.5% oxygen,5.3% carbon dioxide and 76.2% nitrogen
respectively 5.3% carbon dioxide and 94.7% nitrogen.
Stirring was provided by rotating the bags (100 r.p.m.).
After equilibration the blood was analyzed for 2.3-DPG
(NYGAARD AND RØRTH,1969),T50 (the Po_2-value giving 50%
oxygen saturation of hemoglobin)(ASTRUP ET AL.,1965),
actual pH,hematocrit and hemoglobin concentration
(conventional methods).

RESULTS

Using the described incubation procedure,we found,that
the steady-state level of 2.3-DPG and T50 was attained
after a minimum of 3 hours (Fig.1).

    Fig.2 shows the variations of log T50 with pH.
It is clearly seen,that the Bohr-effect (calculated
from the data of ASTRUP ET AL.,1965) is completely
abolished at low pH-values.At higher pH-values,the
oxyhemoglobin dissociation is apparently left unaltered.
At pH 7.40,the difference between results obtained
after incubation with oxygen (more than 95% oxyhemoglobin saturation) and after incubation without oxygen
is about 4-5 mm Hg,the latter giving the highest T50,
i.e.the lowest oxygen affinity.

    Fig.3 shows the pH-dependency of the 2.3-DPG level
in the erythrocytes.The 2.3-DPG concentration decreases
with decreasing pH in the range below pH 7.40.The
maximal linear decrease being about 0.025 molar ratio
per o.ol pH unit.In the pH range above 7.40,there seems
to be a slight decrease in the 2.3-DPG concentration
with increasing pH.In experiments without oxygen at pH
7.40,the 2.3-DPG level was found about 15% higher than
in experiments with oxygenated blood.

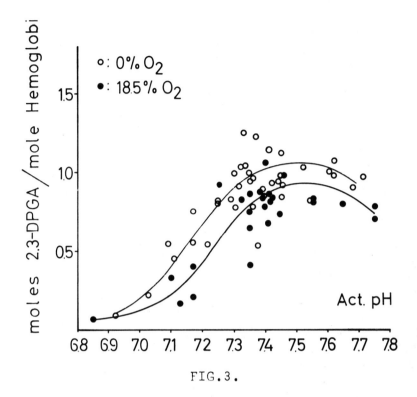

FIG.3.

pH-dependency of the 2.3-DPG level.

These results confirm,at least qualitativelty,the results of ASAKURA ET AL.,1966a(effect of pH) and ASAKURA ET AL.,1966b (effect of deoxygenation).

In some experiments the content of free SH-groups in the erythrocytes was measured,but no significant variation within the pH range 7.00-7.60 was found.

DISCUSSION

As it now seems to be generally accepted,that 2.3-DPG is the most important regulator of T50,it is reasonable to suggest,that the variations in T50 induced in our

experiments were due to variations in the 2.3-DPG level.
Fig.4 shows,that this is probably the case.But it is
noteworthy,that there is a considerable dispersion of
the results in the physiological range,indicating
that other compounds are of importance for the regulation
of the oxyhemoglobin dissociation.

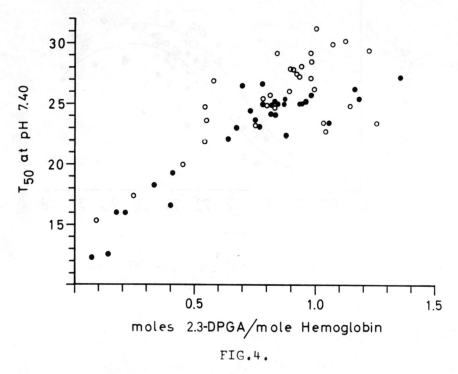

FIG.4.

T50 at pH 7.40 plotted against the 2.3-DPG concentration.

The correlation between 2.3-DPG level and T50 does
of course not necessarily indicate a causal relationship.
It could just be concomitant phenomena.However,when
2.3-DPG is added to hemolysates (hemolysed,packed red
cells),T50 increases ,as shown in Fig.5.

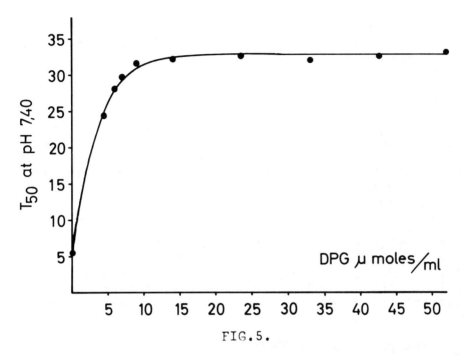

FIG.5.

Effect of addition of 2.3-DPG on T50,corrected
to pH 7.40.
Hemolysates were obtained by repeated freeze and
thawing of packed red cells.

The effect of lowering the pH from 7.40 is remarkably pronounced,though not as pronounced as in
vivo (ASTRUP AND RORTH,1969),but in contrast to in
vivo conditions,an increase of PH above 7.40 does not
lead to an increase in the 2.3-DPG level.

The effect of deoxygenation is in our experiments
far less,than would be expected from the theory of

the level of reduced hemoglobin as regulator of the
2.3-DPG concentration in erythrocytes,and I beleive
that our results are compatible with the assumption,
that the effect of deoxygenation in vitro is due to
a decrease in the pH gradient between plasma and red
cells.

Our in vitro system has,however,not proved to be
a suitable tool for providing an explanation of the
high intraerythrocytic concentration of 2.3-DPG sometimes seen in vivo.It is therefore reasonable to suggest,that an accumulation of 2.3-DPG requires an addition of something more than glucose to the blood,i.e.
a substrate for metabolic reactions or possibly a
hormone,acting as regulator of some enzymatic activity.
Until now we have,however,not been able to find such
"a factor",but it is possible that "the factor" only
operates on reduced blood,in which the level of
"frcc" 2.3-DPG must be lower than in oxygenated blood
(BENESCH AND BENESCH,1969).We are now testing different
relevant compounds on as well oxygenated as reduced
blood samples.

The pronounced effect of pH and the modest effect
of deoxygenation in vitro has led us to the provisio-
nal assumption,that the pH-effects might even be of
regulatory nature.Physiological and pathological
consequences of this hypothesis will be discussed in
the following paper.

SUMMARY

The effect in vitro of pH on the 2.3-DPG level and
oxyhemoglobin dissociation is very pronounced at pH
belove 7.40.The effect of deoxygenation is relatively
small,so that the in vitro effect of deoxygenation
(increase in the 2.3-DPG level)could be due to intracellular pH-changes induced by deoxygenation of hemo-
globin.Other substances may play an important role
in the regulation of the oxygen affinity of blood,as
the correlation between 2.3-DPG level and T50 os not
too good in the physiological range.
It has not been possible in vitro to attain as
high 2.3-DPG levels as sometimes seen in vivo,neither
by increasing pH,by decreasing Po_2 nor by addition of
different compounds to oxygenated blood.
A regulatory influence of pH on the 2.3-DPG level is
proposed.

REFERENCES

Asakura,T.,Sato,Y.,Minakami,S.and Yoshikawa,H (1966)
    Clin.Chim.Acta 14:840
Asakura,T.,Sato,Y.,Minakami,S.and Yoshikawa,H (1966)
    J.Biochem (Tokyo) 5:224
Astrup,P.,Engel,K.,Seweringhaus,J.W. and Munson,E.
    (1965) Scand.J.Clin.Lab.Invest.17:515.
Astrup,P. and Rørth,M. (1969)
    Presented at this meeting.
Benesch,R.and Benesch,R.E. (1969),
    Nature,221:618.
Garby,L. and de Verdier,C.-H..Presented at the Symposium
    on intracellular regulation of Hemoglobin Affinity
    to oxygen (Uppsala,1969).
Lenfant,C.,Torrance,J.,English,E.,Finch,C.A.,Reynafarje
C.,Ramos,J. and Faura J. (1968),
    J.Clin.Invest.,47:2652.
Nygaard,S. and Rørth,M.(1969),
    Scand.J.Clin.Lab.Invest. in press.

DEPENCE OF OXYHEMOGLOBIN DISSOCIATION AND INTRAERY-
THROCYTIC 2,3-DPG ON ACID-BASE STATUS OF BLOOD.
II. CLINICAL AND EXPERIMENTAL STUDIES

P. Astrup

Rigshospitalet

Copenhagen, Denmark

Since our first report (Astrup, 1969) at a symposium in
Uppsala in February 1969 on changes of the oxygen affinity of hemoglobin due to pH-dependent 2,3-DPG changes
we have studied this relationship more extensively in
patients with acid-base disorders and also in normal
individuals with induced changes of the acid-base status of the blood. The results of these investigations
will be presented in this paper.

MATERIAL AND METHODS

The patients with acid-base disorders used for the study were spotted by abnormal results of standard bicarbonate analysis on blood samples sent to out laboratory
for routine examinations. The following morning new
blood samples were drawn for determinations of acid-base
status, intraerythrocytic pH, T_{50} value, concentration
of 2,3-DPG and of other blood constituents. Frequently
the analyses were repeated on following days. All the
records of the patients were seen for evaluation of the
cause of the acid-base disorder and results of clinical
and laboratory investigations of possible interest were
noted. The patients were spread all over the hospital
and did present many types of acid-base disorders. The
more severe cases of metabolic acidosis all had renal
failure.

Furthermore, acid-base disturbances were induced
in normal non-smokers, alkalosis by giving sodium bicarbonate by mouth or intravenously, and acidosis by

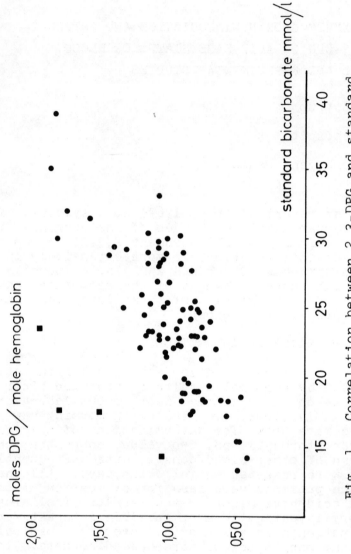

Fig. 1. Correlation between 2,3-DPG and standard bicarbonate in patients with metabolic acid-base disorders. The circles indicate patients with normal or moderately elevated inorganic serum phosphate. Squares indicate patients with high inorganic serum phosphate.

giving ammonium chloride by mouth. In a few anesthetized patients respiratory acid-base changes were induced
by increasing the CO_2 content of the inspiratory air.

The determination of 2,3-DPG was carried out enzymatically (Nygaard and Rørth, 1969). The T_{50} value was
calculated at a pH of 7.40 after determining two points
of the curve by equilibrating the blood at two pO_2 values and at a fixed pCO_2 value. The oxygen saturation
was then determined spectrophotometrically on erythrolysate. Corrections were made for the occurrence of
carboxyhemoglobin. The technique is described in details elsewhere (Astrup et al., 1965). Intraerythrocytic pH was determined by using a capillary glass
electrode directly on erythrolysate, obtained by anaerobic freezing and thawing of packed red cells from
blood equilibrated with a gas mixture having a pCO_2 of
40 mm Hg and a high pO_2. Other determinations of blood
constituents were made by routine methods used in the
department.

RESULTS

Figure 1 illustrates the relation between 2,3-DPG levels and standard bicarbonate levels. The correlation
coefficient was calculated to 0.74. The samples with
standard bicarbonate within the normal range were chosen at random, while all the samples with abnormal
standard bicarbonate values came from patients exclu-
sively with metabolic acid-base disorders. We have
also measured on a few patients with respiratory acidosis having high standard bicarbonate values due to
renal compensation and here found low 2,3-DPG values,
which placed the values in the lower right corner outside the pattern shown in figure 1. The results thus
indicate that it is the blood pH which determines the
2,3-DPG concentration.

It is well known that there is a correlation between standard bicarbonate values and blood pH in all
cases of metabolic disorders depending on the degree
of the respiratory compensation. By correlating pH and
standard bicarbonate values measured on a great number
of samples of capillary blood from patients without respiratory acid-base disorders (correlation coefficient
0.86), and further by correlating to the values in figure 1 it was found, that a pH change of 0.01 corre-
sponded to a change in the 2,3-DPG concentration of
3.8%.

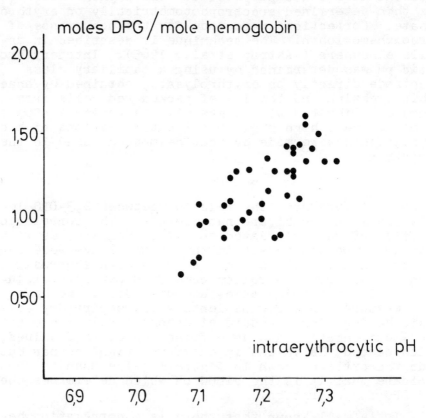

Fig. 2. Correlation between 2,3-DPG and red cell
pH in patients with metabolic acid-base disorders.
Circles and squares: as in fig. 1.

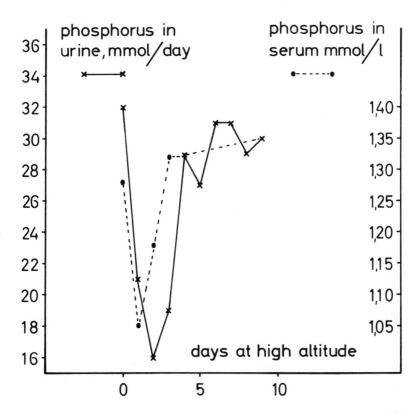

Fig. 3.   Inorganic phosphate values in serum and urine
before and after ascension to high altitude (3500 m).

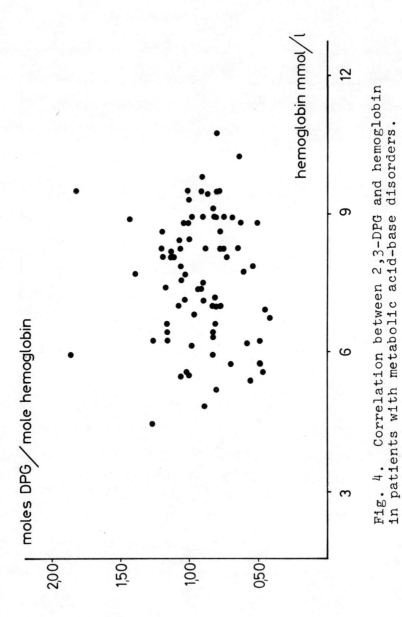

Fig. 4. Correlation between 2,3-DPG and hemoglobin in patients with metabolic acid-base disorders.

Since measured values of blood pH refer to plasma values, it was decided also to measure the red cell pH in samples obtained from a similar group of patients as for figure 1. In figure 2 it is demonstrated that the correlation to the corresponding 2,3-DPG values is good, the correlation coefficient being 0.69. A calculation of the pH/2,3-DPG correlation shows again a 2,3-DPG change of approximately 4% when red cell pH changes 0.01.

Only blood samples from patients with normal or moderately increased concentrations of inorganic serum phosphate (normal range: 0.8-1.5 mmol/liter) were used to give the pH/2,3-DPG correlation indicated by the circles in figure 1 and 2. We found, however, that 4 patients with concentrations of inorganic serum phosphate higher than 3 mmol/liter, all having severe uremic acidosis, had much higher 2,3-DPG values, as shown by the squares in figure 1, than could be expected from their standard bicarbonate values. A connection between the metabolism of inorganic phosphate and of 2,3-DPG, which theoretically might be anticipated, is also illustrated by the very considerable decrease of inorganic phosphate in serum and urine (figure 3) which we in 1967 (Kjeldsen and Damgaard, 1968) found in 8 individuals the first day after ascension to Jungfraujoch (3500 m) in Switzerland. This decrease may probably be explained by the concomitant rise in the intracellular increase in 2,3-DPG concentration, recently measured by us to approximately 20-25% when ascending to Jungfraujoch.

In our patients we found no correlation between the concentration of 2,3-DPG and the concentration in plasma of sodium, potassium, calcium, magnesium, urea and creatinine. Neither was there a correlation to the concentration of hemoglobin as demonstrated in figure 4.

When inducing metabolic alkalosis or acidosis in normal individuals, the concentration of 2,3-DPG increased respectively decreased as demonstrated in figure 5, showing average values for 3 individuals given 200 mmoles sodium bicarbonate daily for 4 days, and for 3 other individuals given the same amount of ammonium chloride. The blood plasma pH was measured every morning and showed a rise respectively a fall in the two groups. Intravenous infusions of sodium bicarbonate in a few individuals did not show any significant change of 2,3-DPG, probably because of only small and transient pH changes. Also in some anesthetized pa-

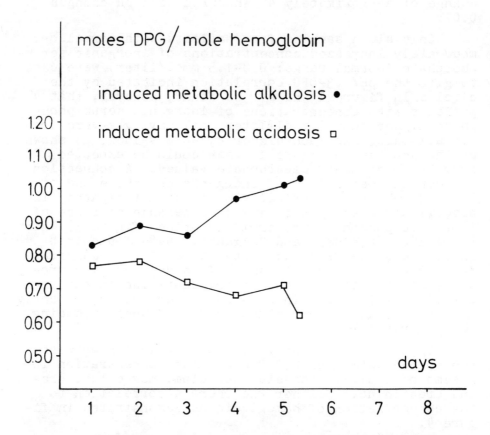

Fig. 5. 2,3-DPG values in normal individuals with induced acid-base disorders. Each curve gives average
values of 3 individuals.

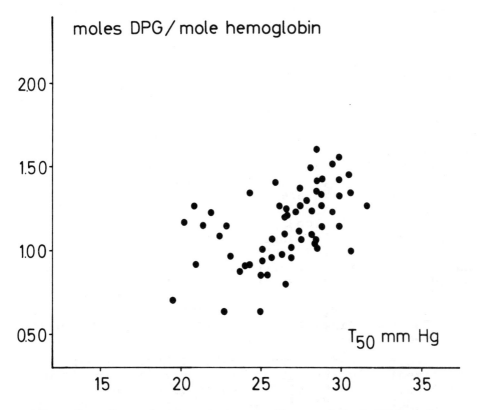

Fig. 6. Correlation between T_{50} and 2,3-DPG values in patients with metabolic acid-base disorders.

tients the induction of respiratory acidosis respectively alkalosis during a few hours was not followed by significant 2,3-DPG changes, except in one case. In the
other patients there was a tendency to obtain the expected 2,3-DPG changes, but obviously the exposure time
was too short.

The results of T_{50} measurements on blood from the
patients with metabolic acid-base disorders are shown
in figure 6. The T_{50} values are related to 2,3-DPG values, and it is obvious, that a correlation between
the two parameters exists.

DISCUSSION AND CONCLUSIONS

Our investigations indicate that the red cell level of
2,3-DPG is controlled by the red cell pH. This is not
a new finding, since Rapoport and Guest (1939) published similar results. Rapoport and coworkers also described the involved enzymatic reactions, now known as
the Rapoport-Luebering pathway. It is, however, remarkable that a change of red cell pH as small as 0.01
will change the 2,3-DPG concentration as much as approximately 4%. We are of the opinion that the 2,3-DPG
changes found at high altitude are caused by the so far
overlooked small blood pH changes which occur there.
Likewise, small pH changes are probably also responsible for the 2,3-DPG changes found in anemia and perhaps also under other circumstances, where the cause of
a 2,3-DPG change so far has been unknown. So, at a altitude of 3500 m the arterial blood pH increases from
7.40 to 7.42-7.43, which should give a 10-15% rise of
2,3-DPG thus being responsible for a great part of the
measured change.

Since a pH-dependent 2,3-DPG change takes place
not immediately, but at optimal conditions in vitro after 3 hours (Rørth, 1969), and in vivo after 12-24
hours (Mulhausen, 1968), and since it is the red cell
pH which has importance, we feel that the concept mean
red cell pH should be introduced.

We should like to emphasize, that the mean red
cell pH theoretically must depend on the relation between the total amount of protons in blood on the venous side and on the arterial side, since the venous
blood is slightly more acid than the arterial blood
and by volume comprises 3-4 times more than the arterial blood. Furthermore it should be realized that
oxyhemoglobin is a stronger acid than reduced hemoglobin, which means that the red cell pH increases 0.08%

0.09%due to the Donnan effect when deoxygenation takes
place at a constant plasma pH. This makes it necessary
also to consider the time factor for obtaining equilibrium of protons between the red cells and plasma, when
the oxygenation is changed. Finally it should be considered that we do not measure pH inside the red cells
themselves, but always after lysis. There might be a
difference between these two values.

Having emphasized the importance of those considerations we shall now try to evaluate how the red cell
pH may change in certain conditions. In anemia we usually have a slight pH increase of arterial blood due to
a tendency to hyperventilation. Furthermore, the relation between the total amount of reduced hemoglobin and
of oxygenated hemoglobin is higher than normal, thus
causing a tendency to a higher red cell pH. The same
occurs under all hypoxic conditions, also at high altitude, due to the decrease of arterial oxygen saturation. If we on the other hand expose individuals to
carbon monoxide or to a high oxygen pressure, so the
5-7% of reduced hemoglobin on the arterial side disap-
tears, we should have a tendency to a decrease of 2,3-
DPG. This is actually what happens, measurements show
a 5-15% decrease of 2,3-DPG in such conditions (Astrup,
1969). We therefore find it reasonable to assume, that
the relation between the total amount of reduced and
oxygenated hemoglobin in the vascular system determines
the 2,3-DPG concentration by a primary influence on
mean red cell pH.

Perhaps the mean red cell pH as measured by the
2,3-DPG concentration will appear to be a useful acid-
base parameter for evaluation of various disturbances
of circulatory, respiratory and metabolic functions,
since it expresses the effect of more sustained acid-
base changes. It could be a valuable supplement to
the usually measured acid-base values and perhaps tell
more about the actual status of the patient.

Our investigations have furthermore shown, that
the 2,3-DPG metabolism is related to the metabolism of
inorganic phosphate. This might also be anticipated
since the formation of 1 mole 2,3-DPG requires 2 moles
of phosphate. The significance of this connection under physiological and pathological conditions needs
further investigations, especially by following patients having changing 2,3-DPG concentrations by determining also inorganic serum phosphate and the phosphate balance. Furthermore, the relations between mean
red cell pH and serum inorganic phosphate for determi-

ning the 2,3-DPG level should be investigated. However, as far as it can be seen from the present observations, only highly elevated serum phosphate levels influence the 2,3-DPG concentration to a considerable degree.

The correlation between the T50 and the 2,3-DPG values in blood from patients with acid-base disorders is less pronounced than after in vitro acid-base changes in blood drawn from normal individuals. This indicates that also other intraerythrocytic components than 2,3-DPG are influencing the oxygen affinity of hemoglobin which, however, does not weaken the theory of 2,3-DPG as having general importance for regulating the oxygen affinity of hemoglobin. If this regulation as indicated by the results reported here is directed by the mean red cell pH, it is reasonable to assume that it forms a feedback control system which makes physiological sense and which increases the security of the regulatory interactions between the uptake of oxygen and the excretion of carbon dioxide, the mechanisms which have challenged the physiologists since the beginning of the century.

It should be stressed however that also other regulatory mechanisms might exist, since very high 2,3-DPG levels are found in patients with red cell mass deficits, but without significant acid-base changes.

Summary

The relationship between intraerythrocytic concentrations of 2,3-diphosphoglycerate and the oxygen affinity of hemoglobin was studied in patients with acid-base disorders and in normal individuals with induced changes of blood acid-base status.

The results indicate that the mean red cell pH is the main determinant of the intraerythrocytic concentration of 2,3-diphosphoglycerate. Furthermore it is shown that relations exist between changes in concentrations of inorganic phosphate in serum and urine and changes in the 2,3-diphosphoglycerate concentrations.

The results are discussed and it is concluded that the regulation of the concentration of the 2,3-diphosphoglycerate by its linkage to the mean red cell pH forms a feed-back control system for maintaining normal oxygen release from hemoglobin.

REFERENCES

Astrup, P. (1969). Forsvarsmedicin. In press.
Astrup, P., Engel, K., Severinghaus, J.W., and Munson, E. (1965). Scand. J. Clin. Lab. Invest. 17:515.
Kjeldsen, K., and Damgaard, F. (1968). Scand. J. Clin. Lab. Invest., Suppl. 103, 22:20.
Mulhausen, R.O., Astrup, P., and Mellemgaard, K. (1968). Scand. J. Clin. Lab. Invest., Suppl. 103, 22:9.
Nygaard, S., and Rorth, M. (1969). Scand. J. Clin. Lab. Invest. In press.

Rapoport, S., and Guest, G.M. (1939). J. Biol. Chem. 131:576.
Rorth, M. (1969). This journal, preceding paper.

ERYTHROCYTE GLYCOLYTIC INTERMEDIATES AND COFACTORS CORRELATED WITH

THE HAEMOGLOBIN CONCENTRATION IN HUMAN NEONATES AND ADULTS

Magnus Hjelm

Department of Clinical Chemistry

University Hospital, Uppsala, Sweden

Human erythrocytes are highly specialized cells containing haemoglobin for the transport of oxygen. It seems reasonable to assume
that their simplified metabolic systems, the glycolytic pathway and
the pentose phosphate shunt, is essential for the maintenance of
this oxygen carrying function. It has previously been reported that
reduced glutathione (GSH) influences the affinity of haemoglobin
to oxygen in intact erythrocytes (cf. Horejsi 1967) and it has
recently been found, that several organic phosphocompounds, some
of which are normally present in human erythrocytes, bind to haemoglobin in vitro (Chanutin & Curnish 1964, Benesch & Benesch 1968,
Garby & de Verdier 1968). Most of the compounds investigated
showed a higher affinity for deoxygenated than for oxygenated haemoglobin. The binding is correlated with an decreased affinity of the
haemoglobin molecule for oxygen (Chanutin & Curnish 1967, Benesch &
Benesch 1967). If these findings are relevant also for the conditions in vivo, then there should be a correlation between the
average amount of deoxygenated haemoglobin and the binding of
organic phosphocompounds, i.e. the molar ratio of phosphocompound
to haemoglobin should increase with increasing average deoxygenation of the circulating haemoglobin. Several pieces of evidence
have also been obtained, that support this concept. An increased
content of phosphocompounds, mainly 2,3-diphosphoglycerate (DPG)
and ATP, has been found in erythrocytes from subjects with a
decrease of the oxygen saturation of the blood (Lenfant et al. 1969)
or where it seems likely to assume that the time average concentra-

This investigation was sponsored by the Swedish Medical Research
Council (Project No. B 66- 19 X -153 -02)

tion of deoxygenated haemoglobin is increased (Eaton & Brewer 1968, Hjelm 1968, 1969, Fortier & Valeri 1969).

Based on these findings in vitro and in vivo a hypothesis concerning the regulation of the tissue oxygen tension has been proposed (de Verdier, Garby & Hjelm 1969, Benesch & Benesch 1969). The hypothesis explains the decreased oxygen affinity in subjects with anaemia (cf. Rodman, Close & Purcell 1960) and may also be essential for the understanding of the relation between the cardiac output and the haemoglobin mass. (cf. Wade & Bishop 1962)

This report deals with the correlation between the content of some organic phosphocompounds in human erythrocytes and the haemoglobin concentration found in healthy neonates and adults and subjects with anaemia. The correlation between the content of erythrocyte glutathione (GSH) and the haemoglobin concentration found in adults (cf Horejsi 1967) and in healthy neonates (Hjelm 1969) will also be discussed as this correlation has been considered important for the oxygen release capacity of the circulating haemoglobin mass.

Materials and Methods

The different types of subjects and methods used have as a rule been described in detail elsewhere (Hjelm 1969 b). DPG was determined by de Verdier's and Killanders's modification (1962) of Bartlett's chromatografic method (1959). ATP was determined by the enzymatic method of Adam 1962 and glucose-6-phosphate (G-6-P) and fructose-6-phosphate (F-6-P) by the enzymatic method of Hohorst 1962. For the determination of GSH the glyoxalase method was used (Racher 1951). Oxidized glutathione (GSSG) was determined by the glutathione reductase method. Standard bicarbonate determinations were performed according to Andersen et al. 1960. Haemoglobin was determined with the cyanmethaemoglobin method and haematocrit determinations according to Garby & Vuille 1961.

Calculations: The content of erythrocyte compounds has been calculated as moles per liter of cells (cf. Hjelm 1969 a). The sum of G-6-P + F-6-P has been used to eliminate the possible conversion of small amounts of G-6-P to F-6-P during the analytical procedure. The sum of GSH + 2 GSSG was used as a measure of GSH for the same reason (cf. Srivastava & Beutler 1968).

Result and Discussion

1. The correlation between the content of erythrocyte DPG and the haemoglobin concentration

In table I constants are given for the correlation between the content of erythrocyte DPG and the haemoglobin concentration - used as

TABLE I
The correlation between the content of erythrocyte DPG (y) and
haemoglobin concentration in blood (x). From Hjelm 1969 (b).

	N	$a^{1)}$	$b^{1)}$	$r^{2)}$	Hb, range $^{3)}$
$y = DPG^{4)}$					
Neonates >80 hours$^{5)}$	16	-.55	15.9	$-.81^{***}$	15 - 21
Healthy males	28	-.64	13.5	$-.65^{**}$	12 - 15
Healthy females	27	-.52	11.1	$-.61^{***}$	11 - 14.5
Nonsperocytic haemolytic anaemia$^{6)}$	13	-.45	10.0	$-.87^{***}$	9 - 14
Iron deficiency anaemia$^{7)}$	16	-.33	8.9	$-.69^{**}$	6 - 10

1) constants for y = ax + b   * $0.05 > p > 0.01$
2) Correlation coefficient, the significance   ** $0.01 > p > 0.001$
   of the values has been tested with Student's *** $0.001 > p$
   t-test.
3) g/100 ml.
4) Calculated as moles x 10^{3}/liter of erythrocytes.
5) All neonates were fullterm, apparently healthy
   and no evidence of pathologically increased
   bilirubin values.
6) The values of erythrocyte hexokinase, phosphofructokinase, diphosphofructoaldolase, glucose
   6-phosphate dehydrogenase and glutathione
   reductase ($NADPH^{+}$ dependent) were within or
   slightly above the normal range.
7) As judged from MCHC (low values) and bone marrow
   smears.

an indirect measure of the haemoglobin mass - in different groups
of subjects. It is evident that highly significant inverse correlations are found between the two variables both in healthy neonates,
adults and subjects with nonspherocytic haemolytic or iron
deficiency anaemia. These correlations can be interpreted, that
the time average concentration of deoxygenated haemoglobin increases
at decreasing haemoglobin concentration in all groups investigated.

It is of interest to notice that the content of erythrocyte DPG in
neonates is nearly twice that in adults at a haemoglobin concentration of 15 grams/100 ml. It has recently been found that haemoglobin
F in vitro binds less DPG than haemoglobin A does (de Verdier &
Garby 1969). This condition is probably of physiological importance
in utero for the oxygen release capacity of the circulating blood

with respect to the low oxygen tension in arterial blood and peripheral tissues as discussed by de Verdier & Garby 1969. However, this property of haemoglobin F is probably a disadvantage after delivery, if the content of DPG was the same in erythrocytes from neonates as in those from adults and if it is assumed of importance to keep the tissue oxygen at the same level as for adults. In this respect the increased content of DPG in neonatal erythrocytes may be looked upon as compensatory. It is suggestive to speculate, that the increased glycolytic rate (cf. Oski & Naiman 1966) found in neonatal erythrocytes compared to adults is of functional significance in this respect and reflects nature's way of regulating the oxygen release from cells with different haemoglobin molecules.

In table I the content of erythrocyte DPG has been calculated per liter of cells (cf. Hjelm 1969 a). The correlations are principally valid also when the content of erythrocyte DPG is calculated as moles per intracellular haemoglobin or per cell in healthy neonates and adults and in subjects with nonspherocytic haemolytic anaemia with a normal mean corpuscular haemoglobin concentration (MCHC). The values increase considerably, when expressed per intracellular haemoglobin or per cell in the group of subjects with iron deficiency anaemia compared with the other groups investigated due to the decreased values of MCHC and the mean corpuscular cell volume (MCV). Thus the content of erythrocyte DPG and also of other compounds in the erythrocytes should probably not be calculated as moles per intracellular haemoglobin in this connection as an increased value will probably not reflect an increased molar ratio of the phospho-compounds (cf. Hjelm 1969 a).

The content of erythrocyte DPG in subjects with nonspherocytic haemolytic anaemia and concommitant pyruvate kinase deficiency correlated with the haemoglobin concentration is shown in fig. 1. Though the number of subjects investigated are too small to allow statistical calculations, there is a tendency towards increased DPG values at a decreased haemoglobin concentration also in this group, though the content of erythrocyte DPG is considerably increased compared with healthy adults at a fixed haemoglobin concentration.

Neonates younger than eighty hours have been excluded from the correlataons in table I as it was found that the content of erythrocyte DPG varied considerably during the first days of life. (Fig. 2). The content of erythrocyte DPG decreased during the first days and increased during the rest of the neonatal period. It seems reasonable to assume that the initially high DPG values can be explained by insufficient oxygenation of the lungs after delivery (Koch 1968) and that the slowly increasing DPG values (Table III) in neonates older than fourty hours are correlated with the increase of relative oxygen consumption during the period (Hill & Robinson 1968)

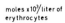

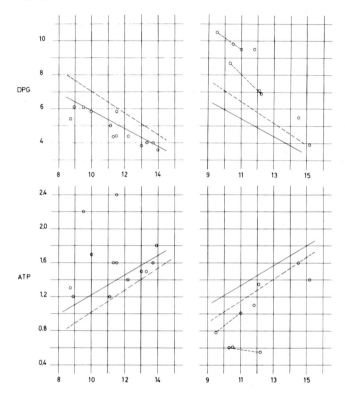

Fig. 1. The correlation between the content of erythrocyte DPG and ATP and the haemoglobin concentration in blood in subjects with nonsperocytic haemolytic anaemia without pyruvate kinase deficient erythrocytes (A) and with decreased activities of the enzyme (B). The regression lines for healthy men (---) and women (——) are also indicated in the figure (Hjelm 1969 (b)).

TABLE II

The correlation between the content of erythrocyte ATP or G-6-P + F-6-P (y) and the haemoglobin concentration in blood (x).[3] Hjelm 1969 b.

	N	a[1]	b[1]	r[2]
y = ATP[4]				
Neonates > 80 hours[5]	13	.070	.09	.80***
Healthy males	25	.13	.27	.60***
Healthy females	26	.11	.08	.53***
y = G-6-P + F-6-P[4]				
Neonates > 80 hours	16	.005	.02	.49*
Healthy males	16	.017	.17	.92***
Healthy females	25	.007	.04	.58***

1, 2, 4, 5) Cf. text to table I.
3) The range of the haemoglobin concentrations was the same as in table I.

TABLE III

Constants for the correlation between the age of the neonate and the content of erythrocyte DPG, ATP and G-6-P + F-6-P. (Cf. Fig. 2)

x	y	n	a[1]	b[1]	r[2]
Age, 40 –120 hours	DPG[4]	20	.024	3.9	.75***
	ATP[4]	20	.0028	1.7	-.47*
	G-6-P + F-6-P[4]	18	.00021	.074	-.48*

1, 2, 4) Cf. text to table I

2. The content of erythrocyte ATP and G-6-P + F-6-P correlated with the haemoglobin concentration.

In table II constants are given for the correlation between the content of erythrocyte ATP or hexosmonophosphates (G-6-P + F-6-P) and the haemoglobin concentration in healthy neonates and adults.

Direct significant correlations are found in all groups. The
correlations also imply, that erythrocytes from neonates contain
about two thirds of the amount of ATP and one third of the amount
of G-6-P and F-6-P compared with adults at comparable haemoglobin
concentrations (14 - 15 g/100 ml).

How these results should be explained is unclear at present. There
is evidence, however, for a competition between organic phosphocompounds in vitro (Garby, Gerber & de Verdier 1969). Thus the
direct correlations found between the content of erythrocyte ATP
or G-6-P + F-6-P and the haemoglobin concentration in vivo in
healthy individuals during standardized conditions may indicate
a competition between these organic phosphocompounds and DPG also in
vivo. This concept is also supported by the finding that the content of erythrocyte DPG increased and that of ATP and G-6-P + F-6-P
decreased with age after delivery in neonates older than 40 hours.
(Fig. 2 and table III).

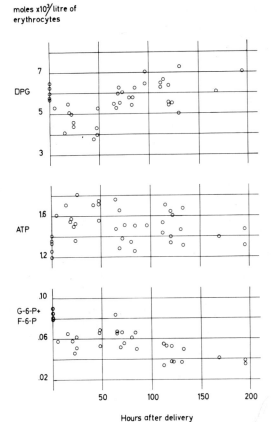

Fig. 2. The content of erythrocyte DPG, ATP and G-6-P + F-6-P in
full-term, healthy neonates during the first week of life.

It has been reported, however, that the content of erythrocyte ATP correlated inversely with the haemoglobin concentration in individuals with anaemia after traumatic injuries (Fortier & Valeri 1969). There is also a tendency for the ATP values to follow the DPG values in erythrocytes from subjects with burns (Arturson & Hjelm 1969) and there is no clear tendency in subjects with anaemia (Hjelm 1969 b). These findings indicate that additional factors are of importance for the content of organic phosphocompounds in the erythrocytes in vivo.

In subjects with nonspherocytic haemolytic anaemia and pyruvate kinase deficiency, the content of erythrocyte DPG and ATP have been found to be increased and decreased respectively. Cf. Fig. 2. These findings have previously been explained by disturbances in the energy balance of the cells (cf. Busch 1964, Nathan et al. 1965), Tanaka & Valentine 1968). An alternative explanation might be, however, that there is an increased competition between DPG and ATP for the haemoglobin molecule in pyruvate kinase deficient erythrocytes, the low ATP values being explained by a decreased binding of ATP to the haemoglobin molecule at a more or less constant level of unbound ATP.

3. The content of erythrocyte glutathione correlated with the haemoglobin concentration.

In table IV constants are given for the correlation between the content of erythrocyte glutathione and the haemoglobin concentration in healthy neonates and adults. There is a close inverse correlation between the content of erythrocyte glutathione and the haemoglobin concentration in neonates older than 50 hours [*] and in accordance

TABLE IV

The correlation between the content of glutathione (y) and the haemoglobin concentration in blood (x).

	n	a[1]	b[1]	r[2]	Hkt[3]
$y = GSH + 2 GSSG$[4]					
Neonates >40 hours[5]	10	-.040	4.3	-.93[***]	46 – 68
Adults(males+females)	25	-.32	4.6	-.43[*]	36 – 46

1, 2, 4, 5) Cf. text to table I
3) The range of the haematocrit values in the two groups investigated.

---

[*] Neonates older than 50 hours have been chosen as the content of glutathione varied slightly during the first days of life.

with previous reports (Tomita 1961. Cernoch & Malinska 1966) a
less pronounced though significant inverse correlation between the
two parameters in adults. It is interesting to notice that the
content of erythrocyte glutathione is considerably increased at a
fixed haemoglobin concentrataon compared to adults. The finding
cannot be explained at present but may have a bearing on the
supposed effect of reduced glutathione on the oxyhaemoglobin dissociation curve (Horejsi 1967).

4. The influence of age on the content of intraerythrocytic compounds.

The content of many compounds differs in young and old erythrocytes
(cf. Oski & Naiman 1966). Thus the increased content of erythrocyte
DPG in subjects with a decreased haemoglobin concentration could
be explained by a decreased mean age of the circulating erythrocytes. However, there is no general agreement at present, concerning the change of the content of erythrocyte DPG with age. Both a
constant (Prankerd 1958, Bernstein 1959) ,(fig. 3) and a decreased
(Bunn, May, Kocholaty & Shields 1969) content of erythrocyte DPG
with increased cell age have been found. Shojana, Israels & Zipursky
in 1968 did not find any significant variation of the content of
erythrocyte DPG with cell age in rabbits.

These discrepancies probably depend both on methodological factors
and the mode of expressing the result (cf. Hjelm 1969). However,
the difference found in the content of erythrocyte DPG with cell
age(Bunn et al. 1969) is under all circumstances too small to
explain the difference in the content of erythrocyte DPG in subjects
with low and normal haemoglobin levels even if it is assumed that
the mean age of the circulating erythrocytes is considerably
decreased in the subjects with low haemoglobin concentrations.

The determination of the content of ATP in young and old erythrocytes
did not reveal any significant variation with age (Prankerd 1958,
Bernstein 1959, Hjelm 1968, 1969). Thus the variations observed in
the content of erythrocyte ATP with the haemoglobin concentration
in healthy neonates and adults cannot possible be explained by
differences in the mean cell age of the circulating erythrocytes
at high and low haemoglobin concentrations.

5. The haemoglobin concentration in whole blood correlated with the content of erythrocyte DPG and the concentration of standardbicarbonate in whole blood.

In fig. 4 the haemoglobin concentration in whole blood has been
correlated with the content of erythrocyte DPG or the concentration of standard bicarbonate in whole blood in subjects with no
apparent signs of impaired kidney or lung function. MCHC did not

---

ᵡ The values recalculated as moles per cell volume.

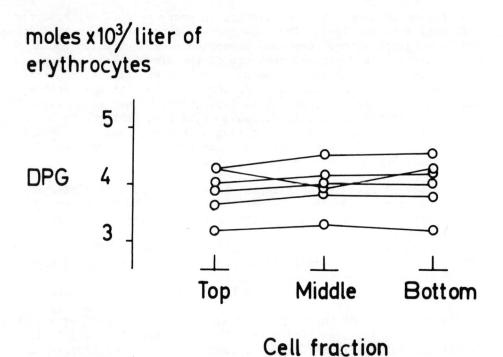

Fig. 3. The content of erythrocyte DPG in erythrocytes separated in age groups Top = younger cells; Bottom = older cells. The cells were fractionated according to Garby & Hjelm 1963.

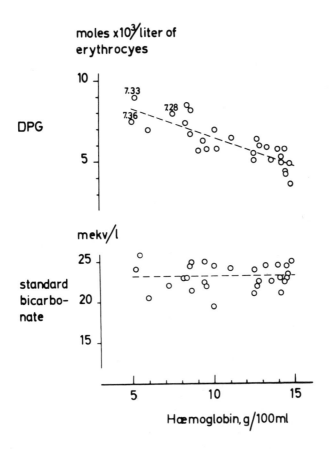

Fig. 4. The correlation between the haemoglobin concentration
(x) in whole blood and the content of erythrocyte DPG
(y) = -.36x + 9.8; r = -.85; n = 28) or the concentration of standard
bicarbonate (y = -.11x + 10.3; r = -.11; n = 28). The subjects
investigated had values of MCHC within the normal range and no
signs of impaired kidney or lung function.

vary with the haemoglobin concentration. Evidently the content of
erythrocyte DPG and not the concentration of standard bicarbonate
varies with the haemoglobin concentration in whole blood. The constant
level of standardbicarbonate indirectly indicates, that arterial pH
also was constant in the subjects investigated. Thus the inverse
correlation between the content of erythrocyte DPG and the haemoglobin concentration strongly indicates, that an increased concentration of deoxygenated haemoglobin and an increased binding
of the phosphocompound at a decreased haemoglobin concentration
is responsible for the increased content of erythrocyte DPG. It
seems reasonable to assume, however, that there is one regression
line between the content of erythrocyte DPG and the haemoglobin

concentration for every pH-value in arterial blood and the intercept
- the content of erythrocyte DPG - on the y-axis probably decreased
at decreased pH-values, though this hypothesis needs further
experimental confirmation.

References:

Adam, H.: 'Adenosin-5'-triphospat und Adenosin-5'-diphosphate'
in H.-U Bergmeyr (ed) Methoden der enzymatischen Analyse. Verlag
Chemie GmbH, Weinheim 1962, p 573.

Andersen, O.S., Endel, K., Jörgensen, K. & Astrup, P.: Scand.
J. Clin. Lab. Invest. 12, 172, 1960.

Arturson, G & Hjelm, M.: in Symposium on intracellular regulation
of hemoglobin affinity to oxygen. Försvarsmedicin 5, 260, 1969.
Swedish Goverrnent Publishing House, Gustaf Adolfs Torg 22-25,
S-111 52 Stockholm, Sweden.

Benesch, R & Benesch, R.E.: Proc.Nat.Acad.Sci. 59,526, 1968.

Benesch, R. & Benesch, R.E.: Nature 221, 618, 1969.

Bernstein, R.E: J.Clin.Invest, 38, 1572, 1959.

Bunn,H.F.,May, M.H., Kocholaty, W.F. & Shields, C.E.: J.Clin.Invest.
48,311,1969.

Busch,D.: Blut 13,109, 1966.

Cernoch,M. & Malinska, J.: Clin.Chim.Acta 14,335,1966.

Chanutin, A. & Curnish, R.R.: Arch.Biochem.Biophys.106,433,1964.

Chanutin,A. & Curnish, R.R.: Arch.Biochem.Biophys. 121,96,1967.

de Verdier, C.-H. & Garby, L.: Scand.J.Clin.Lab.Invest.23,149,1969.

de Verdier, C.-H.,Garby,L. & Hjelm, M.: Acta Soc.Med.Upsaliensis
74, 209,1969.

de Verdier, C.-H. & Killander, J.: Acta Physiol.Scand. 54,346,1962.

Eaton, J.W. & Brewer, G.J.: Proc.Nat.Acad.Sci.61,756,1968.

Fortier, N.L. & Valeri, C.R.:in Symposium on intracellular
regulation of hemoglobin affinity to oxygen. Försvarsmedicin 5,
   1969. Swedish Government Publishing House, Gustaf Adolfs Torg
22-25, S-111 52 Stockholm, Sweden.

Garby, L. & Hjelm, M.: Blut 9, 284,1963.

Garby, L. & de Verdier, C.-H.: Fol.Haemat. 89,421,1968.

Garby, L., Gerber, G. & de Verdier, C.-H.: Eur.J.Biochem. 10, 110, 1969.

Garby, L. & Vuille, J.-C.: Scand.J.Clin.Lab.Invest. 13,642,1961.

Hill,J.R. & Robinson, D.C.: J.Physiol. 199, 685,1968.

Hjelm, M.: Fol.Haemat. 89,392,1968.

Hjelm,M.: Communication in November 1968 at the national meeting of the Swedish Medical Society.

Hjelm, M.: Scand.J.Haemat. 6,56,1969 (a).

Hjelm, M. in Symposium on intracellular regulation of haemoglobin affinity to oxygen. Försvarsmedicin 5,195,1969, (b 1). Swedish Government Publishing House, Gustaf Adolfs Torg 22-25 S-111 52 Stockholm, Sweden.

Hjelm, M. in Symposium on intracellular regulation of haemoglobin affinity to oxygen. Försvarsmedicin 5,219,1969 (b 2). Swedish Government Publishing House, Gustaf Adolfs Torg 22-25 S-11 52 Stockholm, Sweden.

Hohorst, H.-J.: 'D-Glucose-6-phosphat und D-fructose-6-phospate' in H.-U.Bergmeyer (ed.) Methoden der enzymatischen Analyse, Verlag Chemie GmbH, Weinheim 1962, p 134.

Horejsi, J.: Haematologia 1, 35, 1967.

Koch, G: (Thesis) Acta Paediat.Scand.suppl.181, 1960.

Lenfant,C., Torrance, J.,English,E., Finch,C.A., Reynafarje, C., Ramos, J & Faura, J.: J.Clin.Invest. 47,2652, 1968.

Nathan, D.G., Oski, F.A., Sidel, V.W.& Diamond, L.K.: New.Engl. J.Med. 272, 118, 1965.

Oski, F.A. & Naiman, J.L.: Hematological problems in the newborn. W.B.Saunders Company, Philadelphia and London 1966.

Prankerd, T.A.J.: J.Physiol. 143,325,1958.
Racher,E.: J.Biol.Chem. 190,685,1951.

Rall, T.W. & Lehninger, A.L.: J.Biol.Chem. 194,119,1952.

Rodman, T., Close, H.P. & Purcell, M.K.: Ann. Internal Med. 52, 295, 1960.

Rose, J.A. & O´Connell, E.L.:   J. Biol.Chem. 239, 12, 1964.

Shojana, A.M., Israels, L.G. & Zipursky, A.:   J.Lab. & Clin.Med. 71,41, 1968.

Srivastava, S.K. & Beutler, E.:   Anal.Biochem. 25, 70, 1968.

Tanaka, K.R. & Valentine, W.N. in Hereditary Disorders of erythro-cyte metabolism (ed.Beutler).   Grune & Stratton, New York and London 1968 p.229.

Tomia, S.:   Acta Med.Univ. Kioto 37, 393, 1961.

Wade, O.L. & Bishop, J.M.   Blackwell Scientific publications, Oxford, 1962, p. 185.

STUDIES OF RED CELL GLYCOLYSIS AND INTERACTIONS WITH CARBON MONOXIDE, SMOKING, and ALTITUDE

George J. Brewer, John W. Eaton, John V. Weil, and Robert F. Grover
Departments of Human Genetics and Medicine (Simpson Memorial Institute), University of Michigan and Department of Medicine, University of Colorado

INTRODUCTION

The exciting story of the functional association between phosphorylated intermediates of the red cell and hemoglobin may be viewed as beginning in 1963 when Chanutin's laboratory first published data showing that a number of phosphate compounds reacted with hemoglobin to form a complex which had an altered electrophoretic mobility (Sugita and Chanutin, 1963; Chanutin and Curnish, 1964 and 1965). This was followed in 1967 by Chanutin and Curnish's report that certain of these bound phosphorylated intermediates of the red cell, including 2,3-diphosphoglycerate (DPG) and ATP, affect the oxygen dissociation properties of hemoglobin. In the same year, Benesch and Benesch (1967) reported similar effects. Subsequent observations from a number of laboratories have highlighted the importance of these findings. These developments have given great impetus to the whole area of red cell metabolism and function, and to the study of the interrelationships of the red cell with the rest of the organs of gas transport. In 1968, we (Eaton and Brewer, 1968) reported that a correlation exists between levels of red cell DPG and whole blood

This work was supported in part by the United States Public Health Service Research Grants AM 09381 and HE 08728, Career Development Awards 1-K3-AM-7959 (GJB) and 1-K3-HE-29,237 (RFG), Training Grant T01-GM-00071, and in part by the Research and Development Command, Departments of the Army and Navy, under Contract DADA17-69-C-9103.

hemoglobin levels, suggesting that, contrary to the statements of
Benesch et al. (1968), variation of DPG in the physiological
range was of significance in oxygen transport. These findings
have been confirmed and extended in a number of papers reported
at this conference.

It is the aim of this report to present some new findings in
several areas of red cell metabolism and function, and hopefully
thereby to give some idea of the breadth and importance of this
burgeoning interdisciplinary area. The first part of the paper
will deal with some of the factors that may play a role in the
regulation of carbohydrate metabolism in general, and DPG levels
in particular. These factors will be considered at 3 levels:
1) A broad level - are the levels of red cell intermediates
determined by genetic as well as by environmental influences?
2) An intermediate level - what is the general nature of the
mechanisms whereby the levels of the intermediates are changed
under various environmental influences? 3) A more narrow level -
what happens to red cell glucose consumption under varying
environmental influences?

The second part of the paper will be a detailed consideration
of our recent work on the problem of excessive polycythemia of
altitude. This portion of the paper ties in with the first in
that red cell adjustments are made in this hypoxic disorder.
Beyond this however, it serves as an excellent example of the
interrelationships of red cell metabolism with other disciplines.

METHODS

Hemoglobin and hematocrit determinations were carried out by
standard hematologic methods. Assays of levels of ATP in red cells
were carried out as previously described (Brewer and Powell, 1966;
Brewer, 1969). Assays of red cell DPG content were carried out
primarily by the chromatropic acid method of Bartlett (1959),
modified as previously described (Eaton et al., 1969). In
addition, DPG was assayed in some of the samples from each study
by a specific enzymatic method. This method was a modification of
that of Schroter and Winter (1967) and was carried out in the
following way:

The assay mixture for measurement of DPG contained 100 umoles
tris-HCl buffer, pH 9.0, 10 umoles $MgCl_2$, 3.0 umoles phosphoenol
pyruvate, 0.1 mg phosphoglyceromutase (18 units/mg, Boehringer),
0.25 mg enolase (27 units/mg, Boehringer) and 0.1 ml of sample in
a total volume of 3.0 ml. The extract containing DPG was diluted
1:100 to 1:250 before measurement to adjust the DPG concentration
to between 1×10^{-6} and 7×10^{-6} M. The change in absorbancy at
240 (due to removal of phosphoenol pyruvate) was measured. The
enzymatic method was used to check the specificity and accuracy of
the chromatropic acid method, particularly in non-human red cells.

Levels of carboxyhemoglobin were determined by the use of an

Instrumentation Laboratories Co-Oximeter, Model 182. When levels of carboxyhemoglobin were determined in smokers, blood was always drawn in the afternoon with an allowance of at least a 6 hour period of smoking prior to the measurement. Each individual reported smoking at least 6 cigarettes during the day prior to blood drawing. (Our data support the general concept that after approximately 6 cigarettes the smoking technique is much more crucial in determining levels of carboxyhemoglobin than the actual number of cigarettes smoked).

Study of glucose consumption was carried out under conditions which were as physiological as possible. Blood was drawn anaerobically by the use of a vacutainer needle directly into a previously evacuated 3 ml tightly stoppered vial containing dried heparin. After mixing by repeated inversion, a small aliquot was removed through the stopper for glucose measurement. The vial was then incubated under anaerobic conditions at 37°C for 90 minutes and the glucose level redetermined. Results were expressed as milligrams of glucose consumed per hour per gram of hemoglobin. Glucose was assayed by the glucose oxidase method as described in Sigma Technical Bulletin No. 510 (Sigma Chemical Co., St. Louis, Mo.). The percent oxyhemoglobin was determined on each sample to evaluate the effect of variation in saturation on glucose consumption. Saturation values varied to a certain extent between samples (30-70% range), but no detectable correlations between saturation and glucose consumption were found in the various studies.

Study of the rate of oxygen pickup in vitro was carried out with the rogeometer described in an earlier paper in this Conference (Eaton and Brewer, 1969). Equal parts of blood, in one case equilibrated with oxygen and 5.5% CO_2, and in the other case equilibrated with nitrogen and 5.5% CO_2, were mixed. This mixture (of approximately 50% oxyhemoglobin) was pumped through the rogeometer at a previously determined flow rate (selected such that there was an average increment of 10-20% increase in saturation). The gas mixture used to flush the rogeometer, from which the blood was picking up oxygen, was selected such that the oxygen tension would equal approximately the alveolar pO_2 in Leadville, Colorado. (This was a mixture of 14% oxygen, 5.5% CO_2, the balance being nitrogen). Since the rate of oxygen pickup is inversely related to the starting oxygen saturation, the saturation of the blood before passage through the rogeometer was determined and the final saturation results corrected by use of a regression line.

The position of the oxygen dissociation curve was determined by Van Slyke gasometric analysis after equilibration in a tonometer with specific gas mixtures. The pH and pO_2 were determined on the sample after equilibration by means of Radiometer oxygen and pH electrodes, and the percent saturation as determined by the Van Slyke method adjusted to standard conditions (pH 7.4 and a specific pO_2) by the Severinghaus slide rule.

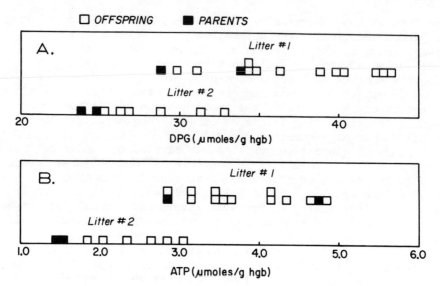

Figure 1. Levels of red cell DPG (part A) and ATP (part B) in rat parents (shaded blocks) and their offspring in 2 litters of equal age. All assays were carried out at the same time after the offspring had reached young adulthood. The higher levels of DPG and ATP in the offspring compared to the parents is attributed to an age effect (young animals have higher levels).

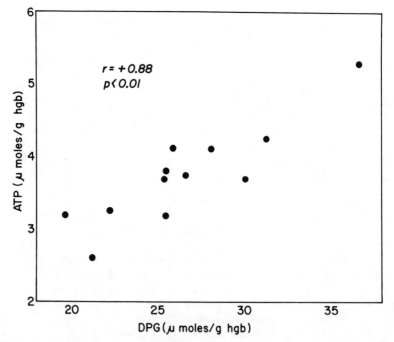

Figure 2. Correlation between red cell DPG and ATP in 12 rat parents.

Arterial blood for blood gas and pH studies was taken anaerobically from the brachial artery and analyzed by Radiometer electrodes.

RESULTS AND DISCUSSION - PART I

1.   Genetic Control of DPG Levels

It is now well recognized that the environment influences levels of DPG in the red cell. Thus, hypoxia of any type, altitude, anemia, pulmonary disease, severe exercise, all cause an increase in levels of DPG. Similarly hyperoxia reduces DPG levels. It is becoming generally accepted that such environmentally-induced changes in the cell's metabolism are crucial to its function.

However, we have previously shown that the level of erythrocyte ATP in the human is under partial genetic control (Brewer, 1967). Therefore it would not be surprising if a similar situation pertains to DPG, and such an influence could be quite important in determining, for example, the possible range of environmentally-induced change in a given individual's DPG levels. Our genetic studies have just begun, and so far are restricted to rats, but we feel that the preliminary results are of interest. The results with our first two litters of Hooded rats are shown in Figure 1, Part A. It is apparent that the offspring of the parents with higher levels of DPG (Litter 1) have higher levels of DPG than the offspring of the parents with lower levels of DPG (Litter 2) ($t = 4.20$; d.f. = 16; $p < 0.01$). It is of interest that the parents of Litter 1 were originally selected for high levels of ATP, and the parents of Litter 2 for low levels of ATP, without prior knowledge of DPG levels. In Figure 1, part B, it can be seen that the offspring in Litter 1 have higher levels of ATP than those of Litter 2 ($t = 4.52$; d.f. = 16; $p < 0.01$). These data imply that ATP and DPG levels are positively correlated in Hooded rats, and this is the case. The correlation coefficient between DPG and ATP in 12 parent rats (Figure 2) used in this study was $+0.88$ ($p < 0.001$) and in 29 offspring rats was $+0.55$ ($p < 0.01$).

We should point out that the correlation between DPG and ATP is much weaker, if it exists, in humans. In our studies of reasonably large samples of people the correlation has not been significant. The higher levels of DPG and ATP in rats than in humans may have something to do with this difference.

Our view then, is that while levels of red cell DPG are responsive to various environmental stimuli such as altitude, exercise, and disease, the levels are also influenced by genetic factors. As in the case of ATP (Brewer, 1967) we suggest that the genetic system is probably multifactorial with many enzymes, and hence many genes, involved. Of course, as in the case of ATP, we may expect major genetic modifiers, that is, single genes with marked influence on DPG levels. Thus, the family reported by

Zurcher et al. (1965) in which the erythrocyte pyruvic kinase activity was quite high and the DPG levels of affected individuals quite low, probably falls into this category.

2.   General Mechanisms of Environmental Influences on DPG Levels

In the preceding section we have considered genetic versus environmental influences on erythrocyte DPG and ATP levels. In this section we wish to consider the general nature of the mechanism or mechanisms by which the environment, hypoxia for example, influences DPG levels. It has been assumed by some that the control operates primarily through a hemoglobin desaturation mechanism. Under conditions of hypoxia, increased desaturation of hemoglobin results in a greater binding of DPG, since deoxyhemoglobin has a greater affinity for DPG than oxyhemoglobin. The mechanism regulating levels of DPG within the cell, presumably sensitive only to unbound DPG, responds with an increased synthesis of DPG, and the total levels increase.

However, in some conditions, such as in anemia, we often see elevations of DPG which are higher than should be accounted for by this mechanism. Further, the notion that DPG levels may be regulated by mechanisms outside simple desaturation of hemoglobin is intuitively appealing. In such a case, the organism could respond to hypoxia with a rise in DPG levels irrespective of the status of hemoglobin desaturation, and to a degree greater than that allowed by the desaturation mechanism.

Most clinical situations have not allowed us to identify with certainty a mechanism other than hemoglobin desaturation. Anemia, pulmonary disease, high altitude hypoxia, and exercise-conditions which show a rise in DPG - all produce both hypoxia and increased hemoglobin desaturation. However, it has occurred to us that a condition in which hypoxia is not associated with increased hemoglobin desaturation is carbon monoxide (CO) loading (Brewer et al., 1969). A substantial amount of CO loading produces hypoxia (1) by virtue of removal of a portion of the hemoglobin from oxygen transport, and (2) by a shift in the oxygen dissociation curve to the left. Since carboxyhemoglobin has the same decreased affinity for DPG as does oxyhemoglobin, and since the dissociation curve is shifted to the left, we have a situation in which hypoxia is not associated with increased levels of desaturated hemoglobin. This system should provide an excellent test for whether or not hypoxia can produce elevations of DPG without hemoglobin desaturation. If DPG levels were regulated primarily through hemoglobin desaturation, we would not expect an increase in the levels of DPG. If anything, DPG levels should decrease.

In a study of CO loading of 10 humans (doses of CO at 0 and 3 hours with carboxyhemoglobin levels between 10 and 25% sustained for 6 hours) an increase in DPG averaging 12% resulted after 6 hours. (DPG levels before treatment vs. after treatment: $t = 2.49$; d.f. $= 18$; $p < 0.05$) (Brewer et al., 1969). The levels were as

high at 3 hours as they were at 6 hours. Extensive studies of
CO loading in rats have also been carried out. The rats were
given CO to the point of symptoms (30-60% carboxyhemoglobin) at 0
and 3 hours, and the DPG levels measured at 0 and 6 hours. The
DPG levels increased an average of about 10%, a significant increase
in comparison to a group of control rats similarly treated except
for CO loading ($t = 3.49$; d.f. = 44; $p < 0.01$). Rats blow off CO
at a rapid rate, for example, 3 hours after CO loading, practically
no carboxyhemoglobin remains in the rat. Interestingly, if CO
levels are maintained at a high level by frequent redosing, DPG
levels do not rise but remain about the same. Similar results are
obtained if high levels of methemoglobin are maintained for a 6
hour period. We interpret these results to indicate that the
hemoglobin binding mechanism operates as vigorously as the hypoxia
mechanism, but in an opposite direction.

These data suggest that in hypoxia, a mechanism exists, beyond
simple desaturation of hemoglobin, capable of stimulating an
increase in levels of red cell DPG. There are many possibilities
for such a mechanism, and we will not consider them here. A
hormone might be released in hypoxia which stimulates red cell
glycolysis. In studies to date (Brewer, J., Brewer, G., and
Eaton, J. - unpublished data) we have not been able to demonstrate
a humoral factor in the plasma of rats exposed to hypoxia which
will cause an increase of DPG levels in rats injected with the
plasma.

3.   Studies of Erythrocyte Glucose Consumption Under Various
     Conditions

Regulation of glucose utilization of the human erythrocyte
may occur in part through regulation of hexokinase activity
(Chapman et al., 1962; Jacobasch, 1968).   Hexokinase of the
intact erythrocyte appears to be in a constantly inhibited state
(deVerdier and Garby, 1965; Chapman et al., 1962).   An early
report by Dische (1941) suggested that DPG inhibits hexokinase.
However, this was not confirmed by deVerdier and Garby (1965).
We have recently reinvestigated this area and have found that under
appropriate circumstances DPG inhibits hexokinase activity, and
that this inhibition is relieved by increasing ATP and magnesium
concentration (Brewer, 1969). It appears possible that this
system may be ideally suited for a functionally related feedback
control of glucose consumption. In such a system, DPG, vital to
hemoglobin function, would help control glucose utilization and
hence its own production, through inhibition of hexokinase.
Irrespective, however, of the mechanism for the regulation of
glucose consumption, it appears likely that the increases in levels
of DPG seen in various hypoxic conditions arise ultimately from
an increase in glucose consumption.

We have carried out studies of glucose consumption of fresh

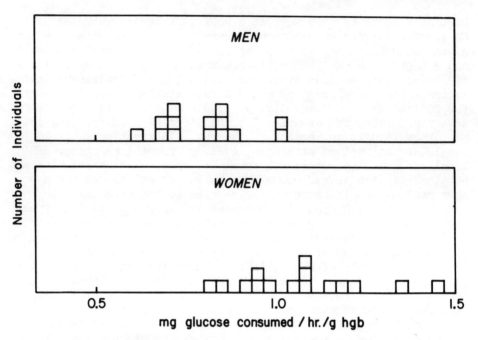

Figure 3. Glucose consumption of fresh whole blood in men and women. Women have a significantly higher rate of glucose consumption than men.

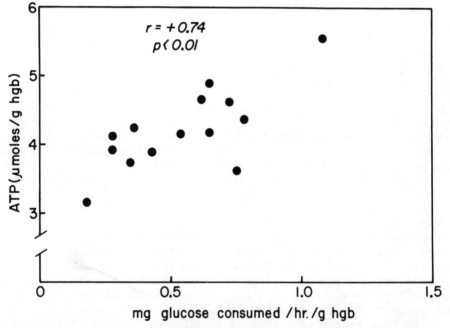

Figure 4. Glucose consumption of fresh whole blood correlated with red cell ATP levels in men after one hour's vigorous exercise.

whole blood taken from persons under a variety of conditions.
First, in normal blood taken from persons during sedentary activity,
there is a sex difference in glucose consumption (Figure 3 and
Table 1, part 1). The reason for the higher consumption of
glucose in erythrocytes of women is not clear. In rather extensive studies we have not been able to show any differences in levels
of erythrocyte ATP between men and women (Brewer, 1967). Levels
of red cell DPG also have not been shown in our studies to differ
significantly between the sexes (Eaton and Brewer, 1968; Eaton et
al., 1969). However, women do have greater rates of desaturation
than men, as studied in the rogeometer (Eaton and Brewer, 1969),
and probably this comes about through some mechanism related to
glycolysis. Another red cell characteristic that is known to show
a sex difference is the level of potassium, which is significantly
higher in females. Presumably this somewhat higher cation gradient
is maintained by expenditure of glycolytic energy. So far as we
are aware, no data have been reported which shows a significant
difference between men and women in the position of the oxygen
dissociation curve.

A significant positive correlation is seen between levels of
red cell ATP and the rate of blood glucose consumption in females
at rest (Table 1, part 1). In men at rest, this correlation was
not significant, but in a study of blood taken from men after an
hour's vigorous exercise a very tight positive correlation between
ATP and rate of glucose consumption was seen (Figure 4 and Table 1,
part 2). Correlations between DPG content and rate of glucose
consumption were non-significant in all studies. This data
suggests that of the two variables, ATP and DPG, variation in ATP
may be more critical in relation to glucose consumption. Presumably ATP could be involved in regulation of glucose consumption by
stimulation of the hexokinase reaction directly, by modulation of
the DPG inhibitory effect on hexokinase, stimulation of the phosphofructokinase reaction, or some combination of these effects.

There is a significant negative correlation between glucose
consumption and hemoglobin level in the Leadville, Colorado,
sample (Table 1, part 3), and a trend in this direction, particularly
in females, in a small sample studied at near sea level (Table 1,
part 1). Anemia from any one of a variety of etiologies (not
characterized by reticulocytosis) produces a marked increase in
glucose consumption, often by 2 or 3 fold (Table 1, part 4). Thus,
in general, there is an inverse relation between hemoglobin level
and glucose consumption. The higher the level of hemoglobin, the
lower the rate of glucose consumption and vice versa.

The hexokinase of the red cell requires magnesium for activity.
We have previously shown that magnesium also markedly relieves
DPG inhibition of hexokinase (Brewer, 1969). Magnesium was included
in several incubation studies, and caused a marked increase in
glucose consumption (Table 1, part 5). The level of free magnesium in the red cell (about 5% of the total) is sufficiently low

so that activity of hexokinase, which requires the magnesium ion, is not optimal, and also DPG inhibition of hexokinase should be pronounced. Possibly the magnesium stimulation of glycolysis operates by stimulating the hexokinase reaction and/or by relieving DPG inhibition of hexokinase.

These studies of glucose consumption raise more questions than they answer. The sex difference is unexplained, and we can't be sure of the reasons between the positive correlations of glucose consumption with ATP levels or the negative correlation with hemoglobin levels. Nor can we do more than speculate on the role of variation in levels of serum magnesium on regulation of glucose metabolism. However, since it appears likely that changes in glucose consumption ultimately must be effected in order to bring about changes in levels of carbohydrate intermediates, it would seem profitable to explore these relationships further.

RESULTS AND DISCUSSION - PART II

Excessive Polycythemia of Altitude

Excessive polycythemia of altitude, also called chronic mountain sickness if symptomatic, is a longstanding and intriguing problem on which we believe our current investigations, centered on the red cell, are beginning to shed new light. As mentioned earlier, it is an excellent example of an interdisciplinary challenge. Our observations have been made in the town of Leadville, Colorado, at an altitude of 10,200 feet. The disorder under consideration may be viewed simply as hypoxia associated with altitude. All of the manifestations, including the polycythemia, can be traced to the hypoxia of arterial blood which exists in this condition. What has not been clear, however, is the etiology of the hypoxia. The condition is much more common in men, perhaps 5 or 10 times as common as in women, and is positively correlated with age. That is, it is rarely seen before the age of 30, but becomes increasingly more common with increasing age. In the town of Leadville, perhaps 5% of the males over the age of 35 have excessive polycythemia, defined for our purposes as a sustained hematocrit over 56 volumes percent.

The polycythemia may be quite striking. Hematocrits of 70 to 80 are not unusual. Usually treatment is directed at keeping the hematocrit below a level of 60 volumes percent by phlebotomy. Among the hypotheses advanced to explain this condition have been hypoventilation, underlying lung disease, and among the local populations of Leadville, a tendency to attribute the condition to drinking alcoholic beverages.

The first study by our combined University of Michigan - University of Colorado team was a survey of DPG levels in 153 normal and 49 polycythemic individuals in Leadville (Eaton et al., 1969). The majority of this sample were men. The polycythemic

Table 1. Studies of Glucose Consumption

	N	Glucose Consumed (Mean ± 1S.D.)	t test (Differences of Means)	Correlation of glucose consumed With ATP	With Hb
Part 1 (Men and women at rest - Ann Arbor, altitude 900 feet)					
A. Men	14	0.80 ± 0.12	t = 4.92	r=-0.22 p<0.1	r=-0.29 p<0.1
B. Women	15	1.08 ± 0.18	p < 0.01	r=+0.48 p<0.05	r=-0.44 p<0.1
Part 2 (Men before and after vigorous exercise - Ann Arbor)					
A. Before	14	0.71 ± 0.28	t = 1.61	r=+0.39 p<0.1	
B. After	14	0.55 ± 0.25	p < 0.2	r=+0.74 p<0.01	
Part 3 (Polycythemic and control men - Leadville, Colorado, altitude 10,200 feet)					
A. Control	18	0.83 ± 0.41	t = 0.89	r=+0.31 p<0.1	r=-0.45 p<0.01
B. Polycythemic	17	0.76 ± 0.39	p < 0.4	(entire group)	(entire group)
Part 4 (Anemic men and women - Ann Arbor)					
A. Control	7	0.68 ± 0.17	t = 5.52		
B. Anemia	6	2.21 ± 0.71	p < 0.01		
Part 5 (Addition of magnesium, 0.01 M, to incubation)					
A. Control	6	0.67 ± 0.18	t = 2.31		
B. Magnesium	6	1.35 ± 0.70	p < 0.05		

Table 2. Blood gas studies in Leadville, Colorado (altitude 10,200 feet)

	N	Arterial pO_2 (Mean ±1 S.D.)	Arterial pH (Mean ±1 S.D.)	Arterial pCO_2 (Mean ±1 S.D.)
1. Polycythemic Group	24	46.8 ± 5.2	7.401 ± 0.021	34.3 ± 4.5
2. Controls - Smokers	8	53.4 ± 5.8	7.422 ± 0.011	34.7 ± 2.0
3. Controls - NonSmokers	12	58.6 ± 4.2	7.421 ± 0.013	32.8 ± 3.3

t test of differences between means:

		$t =$	p
Arterial pO_2	1 vs 2+3	6.04	<0.01
	2 vs 3	2.34	<0.05
Arterial pH	1 vs 2+3	1.20	<0.3
	2 vs 3	0.18	<0.9
Arterial pCO_2	1 vs 2+3	0.60	<0.6
	2 vs 3	1.44	<0.2

group was ascertained primarily from medical records, mostly the clinical records of the Climax Molybdenum Company which employs a large share of the men of Leadville. Our sole criteria for including individuals in the polycythemic category was a history of hematocrits consistently over 56 volumes percent. From this study we learned that the mean DPG level in the polycythemic group was significantly elevated over other altitude acclimatized individuals (Eaton et al., 1969).

We subsequently studied a subgroup of the polycythemic male sample in considerable detail. The polycythemic group was compared to a control group of men of approximately the same age and working primarily in the same industry (mining). Table 2 presents arterial blood gas and pH data from this study. The well known reduction in arterial oxygen tension in the polycythemic group can be readily seen. Most interesting, however, was the rather striking reduction in arterial oxygen tension in normal cigarette smokers contrasted to non-smokers (Table 2). As far as we are aware this effect has not previously been reported. We will return to this subject when we discuss the effects of discontinuation of smoking.

One of our early hypotheses was that the high levels of DPG in polycythemic subjects had shifted the hemoglobin oxygen dissociation curve sufficiently far to the right to prevent adequate hemoglobin saturation in the lungs at the oxygen tension available at 10,200 feet. The arterial desaturation observed in polycythemic individuals would fit with this possibility. However, when studied with the rogeometer in such a way that rate of saturation could be measured, the rate of oxygen pickup was significantly increased, rather than decreased, when the blood was exposed to an oxygen tension approximating the alveolar oxygen tension at 10,200 feet (t = 2.45; d.f. = 36; p < 0.02). The mechanism of this increased rate of saturation in the presence of increased levels of DPG is unknown. However, it became clear that we could not explain the polycythemic syndrome on the basis of a decreased rate of hemoglobin saturation in the lungs.

At this time we became aware of two facts. First, preliminary data on the position of the oxygen dissociation curve in polycythemic individuals determined by reflectance oximetry indicated that in general the curves were not right-shifted with respect, even, to the curves of low altitude residents. This was very surprising in view of the marked elevations of DPG in the red cells of polycythemic individuals (Eaton et al., 1969). Second, we became aware that most of the polycythemic individuals were cigarette smokers. The exceptions (4 out of 24) were individuals with obvious lung disease - silicosis, emphysema, or both.

Cigarette smoke contains significant levels of carbon monoxide (CO). Carboxyhemoglobin is known to cause a left shift in the oxygen dissociation curve and we postulate that the failure of the curve to shift to the right in the polycythemic individuals, in spite of very high DPG levels, results from the presence of significant levels of carboxyhemoglobin. A failure of the curve

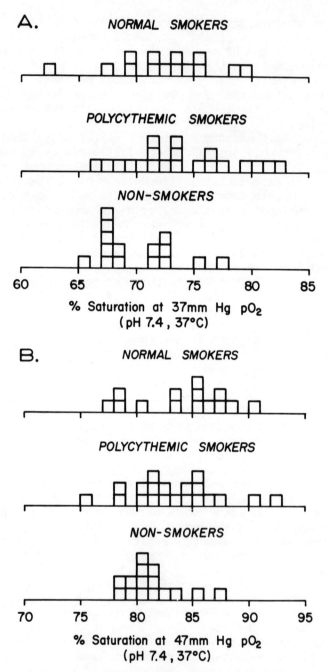

Figure 5. Oxygen dissociation data obtained by the Van Slyke
method at 37 mm Hg (part A) and 47 mm Hg (part B) oxygen tension
on normal smokers, polycythemic smokers, and non-smokers in
Leadville, Colorado (altitude 10,200 feet).

to shift to the right could be a factor in the etiology of the syndrome.

We have subsequently carried out an additional study in Leadville to define more thoroughly the various interrelationships. The study group comprised 20 polycythemic cigarette smokers, 15 non-polycythemic cigarette smokers, and 15 normal non-smokers, all from Leadville. This study has just been completed and only a preliminary analysis of the data is available. However, certain important facts have emerged. It is clear from Table 3 that the mean level of carboxyhemoglobin is significantly higher in smokers at 10,200 feet (6.6%) than in smokers at altitude 1,000 feet (4.7%). The reason for the higher levels of carboxyhemoglobin at altitude could be due to one or more of several factors. The lower oxygen tension may result in more CO production in the burning cigarette, a greater rate of CO uptake by hemoglobin, or a slower rate of CO release by hemoglobin once the CO is bound.

The position of the oxygen dissociation curve in the 3 groups of subjects was measured by Van Slyke gasometric analysis, by an Instrumentation Laboratories Co-Oximeter, and by a micro-gasometric method involving displacement of oxygen with CO. The comparison of oxygen dissociation curves by various methods in the presence of high levels of carboxyhemoglobin is a complicated subject and our comparative data from Leadville will be presented elsewhere. Since the oxygen dissociation curve is traditionally defined by gasometric, such as Van Slyke, analysis, in this paper we will consider only our Van Slyke data.

Data from 2 representative oxygen tensions are shown in Figure 5 and Table 4. Although there is overlap, the mean saturation values of the normal smokers and the polycythemic smokers are significantly higher than that of non-smoking normals at one of the two oxygen tensions (Table 5). This means that, on the average, the oxygen dissociation curve of smokers in Leadville is left-shifted compared to non-smokers. There was no significant difference between the position of the curve in normal smokers and polycythemic smokers at either oxygen tension.

As described earlier, smoking results in a significantly lower arterial oxygen tension (Table 2). Thus, cigarette smokers at altitude would appear to have 3 effects working against oxygen delivery; the binding of a proportion of hemoglobin with CO, a shift to the left of the oxygen dissociation curve resulting from carboxyhemoglobin, and a reduction in arterial oxygen tension. It would appear from this data that smoking could be a significant contributory factor to the syndrome of excessive polycythemia of altitude, although it could not be the sole factor, since many smokers do not develop polycythemia.

Accordingly, an effort was made to persuade a group of 20 polycythemic volunteers to stop smoking for a 3-4 month period, in order to assess possible benefit. This group is now in the second month of this period. Some benefits from the discontinuation of smoking were immediately apparent (Table 5). Carboxyhemoglobin

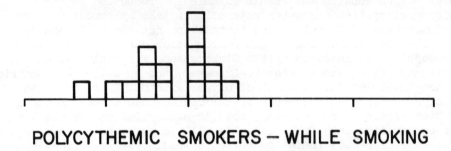

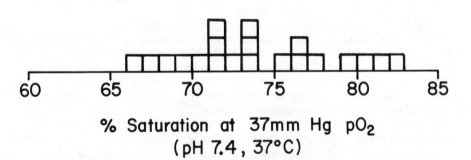

Figure 6. Oxygen dissociation data obtained by the Van Slyke method at 37 mm Hg oxygen tension on polycythemic subjects before and after (1-8 days) smoking was discontinued.

levels dropped (the amount depending probably upon the completeness with which smoking was stopped), and the oxygen dissociation curve shifted to the right, the degree of shift depending on the amount of reduction in carboxyhemoglobin (Table 5 and Figure 6). It is of interest that the mean saturation value obtained on the polycythemics (68.9%) after smoking was discontinued indicates a right shift of the dissociation curve beyond the non-smoking group, whose value was 70.3%. This presumably results from the high levels of DPG unopposed by carboxyhemoglobin.

Table 3. Comparison of carboxyhemoglobin levels in cigarette smokers at 10,200 feet vs. 1,000 feet altitude

	N	CO Hgb Levels (Mean ±1 S D.)	t test (Differences of Means)
Smokers-10,200 feet	34	6.6±2.7	t=3.02 p < 0.01
Smokers- 1,000 feet	28	4.7±2.2	

Table 4. Oxygen dissociation data (Van Slyke Method) at 2 oxygen tensions in normal smokers, polycythemic smokers, and non-smokers in Leadville, Colorado

A. 37 mm Hg pO_2, pH 7.4, 37°C

	N	% Oxyhemo-globin (Mean ±1 S.D.)	t test (Differences of Means)	p
1. Normal Smokers	14	72.4±4.3	1 vs 2 = 1.23	< 0.3
2. Polycythemic Smokers	20	74.4±4.9	2 vs 3 = 2.76	< 0.01
3. Non-smokers	15	70.3±3.4	1 vs 3 = 1.46	< 0.2

B. 47 mm Hg pO_2, pH 7.4, 37°C

	N		t test	p
1. Normal Smokers	14	84.1±4.0	1 vs 2 = 1.85	< 0.1
2. Polycythemic Smokers	20	83.4±4.0	2 vs 3 = 1.59	< 0.2
3. Non-smokers	15	81.5±2.6	1 vs 3 = 2.08	< 0.05

Table 5. Carboxyhemoglobin levels and oxygen dissociation data in
          polycythemic subjects before and after discontinuing
          smoking.

Polycythemic Subjects	N	% Carboxyhemoglobin (Mean ± 1 S.D.)	N	% Oxyhemoglobin 37 mm Hg pO_2 (Mean ± 1 S.D.)
While smoking	20	6.1±2.2	20	74.4±4.9
		t=7.22		t=4.08
After discontinuing (1-8 days)	18	1.8±1.2 p 0.01	16	68.9±2.4 p<0.01

Some evidence was obtained that the factor in smoking which
causes the decrease in arterial oxygen tension is transient (Table
6). In 2 cases (subjects 1 and 5, Table 6) in which it was possible
to recheck the arterial blood gases after smoking had been stopped
for 1 or 2 days, the oxygen tension increased 13 and 7 mm of
mercury respectively. In 3 other cases (subjects 2, 3, and 4,
Table 6), only slight change occurred in the arterial oxygen
tension after smoking had been supposedly discontinued for 1 to 2
days, but in all 3 cases there was evidence that smoking had not
been stopped completely.

Table 6. Arterial oxygen tensions and carboxyhemoglobin levels in
          5 polycythemic subjects before and after discontinuing
          smoking.

Polycythemic Subjects	Number of days Between Studies*	Arterial pO_2		% Carboxyhemoglobin	
		1st Study	2nd Study	1st Study	2nd Study
1	2	44.0	57.0	9.0	0.8
2	2	44.0	43.8	4.2	3.7
3	2	48.0	49.5	6.8	2.3
4	1	45.0	47.0	7.6	2.6
5	1	41.0	48.0	11.0	2.8

*This column indicates number of days smoking supposedly stopped

SUMMARY

There appear to be genetic influences on DPG levels, at least
in Hooded rats. Environmentally induced changes in DPG seem to be
mediated through at least two mechanisms - deoxyhemoglobin binding
of DPG, and in addition, another mechanism triggered by hypoxia,

perhaps humoral in nature. Glucose consumption is higher in erythrocytes of women than men, correlates positively with ATP levels, correlates negatively with hemoglobin levels, and is stimulated by addition of magnesium.

At the present time the studies of polycythemic subjects in Leadville (altitude, 10,200 feet) can be summarized as follows: A significant proportion of the male population over age 30 develop excessive polycythemia. These individuals have low arterial oxygen tensions and saturations and are usually cigarette smokers. They have high levels of carboxyhemoglobin, high levels of red cell DPG, and an oxygen dissociation curve which is not right-shifted, even though they live at 10,200 feet altitude and have high DPG levels. These studies have also revealed that normal smokers have significantly reduced arterial oxygen tensions compared to non-smokers. The cause of the lowered arterial oxygen tension in smokers is unknown. It may be due to effects on the lung or possibly due to CO, since under some circumstances CO is reported to cause arterial hypoxemia (Brody and Coburn, 1969). Whatever the cause, our preliminary data suggests that it is transient in that cessation of cigarette smoking for 1 to 2 days is capable of producing rather marked improvement in the arterial oxygen tension.

These studies have meaning well beyond the town of Leadville, Colorado. For example, patients with lung disease are, in a sense, functioning at high altitude. All of the harmful effects of smoking on oxygen transport described here apply to such individuals, as well as to those living at high altitudes, and those functioning at reduced oxygen tensions.

REFERENCES

Bartlett, G.R. (1959). J. Biol. Chem. 234:469.

Benesch, R. and Benesch, R.E. (1967). Biochem. Biophys. Res. Comm. 26:162.

Benesch, R., Benesch, R.E. and Yu, C.I. (1968). Proc. Nat. Acad. Sci. 59:526.

Brewer, G. (1967). Biochem. Gen. 1:25.

Brewer, G.J. (1969). In "Biochemical Methods in Red Cell Genetics" (J. Yunis, ed.) pp. 201-230. Academic Press, New York.

Brewer, G.J. (1969). Biochem. et Biophys. Acta. In press.

Brewer, G.J. and Powell, R.D. (1966). J. Lab. & Clin. Med. 67:726.

Brewer, G.J., Eaton, J.W. and Dinman, B. (1969). J. Lab. & Clin. Med. In press.

Brody, J.S. and Coburn, R.F. (1969). Science 164:1297.

Chanutin, A. and Curnish, R.R. (1964). Arch. Biochem. Biophys. 106:433.

Chanutin, A. and Curnish, R.R. (1965). Proc. Soc. Exptl. Biol. Med. 120:291.

Chanutin, A. and Curnish, R.R. (1967). Arch. Biochem. Biophys. 121:96.

Chapman, R.G., Hennessey, M.A., Waltersdorph, A.M., Huennekins, F.
      N.; and Gabrio, B.W. (1962). J. Clin. Invest. 41:1249
DeVerdier, C.-H. and Garby, L. (1965). Scand. J. Haemat. 2:305.
Dische, Z. (1941). Bull. Soc. Chim. Biol. 23:1140.
Eaton, J.W. and Brewer, G.J. (1968). Proc. Nat. Acad. Sci. 61:756.
Eaton, J.W. and Brewer, G.J. (1969). This Conference
Eaton, J.W., Brewer, G.J. and Grover, R.F. (1969). J. Lab. & Clin.
      Med. 73:603.
Jacobasch, G. (1968). Folia Haematologica 89:376.
Schroter, W. and Winter, P. (1967). Klin. Wochenschrift 45:255.
Sugita, Y. and Chanutin, A. (1963). Proc. Soc. Exptl. Biol. Med.
      112:72.
Zurcher, C., Loos, J. and Prins, H. (1965). Proc. 10th Congr.
      Intern. Soc. Blood Transfusion (S. Karger, ed.) p. 549.

II

METABOLIC CONTROL MECHANISMS IN THE RED CELL

SESSION 3 - A. Chanutin, Chairman

GENERAL FEATURES OF METABOLIC CONTROL AS APPLIED TO THE ERYTHROCYTE

John R. Williamson

Johnson Research Foundation, University of Penna.,

Philadelphia, Penna. 19104

The purpose of this paper is to review the background and principles used to elucidate control mechanisms in multienzyme sequences. Examples are taken from the literature to illustrate the sites of control of erythrocyte glycolysis observed under different conditions, and the possible nature of the control chemicals. Emphasis will be placed on control of the 2,3-diphosphoglycerate (DPG) level in erythrocytes and possible feedback relationships between the concentration of free DPG, as determined by its differential binding to oxy- and deoxyhemoglobin, and the regulation of glycolysis. For a more extensive treatment of erythrocyte glycolysis, the reader is referred to several recent reviews (1-3).

Kinetic Properties of Enzymes

Figure 1 shows some of the basic features of the glycolytic pathway. The pentose phosphate pathway of glucose metabolism, which has been estimated to represent about 10% of the glycolytic rate (4), is not shown in the diagram. Its activity is probably controlled by the glucose-6-P and NADP concentrations (5,6).

Hexokinase is inhibited by glucose-6-P and this inhibition is reversed by inorganic phosphate (7). Phosphofructokinase from erythrocytes has not been extensively studied. Apparently, it is subject to similar allosteric interactions as those observed with phosphofructokinase from other cells (1). Inhibition by ATP is strongly pH dependent, increasing rapidly at lower pH values. The inhibition is reversed by fructose-6-P and inorganic phosphate. The $\underline{Km}$ for fructose-6-P is also strongly influenced by pH over the physiological range, and falls with an increase of pH. These pH

117

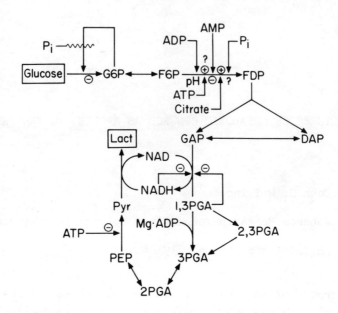

Figure 1. Scheme showing the pathway and postulated controls of erythrocyte glycolysis.

---

dependencies of phosphofructokinase are of great importance in the overall regulation of the glycolytic rate, as will become apparent in later discussions.

The kinetic properties of purified red cell glyceraldehyde-P dehydrogenase are not known in detail, but the enzyme is probably similar to that from muscle. The most interesting features of the muscle enzyme are the pH dependencies of its substrate affinities and its strong product inhibitions (8). Thus, the $\underline{Km}$ for glyceraldehyde-3-P increases from 2.5 μM at pH 7.4 to 90 μM at pH 8.6, while the $\underline{Km}$ for NAD decreases from 90 to 13 μM. The $\underline{Ki}$ values for NADH and 1,3-di-P-glycerate at pH 7.4 are 0.3 μM and 0.8 μM, respectively, but increase with increasing pH.

The kinetic properties of P-glycerate kinase, diphosphoglycerate mutase and diphosphoglycerate phosphatase will be described in a later section. It will suffice to mention at this point that the concentration of magnesium bound ADP probably controls P-glycerate kinase activity, and that diphosphoglycerate phosphatase must be under strong inhibition because of the low $\underline{Km}$ for DPG. Pyruvate kinase is strongly inhibited by ATP ($\underline{Ki}$ of 35 μM), which increases the $\underline{Km}$ for P-enolpyruvate (7), and according to Rose and Warms (9) is controlled by the intracellular concentration of P-enolpyruvate.

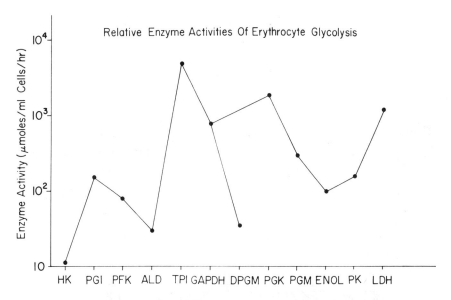

Figure 2. Enzyme activities in human red cells (10,11). Abbreviations used: HK, hexokinase; PGI, phosphoglucose isomerase; PFK, phosphofructokinase; ALD, aldolase; TPI, triose phosphate isomerase; GAPDH, glyceraldehyde-3-P dehydrogenase; DPGM, diphosphoglycerate mutase; PGK, 3-phosphoglycerate kinase; PGM, phosphoglycerate mutase; ENOL, enolase; PK, pyruvate kinase; LDH, lactate dehydrogenase.

Enzyme Contents, Equilibria and Disequilibria

The maximum capacities of the enzymes of glycolysis measured under artificial in vitro conditions reveal little about the control properties of the pathway. Values obtained for human erythrocytes (10,11) are shown in Fig. 2. Hexokinase has the lowest enzyme activity, but even so its capacity is several times greater than the observed glycolytic flux, indicating that it must be under strict control in the intact cell. The teleological reason for high activities of certain enzymes may be to ensure near equilibrium at those steps having a small free energy change, thereby insuring smooth feedback or feedforward metabolite control between control sites.

Another approach to the location of possible control sites in the glycolytic sequence is to calculate the deviation from equilibrium at each step (12). Fig. 3 shows the results of such calculations for human erythrocytes incubated in the presence of 5 to 10 mM glucose, using published data (3) together with unpublished data of Dr. I. A. Rose on 1,3-di-P-glycerate values. The enzymes

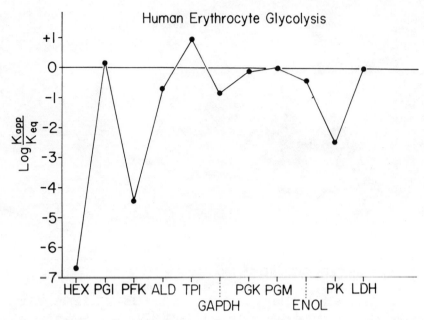

Figure 3. Deviations of glycolytic reactions from equilibrium.
Kapp, observed mass action ratio; Keq, equilibrium constant. Abbreviations as in Fig. 2.

of the glycolytic pathway are plotted along the abscissa while the
ordinate gives the logarithm of the ratio of the measured mass
action distribution of the reactants and products of the enzyme
step compared with the thermodynamic equilibrium constant (12,13).
Despite ambiguities and uncertanties in the approach, it is clear
that hexokinase, phosphofructokinase and pyruvate kinase are displaced from equilibrium by 3 to 7 orders of magnitude, while all
the other enzymes are within one order of magnitude of equilibrium.
The velocity of an enzyme which is far removed from equilibrium is
more susceptable to control than a near equilibrium enzyme; a conclusion which is reinforced by the allosteric properties of many
enzymes catalyzing nonequilibrium reactions.

Use of the Crossover Theorem to Identify Sites of Interaction
in the Glycolytic Sequence

     The crossover theorem provides a method for localizing inter-
action or regulatory sites in complex enzyme systems. Chance and
Williams (14) observed crossover points for the interaction of .
adenosine diphosphate with the respiratory chain of coupled mitochondria under different conditions, and together with Higgins and
Holmes (15) proposed a crossover theorem for the identification of
phosphorylation sites. Later, Chance et al. (16) constructed an

analogue computer model, based on the assumption that the law of
mass action applied to a linear sequence of reactions. It was
also recognized that this theorem also applied to linear sequences
where intermediates could either accumulate or become depleted.
Mathematical proof of the theorems as originally stated was provided by Holmes (17). Recently, using more general mathematical
techniques, it has been possible to provide a broader theoretical
basis for the crossover theorem, together with extensions to systems involving feedback, branched, and closed loop reactions (18).
A brief outline of this treatment, together with summaries of the
most important conclusions, are presented here.

Generalized reactions. The theoretical foundation for the
crossover theorem finds its basis in the concept of generalized
reactions, for which only the monotonic properties of the rate law
are required. For example, $A \underset{k_{-1}}{\overset{k_1}{\rightleftharpoons}} B$ is a first order monomolecular

reaction; its specific rate law is given as $v = k_1 a - k_{-1} b$, where
v is the net reaction rate (to the right), a and b are concentrations, and k_1 and k_{-1} are rate constants. A generalized monomolecular reaction is designated by O - O and has the rate law:
$$\overset{a \quad b}{v = f\,[a/b]} \qquad \text{(Equation 1)}$$

This indicates that the net rate v is some function of a and b,
such that it increases with increasing a and decreases with increasing b. The generalized monomolecular reaction applies to a
variety of detailed reaction mechanisms, and it is only necessary
that the monotonic properties prevail. Thus, even for a complex
enzyme reaction, the generalized net steady state rate (v) is of
the form given by Eq. 1.

A generalized bimolecular reaction is designated by

with the rate law $v = f\,[ab/cd]$ (Equation 2)

which indicates that v is an increasing function of a and b and a
decreasing function of c or d. Generalized reactions involving
inhibitors or activators are indicated as:

inh $v = f\,[a/bc]$ (Equation 3)

$$
\begin{array}{c}
O\ c \\
\downarrow act \qquad v = f\,[ac/b] \qquad\qquad \text{(Equation 4)}\\
O \underline{\quad\quad} O \\
a \qquad b
\end{array}
$$

Increasing $\underline{c}$ causes a decrease in the net flux (inhibition) or an increase in the net flux (activation).

$\underline{\text{Crossover logic.}}$ Based on the generalized rate laws, a simple logic describes "allowed" changes in flux and concentration, as given below for a generalized monomolecular reaction (+ signs indicate an increase and - signs indicate a decrease).

Δv	Δa	Δb	
+	+	+	
+	+	-	
+	-	-	
+	-	+	"fault"
-	+	+	
-	-	-	
-	+	+	
-	+	-	"fault"

(Equation 5)

Since the magnitude of the change is not considered, all changes except those indicated as "faults" are consistent with the monotonic properties of the generalized rate law, whereas those listed as "faults" are inconsistent.

For a bimolecular reaction with the rate law $v = f\,[ab/cd]$ all possible changes in concentrations and flux are allowed except

Δv	Δa	Δb	Δc	Δd
+	-	-	+	+
-	+	+	-	-

, while for an inhibitory interaction (Eq. 3) all changes are allowed except

Δv	Δa	Δb	Δc
-	+	-	-
+	-	+	+

.

The implications of this simple logical treatment may be summarized in the Fault Theorem:

$\underline{\text{If a generalized rate law is postulated for a certain}}$ $\underline{\text{reaction step and, the measured changes in flux and concen-}}$ $\underline{\text{tration of the reactants are experimentally inconsistent,}}$ $\underline{\text{then it follows that there is a logical "fault" in the pos-}}$ $\underline{\text{tulate. The generalized rate law, therefore, is incomplete}}$; $\underline{\text{i.e. some other agent must be affecting the rate of that}}$ $\underline{\text{reaction.}}$

The Fault Theorem is applicable regardless of the complexity of the entire reaction sequence ($\underline{e.g.}$ glycolysis and gluconeogenesis) and is independent of any other other reactions in which the components may be engaged.

Crossover points and plots. Unlike the Fault Theorem, which
applies to single reaction steps, the crossover theorems are dependent on the topology of the entire system. The reaction topology eliminates many of the "allowed" changes, so that of the many
theoretically possible combinations of changes, only a few can
actually occur. Consider a sequence of generalized monomolecular
reactions indicated by:

(Equation 6)

$$[0] \xrightarrow[a_0]{v_1} 0 \xrightarrow[a_1]{v_2} 0 \xrightarrow[a_2]{v_3} 0 \xrightarrow[a_3]{v_4} 0 \xrightarrow[a_4]{v_5} 0 \xrightarrow[a_5]{v_6} 0 \xrightarrow[a_6]{v_7} 0 \xrightarrow[a_7]{v_8} 0 \xrightarrow{} v$$

$$\underset{K}{\overset{act}{\uparrow}}$$

The first intermediate (a_0) is maintained constant (or considered
in great excess) and the final reaction step is considered to be
irreversible (or the final product is considered to be removed).
In a stationary state, the flux through each step is the same. If
the system is then subjected to an interaction with some agent (K),
which is assumed to activate the reaction shown in equation 6, the
system will proceed to a new stationary state having different
concentrations of the intermediates a_1 to a_7 and a new net flux.
Although only the direction of changes is of importance in the
crossover theorem, typical "crossover plots" give the percentage
change in the concentration of each intermediate plotted on the
ordinate, with the individual chemicals of the sequence plotted on
the abscissa, as shown in subsequent figures of this paper.
Points at which the graph crosses the axis are called "crossover
points". Crossovers with the sign of the slope in the same direction as the sign of the flux change, are called "forward crossovers" and the crossover point is located between the two intermediates of the abscissa. Alternatively, a slope with sign
opposite to that of the flux change is called a reverse crossover.
Forward crossovers are identical with "faults", and hence identify
sites of interaction with other agents.

The following brief proof is presented. Assuming an increased
flux, and applying Eq. 1 to the last step in the sequence, it follows from the relationship $v_8 = f[a_7/a_8]$ that if the flux increases, then a_7 must increase since the final product (a_8) does
not affect the reaction. Similarly, from the relationship $v_7 = f[a_6/a_7]$, it follows that if the flux and a_7 increase, then a_6
must also increase. This process may be carried back to the site
of interaction, when a logical "fault" is obtained. For the first
step of the sequence, it follows from the relationship $v_1 = f[a_0/a_1]$, that a_1 must decrease with increased flux, since a_0 is
considered to be constant. Similarly, a_2, a_3 etc. also decrease
up to the site of interaction. Thus, for the sequence shown in
Eq. 6, the intermediates change as follows when flux is increased
by the activator, K:

$$[0] - 0 - 0 - 0 - 0 - 0 - 0 - 0 - 0 - v$$

$$a_0 \quad a_1 \quad a_2 \quad a_3 \quad a_4 \uparrow \quad a_5 \quad a_6 \quad a_7 \quad a_8 \qquad \text{(Equation 7)}$$

$$\text{act}$$

$$- \quad - \quad - \quad - \quad - \mid + \quad + \quad + \quad + \quad +$$

$$K$$

As already pointed out, the topology of the reaction system imposes additional restrictions on the possible sign changes which occur at any particular reaction step. Thus, of the six allowed changes given for individual monomolecular reaction steps (Eq. 5), only one can occur in the system described by Eq. 6. The experimental finding of a reverse crossover or additional forward crossovers would imply an incorrectly proposed topology, an additional interaction, the presence of feedback sites, or any combination of these possibilities. A similar treatment based on generalized rate laws, together with the known topology and reaction kinetics of the system can be applied to determine the significance of observed crossovers in highly complex systems involving branched reactions and loops, as occur in practice for the glycolytic pathway (18).

Effects of pH on Glycolysis

It has been recognized for many years that the rates of glucose utilization and lactate production by erythrocytes are dependent on the pH of the incubation medium. Fig. 4 shows that the pH optimum was about 8.7 for oxygenated erythrocytes and was shifted to a slightly more acid pH upon deoxygenation (19). At physiological pH values, therefore, deoxygenation of the hemoglobin may be associated with an increase of glycolysis. This change is probably attributed to the Bohr effect (20) since oxyhemoglobin takes up a proton when an oxygen molecule is released, thereby causing an increase of the intracellular pH:

$$HbO_2 + H^+ \rightleftarrows H^+Hb + O_2$$

Similarly, the increase of the DPG level upon deoxygenation of the hemoglobin when the initial pH was 7.4 can be explained on the basis of the pH change, since the DPG level is markedly affected by pH over the range of 6.5 to 8.5 (21, Fig. 4).

A crossover plot of the change of the glycolytic intermediates as the pH was increased from 7.0 to 7.4 and then to 7.8 is shown in Fig. 5 (22). Since flux increases, a forward crossover is identified at the phosphofructokinase step. An activation of phosphofructokinase for the pH 7.0 to 7.4 transition cannot be explained by changes of the ATP and ADP contents since these showed little change, but could be caused by the altered kinetic properties of the enzyme at the more alkaline pH, as discussed earlier. At pH 7.8, the ATP levels were lower and the ADP levels higher than at pH 7.0.

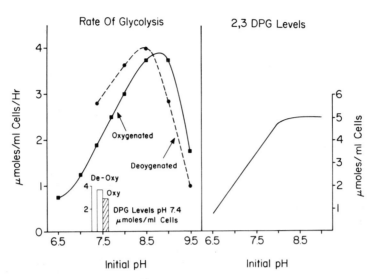

Figure 4. Effect of pH on glycolysis and the content of 2,3-di-P-glycerate (DPG) in human erythrocytes (19,21).

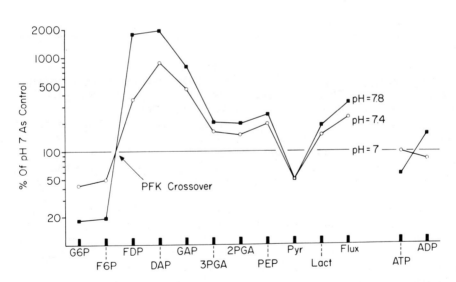

Figure 5. Crossover plot showing the interactions caused by increasing the pH on erythrocyte glycolysis. Data replotted from Minakami and Yoshikawa (22).

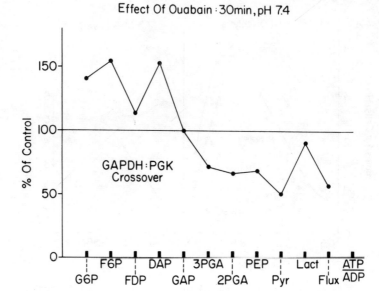

Figure 6. Effect of ouabain on intermediates of glycolysis in erythrocytes (22).

Control at Glyceraldehyde-3-P Dehydrogenase and P-Glycerate Kinase

Inhibition of the energy utilization of the erythrocyte by addition of ouabain to inhibit the ATP driven Na^+ pump also results in an inhibition of glycolysis (22). Fig. 6 shows a crossover plot of the data obtained in a particular experiment, and it is seen that the site of inhibition is located between the triose phosphates and 3-P-glycerate, suggesting an interaction either at glyceraldehyde-3-P dehydrogenase (GAPDH) or at P-glycerate kinase (PGK). The observed increase of the ATP/ADP ratio suggests the possibility of an ADP limitation at the P-glycerate kinase site.

Further evidence of the nature of the factors controlling flux through the GAPDH and PGK steps and their influence on the DPG level is obtained from experiments with erythrocytes incubated in media containing a high phosphate concentration (9). Fig. 7 shows a comparison of the changes of the glycolytic intermediates in erythrocytes incubated in low (1.5 mM) and high (50 mM) phosphate. The high phosphate medium produced an increase of glycolytic flux, a decrease of glucose-6-P and a large accumulation of fructose-1,6-di-P and triose-phosphates. These changes indicate a stimulation of phosphofructokinase. Since the intracellular

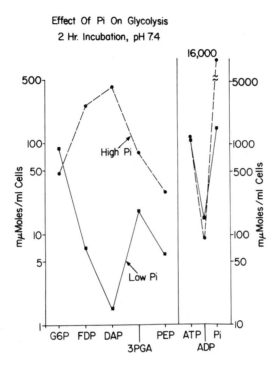

Figure 7. Response of normal human red cells to low (1.5 mM) and high (50 mM) phosphate media. Data replotted from Rose and Warms (9).

phosphate concentration increased to about 20 mM, this effect is probably caused by a direct activational effect of phosphate on phosphofructokinase. The increased phosphate concentration also produces an activation of hexokinase (22), possibly by relief of glucose-6-P inhibition.

The increases of dihydroxyacetone-P and fructose-1,6-di-P in the high phosphate medium were continuous with time, while the levels of 3-P-glycerate and P-enolpyruvate not only were much lower, but also did not change after the first 30 minutes of incubation (Fig. 8). These data suggest that flux through the P-glycerate kinase and glyceraldehyde-3-P dehydrogenase steps is less than that through the phosphofructokinase step.

One possible explanation for the observed metabolic changes is that the elevated phosphate concentration shifts the mass action ratio of glyceraldehyde-3-P dehydrogenase in favor of 1,3-diphosphoglycerate and NADH, which results in a relative inhibition of glyceraldehyde-3-P dehydrogenase. This explanation is indicated by addition of pyruvate to cells incubated for 1 hour in 50 mM

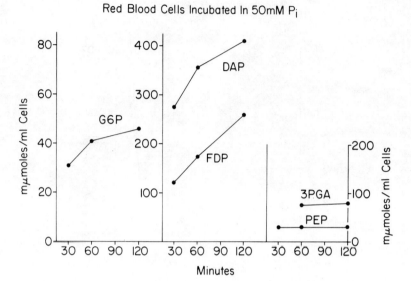

Figure 8. Effect of time of incubation in medium containing 50 mM inorganic phosphate on glycolytic intermediates (9).

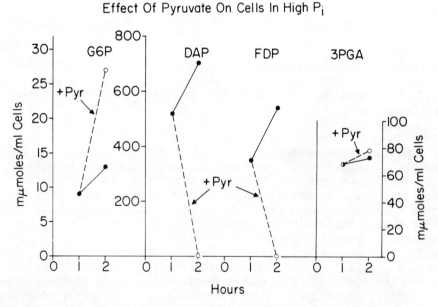

Figure 9. Effect of 3 mM pyruvate on glycolytic intermediates after a 1 hour incubation in 50 mM phosphate (9).

Table I

Effects of Pyruvate at High Pi

Data from (9, 23).

Metabolite	Control	+Pyruvate	Difference
	μmoles/ml cells		
Lactate formed	9.70	11.70	+2.00
Pyruvate used	0.0	2.14	-2.14
2, 3PGA	3.46	5.91	+2.45
	mμmoles/ml cells		
1, 3PGA	0.3	1.5	+1.2
3PGA	68	94	+26
ADP	76	43	-33

phosphate medium, which results in a large and rapid depletion of dihydroxyacetone-P and fructose-1,6-di-P (Fig. 9). Conversely, glucose-6-P levels increased upon addition of pyruvate, suggesting a diminished flux through phosphofructokinase, possibly caused by a loss of the activational effect of fructose-1,6-di-P combined with increased inhibition by the elevated ATP levels. 3-P-Glycerate levels did not change appreciably after addition of pyruvate, and the loss of carbon from the triose-P and fructose diphosphate pool can be accounted for by an increase of DPG (Table I). Similar results were found by Eckel et al. (24) upon addition of pyruvate to stored defibrinated erythrocytes which have accumulated triose phosphates. Table I also shows that the pyruvate removed from the system was quantitatively converted to lactate. The levels of 1, 3-di-P-glycerate increased five-fold, while 3-P-glycerate increased by 40%.

From the available data, and with reference to the scheme shown in Fig. 10, the following explanation may be advanced to explain the effect of pyruvate on DPG levels. The primary effect of pyruvate is as an oxidant for the removal of NADH. This re-leases glyceraldehyde-3-P dehydrogenase from inhibition by NADH and accelerates the formation of 1,3 di-P-glycerate from the large triose phosphate pool. Increased phosphorylation of ADP at the P-glycerate kinase step causes a depletion of ADP (Table I) so that flux through the P-glycerate kinase and pyruvate kinase steps become controlled by ADP. The increase of 1,3 di-P-glycerate over the Km range for di-P-glycerate mutase allows increased conversion to DPG. Apparently this reaction can proceed despite the very low Ki for DPG on the mutase (Fig. 10). In this respect, it may be pointed out that from Michaelis-Menton kinetics for a non-compet-itive inhibitor;

Diphosphoglycerate Bypass

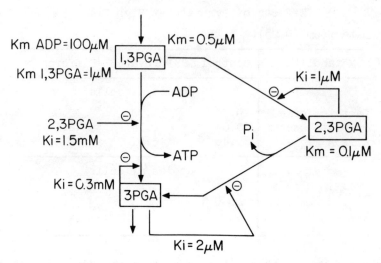

Figure 10. Scheme showing the kinetic constants of the enzymes converting 1,3-di-P-glycerate to 3-P-glycerate. Data from (1,23, 25).

$$v = \frac{V_{max}}{(1 + \frac{Km}{S})(1 + \frac{I}{Ki})} ,$$

when I $\gg$ Ki, the expression reduces to $v \propto \frac{1}{I}$. In other words, the forward velocity of the reaction is progressively inhibited as the concentration of the inhibitor increases. A similar relationship holds for competitive inhibition when S is approximately equal to Km and I $\gg$ Ki. It is clear, therefore, that the rate of conversion of 1,3-di-P-glycerate to DPG will be critically dependent on the concentration of free DPG. Likewise, flux through DPG phosphatase will depend not only on the levels of DPG (its substrate) and 3-P-glycerate (its product and inhibitor), but also on the phosphatase activity associated with P-glycerate mutase. The very low activity of the diphosphoglycerate phosphatase enzymes (26) presumably limits DPG breakdown despite the low Km for DPG.

Estimates of up to 50°/o have been made for the contribution of glycolytic flux through the DPG bypass (27). However, the relative rates of disposal of 1,3-di-P-glycerate through the alternative route clearly will depend on the nature of the metabolic environment to which the erythrocytes are exposed, and may also be critically dependent on the concentration of free DPG. Thus, at high DPG levels, flux through the DPG bypass should be minimal.

Table II

Dissociation Constants of Mg Complexes

Data from (32).

Reaction	K_D (mM)
$ATP \cdot Mg^{2-} \rightarrow ATP^{4-} + Mg^{2+}$	0.019
$ATP \cdot Mg^{-} \rightarrow ATP^{3-} + Mg^{2+}$	1.35
$ADP \cdot Mg^{-} \rightarrow ADP^{3-} + Mg^{2+}$	0.30
$ADP \cdot Mg \rightarrow ADP^{2-} + Mg^{2+}$	7.6
$AMP \cdot Mg \rightarrow AMP^{2-} + Mg^{2+}$	10.0
$2,3PGA \cdot Mg^{2-} \rightarrow 2,3PGA^{4-} + Mg^{2+}$	0.9

The importance of an oxidizing environment for the accumulation of
DPG is revealed by comparable experiments of Saito and Minakami
(28), who found that addition of methylene blue to red cells metabolizing glucose resulted in an accumulation of DPG at the expense
of triose-P and fructose-1,6-di-P, but no increase of lactate and
pyruvate. On the other hand, addition of xylitol to erythrocytes,
which produces NADH by its oxidation to D-xylulose, causes a large
accumulation of triose phosphates, a decrease of pyruvate, an increase of lactate, and practically no change on the DPG levels (29).

Free and Bound Magnesium in Erythrocytes

Since ADP complexed with magnesium is the nucleotide species
reacting with P-glycerate kinase (30) or pyruvate kinase (31),
while free ATP is much more inhibitory than [Mg·ATP] on phosphofructokinase, it is evident that a more complete understanding of
the control interactions of adenine nucleotides with the glycolytic
enzymes can only be achieved by determining the distribution of
the adenine nucleotides between free and complexed forms. Rose
(32) has recently suggested a method for performing such calculations based on the dependence of the adenylate kinase equilibrium
on the Mg^{++} concentration. Table II shows that ATP binds to magnesium much more strongly than either ADP or AMP. With minor
corrections for K^+ and pH effects, it is possible to derive a
relationship between the apparent equilibrium constant of adenylate kinase and the concentration of free Mg^{++} in equilibrium with
the individual nucleotides at any given pH. This relationship is
of the form shown in Fig. 11 at pH 7.0, where it is seen that $\underline{K_{eq}}$
ranges from about 0.4 to 1.1, with a maximum at about 0.3 mM Mg^{++}.
Measured values of the mass action ratio outside these limits is
indicative either of a lack of equilibrium or compartmentation of
the nucleotides, assuming correct analytical measurements. Since

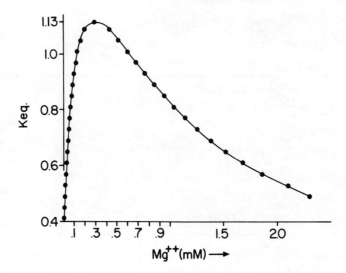

Figure 11. Effect of Mg^{++} concentration on the mass action ratio
of the adenylate kinase equilibrium (32).

the curve is biphasic, a given value of Kapp can be read off as
indicating a low or a high Mg^{++} concentration. Therefore, for
each tissue the directional change of calculated Mg^{++} has to be
determined, as ATP, which is the strongest chelator, is made to
fall experimentally.

This method was evaluated experimentally by Rose by addition
of 5 mM 2-deoxyglucose to red blood cells previously incubated in
isotonic saline containing iodoacetate to inhibit glycolysis at
the glyceraldehyde-P dehydrogenase step (32). Pertinent data from
this experiment are shown in Fig. 12. The left hand side of the
figure shows the measured changes of the individual nucleotides
during a 60 minute incubation with 2-deoxyglucose. The free Mg^{++}
concentration, calculated from the adenylate kinase mass action
ratio, apparently is in the range of 100 μM at normal ATP levels.
The right hand side of the figure shows that ATP is 70 to 80%
complexed with magnesium, while only about 20 to 30% of the ADP
is bound. These percentages are relatively insensitive to the
total ATP or ADP contents. The conclusion is drawn that the concentration of [Mg·ADP] in the erythrocyte is probably below the Km
for P-glycerate kinase and therefore may exert effective control
of the enzyme velocity. Apparently, the total ADP reflects the
[Mg·ADP] reasonably accurately. According to Rose (9), pyruvate
kinase is controlled more by the P-enolpyruvate concentration than
the [Mg·ADP] concentration.

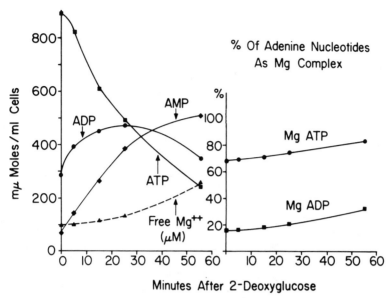

Figure 12. Effect of 2-deoxyglucose on adenine nucleotide contents of red blood cells in relation to the change of free Mg^{++}
concentration. See (32) for experimental details.

Since glyceraldehyde-3-P dehydrogenase and P-glycerate kinase
are near equilibrium reactions (Fig. 3), while pyruvate kinase is
far displaced from equilibrium, the activity of pyruvate kinase
will strongly influence the levels of intermediates between fruc-
tose-1,6-di-P and P-enolpyruvate. However, since the dehydrogenase
and kinase steps are bimolecular, with the concentrations of the
adenine and pyridine nucleotides in the erythrocyte within the $\underline{Km}$
and $\underline{Ki}$ regions of the enzymes, feedback control at the GAPDH and
PGK sites is exerted both by the NAD oxidation-reduction state and
by the phosphate potential. Phosphorylation at the pyruvate kinase
step is of particular significance in the erythrocyte because of
glucose rather than glycogen being the substrate, so that net ATP
production does not occur prior to the pyruvate kinase reaction.
Hence this enzyme step effectively controls both the phosphate
potential by the rate of formation of ATP and the NADH level via
the rate of formation of pyruvate.

Binding of Adenine Nucleotides and 2,3-di-P-Glycerate to Hemoglobin

It is now well established that organic phosphates have the
capacity to bind to hemoglobin, and that the ligand binding in the
presence of 0.1 M salt shows an overwhelming preference for deoxyhemoglobin (33,34). This effect causes the oxygenation curve of

hemoglobin to be shifted to the right in the presence of DPG, so
that a larger percentage of oxygen is unloaded at a given venous
oxygen tension (33-35). The most important physiological organic
phosphate ligands are DPG and ATP, having binding constants to
deoxyhemoglobin of 1.3×10^5 (34) and 2.3×10^4 (36), respectively.
However, since the binding of ATP to magnesium is approximately
forty times stronger than to deoxyhemoglobin, while the binding of
DPG to magnesium is one hundred times less than to deoxyhemoglobin,
it is apparent that oxygenation of hemoglobin will affect the free
DPG concentration to a much greater extent than the free ATP concentration. According to Benesch et al. (34,35), deoxyhemoglobin
has one strong binding site for DPG. Hence when DPG and hemoglobin
are present in equimolar concentrations, as they approximately are
in normal erythrocytes, the free DPG may be expected to vary
greatly from μM amounts when the hemoglobin is deoxygenated to mM
amounts when it is saturated with oxygen. A rapid oscillation of
the free DPG level in blood as it passes from the lungs to the
capillaries may cause periodic alterations in the activities of
diphosphoglycerate mutase and diphosphoglycerate phosphatase (see
Fig. 10), but no experimental data is available concerning fluc-
tuations of the glycolytic intermediates with periodic oxygenation
and deoxygenation of the hemoglobin. Presumably in vivo, the
relatively low turnover times of the glycolytic enzymes provide a
high damping factor on the oscillations expected from alterations
of the free DPG level. However, since the pH also changes with
hemoglobin oxygenation, complex interactions at each of the major
control sites of erythrocyte glycolysis, namely hexokinase, phosphofructokinase and pyruvate kinase are to be expected. Finally,
formation and breakdown of DPG, by eliminating ADP phosphorylation
at the P-glycerate kinase step, will tend to increase glycolysis
by making more ADP available to pyruvate kinase. Clearly, more
work is needed on careful and complete measurements of all the
intermediates of the glycolytic pathway under suitable experimental
conditions before a fuller understanding of the details of control
of erythrocyte glycolysis will be achieved.

ACKNOWLEDGMENTS

Supported by grants from the U. S. Public Health Service
12202 and the American Heart Association. The author is an Established Investigator of the American Heart Association. Helpful
discussions with Drs. I. A. Rose and T. Asakura are gratefully
acknowledged. The reviewer is indebted to Dr. J. Higgins for the
theoretical treatment of the fault theorem. Interpretations of the
data presented represent the views of the reviewer, and may not be
identical with those belonging to the authors of the original
papers from which the data was obtained.

REFERENCES

1. RAPOPORT, S., in P. N. CAMPBELL AND G. D. GREVILLE (Editors), Essays in biochemistry, Vol. 4, Academic Press, New York, 1968, p. 69.
2. MURPHY, J. R., J. Lab. Clin. Med., 55, 286 (1960).
3. YOSHIKAWA, H., AND MINAKAMI, S., Folia Haemat., 89, 357 (1968).
4. DE VERDIER, C. H., Folia Haemat., 78, 184 (1962).
5. TSUTSUI, E. A., MARKS, P. A., AND REICH, P., J. Biol. Chem., 237, 3009 (1962).
6. KAUFFMAN, F. C., BROWN, J. G., PASSONNEAU, J. V., AND LOWRY, O. H., J. Biol. Chem., 244, 3647 (1969).
7. ROSE, I. A., WARMS, J. V. B., AND O'CONNELL, E. L., Biochem. Biophys. Res. Commun., 15, 33 (1964).
8. VELICK, S. F., AND FURFINE, C., in P. D. BOYER, H. LARDY, AND K. MYRBACK (Editors), The enzymes, Vol. 7, Academic Press, New York, 1963, p. 243.
9. ROSE, I. A., AND WARMS, J. V. B., J. Biol. Chem., 241, 4848 (1966).
10. CHAPMAN, R. G., HENNESSEY, M. A., WALTERSDORPH, A. M., HUENNEKENS, F. M., AND GABRIO, B. W., J. Clin. Invest., 41, 1249 (1962).
11. PENNELL, R. B., in C. BISHOP AND D. M. SURGENOR (Editors), The red blood cell, Academic Press, New York, 1964, p. 26.
12. HESS, B., in B. WRIGHT (Editor), Control mechanisms in respiration and fermentation, Ronald Press Company, New York, 1963, p. 333.
13. WILLIAMSON, J. R., J. Biol. Chem., 240, 2308 (1965).
14. CHANCE, B., AND WILLIAMS, G. R., J. Biol. Chem., 217, 409 (1955).
15. CHANCE, B., WILLIAMS, G. R., HOLMES, W. F., AND HIGGINS, J., J. Biol. Chem., 217, 439 (1955).
16. CHANCE, B., HOLMES, W. F., HIGGINS, J., AND CONNELLY, C. M., Nature, 182, 1190 (1958).
17. HOLMES, W. F., Trans. Farad. Soc., 55, 1122 (1959).
18. HIGGINS, J. In preparation.
19. ASAKURA, T., SATO, Y., MINAKAMI, S., AND YOSHIKAWA, H., J. Biochem. (Tokyo), 59, 524 (1966).
20. BOHR, C., HASSELBALCH, K., AND KROGH, A., Skand. Arch. Physiol., 16, 402 (1904).
21. ASAKURA, T., SATO, Y., MINAKAMI, S., AND YOSHIKAWA, H., Clin. Chim. Acta, 14, 840 (1966).
22. MINAKAMI, S., AND YOSHIKAWA, H., J. Biochem. (Tokyo), 59, 145 (1966).
23. ROSE, I. A. Unpublished observations.
24. ECKEL, R. E., RIZZO, S. C., LODISH, H., AND BERGGREN, A. B., Amer. J. Physiol., 210, 737 (1966).
25. ROSE, Z. A., J. Biol. Chem., 243, 4810 (1968).
26. ROSE, Z. A. This monograph.
27. REICH, J. G., Europ. J. Biochem., 6, 395 (1968).

28. SAITO, T., AND MINAKAMI, S., J. Biochem. (Tokyo), 61, 211
    (1967).
29. ASAKURA, T., ADACHI, K., MINAKAMI, S., AND YOSHIKAWA, H.,
    J. Biochem. (Tokyo), 62, 184 (1967).
30. LARRSON-RAZHKIEWICZ, M., Biochim. Biophys. Acta, 132, 33 (1967).
31. MELCHIOR, J. B., Biochemistry, 4, 1518 (1965).
32. ROSE, I. A., Proc. Nat. Acad. Sci. U.S.A., 61, 1079 (1968).
33. BENESCH, R., AND BENESCH, R. E., Nature, 221, 618 (1969).
34. BENESCH, R. E., BENESCH, R., AND YU, C. I., Biochemistry, 8,
    2567 (1969).
35. BENESCH, R., BENESCH, R. E., AND YU, C. I., Proc. Nat. Acad.
    Sci. U.S.A., 59, 526 (1968).
36. LO, H. H., AND SCHIMMEL, P. R., J. Biol. Chem., 244, 5084
    (1969).

THE ENZYMES OF 2,3-DIPHOSPHOGLYCERATE METABOLISM IN THE HUMAN RED CELL

Zelda B. Rose

The Institute for Cancer Research, Fox Chase

Philadelphia, Pennsylvania 19111

Summary

2,3-Diphosphoglycerate is synthesized in red cells by a
specific mutase and hydrolyzed by a specific phosphatase. Diphosphoglycerate mutase catalyzes the synthesis of 2,3-diphospho-
glycerate from 1,3-diphosphoglycerate and 3-phosphoglycerate. The
maximum activity of the enzyme in the mature human erythrocyte is
4 μmoles per minute per ml of cells at 37°. Studies with the
purified enzyme showed activation by 2-phosphoglycerate and
glycolate 2-P. 2,3-Diphosphoglycerate is a competitive inhibitor
of 1,3-diphosphoglycerate (K_m 0.5 μM) with a K_i of 0.8 μM. Due
to the high level of 2,3-diphosphoglycerate in the mature red

---

[1] This investigation was supported by Public Health Service
Research grant no. CA-07819 from the National Cancer Institute,
and also by grants awarded to this Institute: NIH grants CA-06927
and FR-05539, and by an appropriation from the Commonwealth of
Pennsylvania.

137

cell (4-6 mM), the rate of the diphosphomutase will be described
by the equation for competitive inhibition:

$$\frac{v}{V} = 1 \Big/ 1 + \frac{0.5 \ \mu M}{[1,3\text{-diPGA}]} \left(1 + \frac{[2,3\text{-diPGA}]}{0.8 \ \mu M} \right)$$

The activity of 2,3-diphosphoglycerate phosphatase in human
red cells is 1 mμmole per minute per ml of red cells at 37°. The
rate is increased in the presence of certain activators. The
system activated by phosphate and chloride (0.1 M) has a maximal
velocity 14 times higher. Glycolate 2-P activates 1350-fold and
does not require chloride. Since the K_a for phosphate, 0.7 mM, is
higher than the normal intracellular level of 0.4 mM, changes in
inorganic phosphate in the cell will change the rate. The data
are compatible with the following velocity equation:

$$\frac{v}{V} = 0.07 + \left(\frac{0.93}{1 + \frac{0.7 \ mM}{[Pi]}} \right)$$

The presence in the red blood cells of many mammals of high
concentrations of 2,3-diPGA[2] has long been recognized. Recent
work has indicated the central role of this compound in the
functioning of the cell. The importance of the binding of
2,3-diPGA to deoxy hemoglobin is a central subject at this
meeting. Some of the earliest work on this subject was done in
the laboratory of Dr. Chanutin (1). These studies and those of
Benesch (2,3) gave impetus to a surge of fruitful research on the

---

[2] Abbreviations: PGA (phosphoglycerate); Pi (inorganic
phosphate).

physiology of the red cell. 2,3-DiPGA has been reported to be an

inhibitor of several red cell enzymes, AMP· deaminase (4), phos-

phoribosyl pyrophosphate synthetase (5), and several enzymes of

carbohydrate metabolism (6), indicating the importance of the

level of 2,3-diPGA to the energy metabolism of the cell. In

order to understand how the level of 2,3-diPGA is controlled in

the cell, the enzymes involved in its synthesis and breakdown were

studied.

The reactions involved in 2,3-diPGA metabolism were recog-

nized by Rapoport and his co-workers (7,8,9). The synthesis is

catalyzed by diphosphoglycerate mutase and the hydrolysis by a

specific phosphatase. These reactions are closely associated with

the glycolytic pathway, the only energy producing path in the

mature red cell. As in all animal tissues, 2,3-diPGA functions in

these cells as the cofactor of the glycolytic enzyme phospho-

glycerate mutase (Fig. 1).

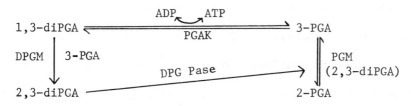

FIG. 1.   Metabolism of 2,3-diPGA in red cells. The
abbreviations are: PGAK, phosphoglycerate kinase; DPGM,
diphosphoglycerate mutase; DPG Pase, diphosphoglycerate
phosphatase; PGM, phosphoglycerate mutase.

Estimates of the rates of the enzymes of diphosphoglycerate

metabolism require a knowledge of the levels of some of the gly-

colytic intermediates. The glycolytic reactions between fructose

1,6-diP and P-enolpyruvate are at equilibrium in the red cell,

with the pyruvate kinase rate determined by the concentration of

P-enolpyruvate and ADP as well as the amount of enzyme (10).

DIPHOSPHOGLYCERATE MUTASE

We have demonstrated that the synthesis of 2,3-diPGA follows

the equation shown (11).

$$1,3\text{-diPGA} \quad + \quad 3\text{-PGA} \longrightarrow 2,3\text{-diPGA} \quad + \quad 3\text{-PGA}$$

The acyl phosphate group of 1,3-diPGA is transferred to C-2 of

3-PGA. The reaction requires added 3-PGA. The addition of 2-PGA

in the presence of sub-optimal 3-PGA increases the rate of the

reaction and also increases the maximum velocity to a higher level

than that found when only 3-PGA is present (Fig. 2). The K_m's

found were 1.45 µM for 3-PGA and 0.74 µM for 2-PGA. 2-PGA can

also act as a phosphoryl acceptor according to the reaction shown.

$$1,3\text{-diPGA} \quad + \quad 2\text{-PGA} \longrightarrow 2,3\text{-diPGA} \quad + \quad 3\text{-PGA}$$

However, 3-PGA is always the major phosphoryl acceptor and this

reaction never accounts for more than 1/3 of the total reaction

(11). Thus the increase in 2,3-diPGA synthesis caused by 2-PGA

is largely due to a stimulation of 3-PGA phosphorylation. It

will be noted that 3-PGA is produced in the reaction and due to

its presence as a contaminant of 1,3-diPGA and its low K_m, it is

an inexhaustable substrate. To show the activator effect, sepa-

rated from the phosphorylation, we examined the effect of

glycolate 2-P. The overall reaction is activated by glycolate 2-P

(Fig. 3). Pi is inhibitory and competitive with 3-PGA, 2-PGA or

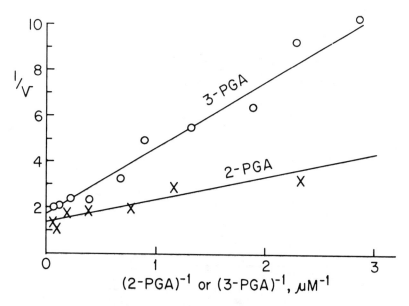

FIG. 2.   A comparison of the K_m and V_{max} observed with 2-PGA
or 3-PGA as the predominant monophosphoglycerate present.
Diphosphoglycerate mutase reaction mixtures contained glycylglycine buffer, pH 7.5 (10 mM), 2-mercaptoethanol (5 mM),
enzyme sufficient for 15% reaction, and additions as noted
in a volume of 0.2 ml.   Incubations were for 10 min at 25°.
1,3-diPGA-1-^{32}P was constant at 0.61 µM (1.6 x 10^4 cpm per
mµmole) and contained 3-PGA at 0.39 µM.   The concentration of
1,3-diPGA was low in order to have as little 3-PGA contamination as possible.   In all double reciprocal plots for this
enzyme the velocities are ratios of the observed rate to the
rate in an assay containing Pi (10 mM), 3-PGA (60 µM);
1,3-diPGA-1-^{32}P (1 µM).   The values shown are calculated from
the total counts fixed into the product.   The apparent K_m
values are 1.45 µM for 3-PGA and 0.74 µM for 2-PGA [from
Rose (11)].

glycolate 2-P.   Pi has a K_i of 0.3 mM whether measured in the

presence of 3-PGA or 2-PGA.   Fig. 4 shows the data obtained with

3-PGA.   A similar picture is found with 2-PGA.   The level of 3-PGA

in the cell is 50-80 µM (12), sufficiently high that the effect

of Pi, although in the physiological range of concentration, should

not be rate-determining.

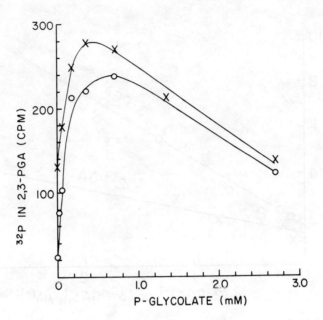

FIG. 3. Effect of glycolate 2-P on the rate of the reaction.
In all cases 10 mM Pi was present and 1,3-diPGA-1-^{32}P (1.3 x
10^4 cpm per mμmole) was at 2 μM. Diphosphoglycerate mutase
was 10^{-4} unit per ml of incubation. 3-PGA 0.3 μM (o) and
2.3 μM (x). Values plotted are observed counts per min.
With saturating 3-PGA, 870 cpm could be obtained [from
Rose (11)].

The enzyme has a high affinity for 1,3-diPGA (K_m 0.53 μM).

The concentration of this metabolite is normally low, and possibly

of this order of magnitude in the mature red cell. 2,3-DiPGA is

a competitive inhibitor (K_i 0.8 μM) (Fig. 5). Since the usual

level of 2,3-diPGA in the cell is 4000 to 6000 μM (12), the

apparent K_m of 1,3-diPGA is greatly increased and the velocity

of the reaction should follow the equation for competitive

inhibition:

$$\frac{v}{V} = 1 \left/ 1 + \frac{0.5 \ \mu M}{[1,3\text{-PGA}]} \left(1 + \frac{[2,3\text{-PGA}]}{0.8 \ \mu M} \right) \right.$$

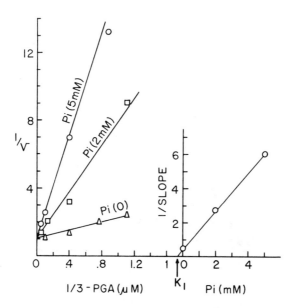

FIG. 4. Effect of Pi on the K_m of 3-PGA. Incubation conditions are given with Fig. 2. 1,3-diPGA-1-^{32}P (1.1 x 10^5 cpm per mμmole) was constant at 1 μM. K_i of Pi is 314 μM [from Rose (11)].

The maximum velocity of the enzyme in normal red cells is 4 μmoles per minute per ml of cells at 37°. Oski et al. (13) have shown that normal erythrocytes contain 44% more 2,3-diPGA after incubation under anaerobic conditions than cells similarly incubated aerobically. Since the anaerobic cells would contain less free 2,3-diPGA because of the specific binding to deoxyhemoglobin, the effect is probably due to a release of the inhibition by 2,3-diPGA of the diphosphomutase of these cells. The rate of the isolated enzyme was not affected by other cellular constituents, including adenine nucleotides, pyridine nucleotides or other glycolytic intermediates.

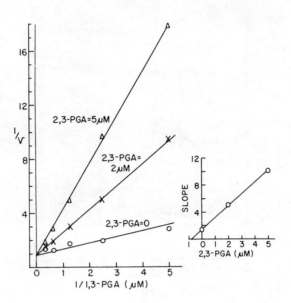

FIG. 5. Effect of 2,3-diPGA on the K_m of 1,3-diPGA. Incubation conditions are given with Fig. 2. Reaction mixtures contained 3-PGA (20 µM); 1,3-diPGA-1-^{32}P (1.25 x 10^5 cpm per mµmole). K_m of 1,3-diPGA is 0.53 µM; K_i of 2,3-diPGA is 0.85 µM [from Rose (11)].

DIPHOSPHOGLYCERATE PHOSPHATASE

The activity of diphosphoglycerate phosphatase in red cells is sufficient to convert 1 mµmole of substrate to products per minute per ml of cells at 37°. This very low rate is increased appreciably in the presence of certain anions (14). Chloride gives a slight increase in the rate of the reaction. Pi also stimulates slightly. Together they give a more than additive increase in the rate (Fig. 6). With Pi at 1 mM, chloride produces an optimal effect at 0.1 M, its physiological level. With chloride at 0.085 M, Pi stimulates at concentrations up to 30 mM. Higher concentrations of either anion inhibit. The effect of

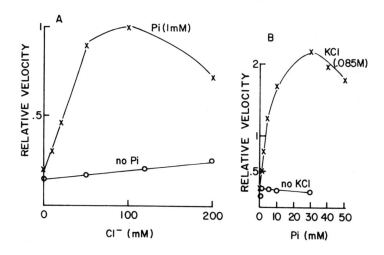

FIG. 6. A. Effect of increasing KCl. B. Effect of
increasing Pi. All diphosphoglycerate phosphatase reaction
mixtures contained glycylglycine buffer, pH 7.5 (10 mM),
2-mercaptoethanol (5 mM), enzyme sufficient for 15% reaction,
and additions as noted in a volume of 0.2 ml. Incubations
were for 15 min at 37°. 2,3-diPGA-^{32}P was 6 μM (3 x 10^4 cpm
per mμmole) in A and 20 μM (1.7 x 10^4 cpm per mμmole) in B.
Relative velocities are ratios of the observed rate to the
rate in an assay containing KCl (0.1 M) and Pi (1 mM).

chloride is shown by the sodium, potassium or magnesium salts but

not by equal concentrations of the acetates. Pi at 0.7 mM gives

a half optimal rate at levels of chloride from 10-100 mM.

Pi-dependent activation is found with fluoride and bromide

(Table 1). Each has the same K_a as found for chloride (about

22 mM when determined with 1 mM Pi). Bromide gives the same rate

as chloride but with fluoride the maximum velocity is decreased

by two-thirds. Iodide is inhibitory. Bicarbonate can replace

chloride (K_a 20 mM) giving a velocity about 70% of that with

Table 1

Substances Effective as Activators of Diphosphoglycerate
Phosphatase in the Presence of Phosphate

Incubation conditions are given with Fig. 6.   2,3-diPGA-^{32}P
was 4 μM.

Activator	K_a	Relative Velocity (no Pi)	Relative V_{max} (10 mM Pi)
None		0.15	0.20
F$^-$	32 mM		0.56
Cl$^-$	31 mM	0.20	2.03
Br$^-$	31 mM		1.90
I$^-$			0.10
			(1 mM Pi)
Cl$^-$	19 mM	0.26	1.0
HCO$_3^-$	20 mM	0.10	0.7

chloride.   Acetate at 0.1 M had no effect on the rate.

Several anions can substitute for Pi to activate the phosphatase in the presence of chloride (Table 2).   Sulfate is a poor
activator.   Arsenate and fluorophosphate give rates closer to Pi.
Sulfite activates with a maximum velocity about 4 times that of Pi
(15,16).   These activators appear to be competitive with Pi.

Glycolate 2-P induces the largest increase in the rate of the
phosphatase.   The maximal velocity is almost 1500 times the rate of
the non-activated enzyme.   Chloride is a non-competitive inhibitor
with respect to glycolate 2-P in the reaction activated by

Table 2

Substances Effective as Activators of Diphosphoglycerate
Phosphatase in the Presence of Chloride

Incubation conditions are given with Fig. 6.   2,3-diPGA-^{32}P
was 4 μM.

Activator	K_a	Relative Velocity (no Cl$^-$)	Relative V_{max} (0.1 M KCl)
None		0.14	0.26
SO$_4^{--}$	0.2 mM	0.04	0.35
HAsO$_4^{--}$	3.0 mM		1.25
Pi^{--}	0.7 mM	0.15	2.38
FPO$_3^{--}$	1.3 mM		3.33
SO$_3^{--}$	1.6 mM	0.20	9.27

glycolate 2-P. As the chloride concentration is raised from 0 to
100 mM, the apparent K_a of the glycolate 2-P changes from 22 μM to
64 μM (Fig. 7). Pi alone added to the glycolate 2-P activated
system is a competitive inhibitor of glycolate 2-P (Fig. 8). When
concentrations of Pi up to 2 mM are added to incubations containing
glycolate 2-P and 0.1 M KCl, there is increased activity. The
stimulation obtained is many times the maximum velocity for Pi
and chloride in the absence of glycolate 2-P (Fig. 9). Higher
levels of Pi are inhibitory. These data indicate that glycolate
2-P, Pi and chloride can all be bound to the enzyme at the same
time and therefore occupy separate sites.

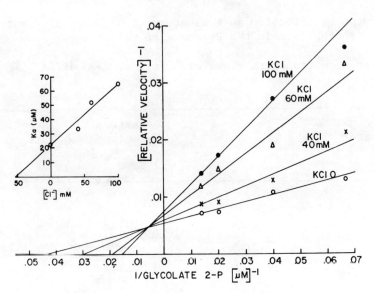

FIG. 7. Effect of Cl⁻ on the K_a of glycolate 2-P. Incubation conditions are given with Fig. 6. 2,3-diPGA-^{32}P (1 x 10⁴ cpm per mμmole) was 30 μM. Apparent K_a values with increasing KCl are (μM): 23, 33, 52, 65.

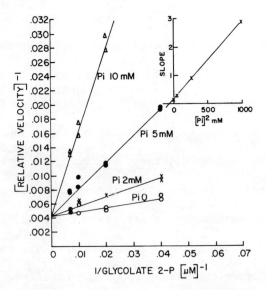

FIG. 8. Effect of Pi on the K_a of glycolate 2-P. Incubation conditions are given with Fig. 6. 2,3-DiPGA-^{32}P (4.4 x 10⁴ cpm per mμmole) was 4 μM. Apparent K_a values with increasing Pi are (μM): 15, 33, 94, 313.

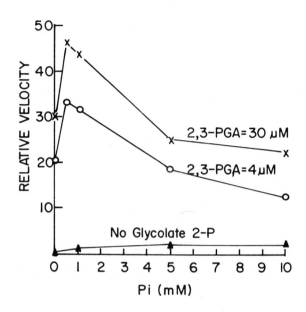

FIG. 9. Effect of Pi and Cl⁻ in the presence of glycolate
2-P. Incubation conditions are given with Fig. 6. Specific
activity of 2,3-diPGA-^{32}P was 0.6 x 10^4 cpm per mμmole.

The K_m of 2,3-diPGA varies over a wide range as the conditions of the assay are changed (Table 3). In the Pi and chloride
activated system, the K_m is very low, with a value of 0.08 μM.
The glycolate 2-P activated system has a K_m of 0.6 μM which
increases to more than 3 μM when 0.1 M chloride is present. The
monophosphoglycerates, added in the proportions present in an
equilibrium mixture, increase the K_m of 2,3-diPGA. This is true
of either the Pi and chloride activated or glycolate 2-P and
chloride activated systems. In either case the K_i observed for
PGA is about 1 μM. With one earlier preparation of the purified
enzyme both 2-PGA and 3-PGA were found to be highly effective
activators (14). They appeared to be acting similarly to

Table 3

K_m of 2,3-DiPGA for Diphosphoglycerate Phosphatase

Conditions	K_m	Relative V_{max}
Pi (1 mM) + KCl (0.1 M)	0.080 μM	1.18
Glycolate 2-P 20 μM	0.61 μM	133
Glycolate 2-P 60 μM	0.61 μM	200
Glycolate 2-P (60 μM) + KCl (0.1 M)	3.12 μM	50

glycolate 2-P. All other properties of this preparation were the same, both qualitatively and quantitatively, as those of preparations showing only inhibition by PGA. The inhibitory situation appears to be the commoner one since several samples of normal blood have shown only inhibition. However the stimulation may be due to a variant molecule and requires further investigation. Such extraordinary stimulation, coming within the normal range of PGA concentration, would certainly result in an abnormally high turnover rate for 2,3-diPGA and a consequent loss to the cell of glycolytic ATP yield.

A summary of the maximum velocities attained under a variety of activating conditions, compared to the non-activated rate, is given in Table 4. Pyrophosphate (K_a about 1 mM), which activates the 2,3-diPGA phosphatase activity of phosphoglycerate mutase (16,17,18), is a weak activator here. It is similar to glycolate 2-P in that there is no chloride requirement. Like glycolate 2-P

Table 4

Activators of Diphosphoglycerate Phosphatase

Activator	Maximum Activity	Requirement for KCl
None	1	
KCl (0.1 M)	1.8	
Pyrophosphate	8	No
Pi (1 mM) + KCl (0.1 M)	7	Yes
NaHSO$_3$ (5 mM) + KCl (0.1 M)	47	Yes
Glycolate 2-P	1350	No

it has a charge of minus 3 at pH 7.5. The glycolate 2-P activated

system shows inhibition by physiological levels of P-enolpyruvate

and ATP. The Pi and chloride activated system was not affected by

these compounds. Fructose di-P, ADP, and AMP at near-cellular

levels were not inhibitors in either system. These studies suggest

that the important regulator of the velocity of the phosphatase in

the cell is the Pi level. Using the data presented for the Pi and

chloride (0.1 M) activated system in which the maximum velocity is

14 mμmoles per min per ml of cells, the rate equation is:

$$\frac{v}{V} = 0.07 + \left(\frac{0.93}{1 + \frac{0.7 \text{ mM}}{[Pi]}} \right)$$

The significance of the glycolate 2-P activation is difficult

to assess. The activated rate would allow the breakdown of

1.5 μmoles of 2,3-diPGA per minute by one ml of red cells at 37°, which is greatly in excess of what is found or would ordinarily be considered desirable. There is a report in the literature that glycolate 2-P is a normal component of red cells and is present at 100 μM (19). The suggestion was made by Dr. A. Mildvan that this tremendous activation could be important in the aging cell. If glycolate 2-P forms in such cells, there is the possibility that it could set off a series of catabolic reactions.

These studies suggest that, barring the presence of glycolate 2-P in the average cell, the diphosphoglycerate mutase is the more important enzyme for regulating the level of 2,3-diPGA in the cell and the most important factors are the concentration of free 2,3-diPGA and of 1,3-diPGA. In intact cells, increased synthesis attributable to increased 1,3-diPGA has been found (11,20). The phosphatase appears to be adapted to the conditions of the red cell since it requires the high chloride level found there to show the activation by Pi. Increases in Pi would stimulate the phosphatase and would be important for the regeneration of ATP by pyruvate kinase.

References

1. Chanutin, A. and Curnish, R. R., Arch. Biochem. Biophys. 121, 96 (1967).

2. Benesch, R. and Benesch, R. E. Biochem. Biophys. Res. Commun. 26, 162 (1967).

3. Benesch, R., Benesch, R. E. and Yu, C. I. Proc. Natl. Acad. Sci. 59, 526 (1968).

4. Askari, A. and Rao, S. N. Biochim. Biophys. Acta <u>151</u>, 198 (1968).

5. Hershko, A., Razin, A. and Mager, J. Biochim. Biophys. Acta <u>184</u>, 64 (1969).

6. Dische, Z. In: <u>The Red Blood Cell</u>, edited by C. Bishop and D. M. Surgenor. New York: Academic Press, 1964, p. 208.

7. Rapoport, S. and Luebering, J. J. Biol. Chem. <u>183</u>, 507 (1950).

8. Rapoport, S. and Luebering, J. J. Biol. Chem. <u>189</u>, 683 (1951).

9. Rapoport, S. and Luebering, J. J. Biol. Chem. <u>196</u>, 583 (1952).

10. Rose, I. A. and Warms, J. V. B. J. Biol. Chem. <u>241</u>, 4848 (1966).

11. Rose, Z. B. J. Biol. Chem. <u>243</u>, 4810 (1968).

12. Bartlett, G. R. J. Biol. Chem. <u>234</u>, 449 (1959).

13. Oski, F. A., Gottlieb, A., Miller, W. W. and Delivoria-Papadopoulos, M. J. Clin. Invest., in press.

14. Rose, Z. B. Fed. Proc., Symposium: Control Mechanisms for Oxygen Release by Hemoglobin, 1969, in press.

15. Mányai, S. and Várady, Zs. Biochim. Biophys. Acta <u>20</u>, 594 (1956).

16. Harkness, D. R. and Roth, S. Biochem. Biophys. Res. Commun. <u>34</u>, 849 (1969).

17. Zancan, G. T., Recondo, E. F. and Leloir, L. F. Biochim. Biophys. Acta <u>110</u>, 348 (1965).

18. Rose, I. A. and Rose, Z. B. In Comp. Biochem. <u>17</u>, 93 (1969), edited by M. Florkin and E. H. Stotz.

19. Örström, A. Arch. Biochem. Biophys. <u>33</u>, 484 (1951).

20. Eckel, R. E., Rizzo, S. C., Lodish, H. and Berggren, A. B. Am. J. Physiol. <u>210</u>, 737 (1966).

METABOLISM OF 2,3-DIPHOSPHOGLYCERATE IN RED BLOOD CELLS

UNDER VARIOUS EXPERIMENTAL CONDITIONS[*]

E. Gerlach, J. Duhm, and B. Deuticke

Department of Physiology, Medical Faculty

Technical University, Aachen (Germany)

It took about forty years after GREENWALD discovered in 1925 (1) 2,3-diphosphoglycerate (2,3-DPG) to be a major constituent of red blood cells (RBC) before the first reports were published concerning the functional significance of this compound. While CHANUTIN and CURNISH detected the binding of 2,3-DPG to hemoglobin (2), BENESCH and BENESCH (3) as well as CHANUTIN (4) almost simultaneously demonstrated the effects of this binding on the oxygen affinity of hemoglobin.

These important findings initiated numerous investigations on the mechanisms and on the biological importance of the 2,3-DPG induced shift of the oxygen dissociation curve of hemoglobin. All the results obtained so far strongly suggest that 2,3-DPG in RBC plays an important role in maintaining a sufficient oxygen supply of tissues. In view of this concept it becomes more and more necessary to extend our knowledge concerning the mechanisms of the metabolic control of the 2,3-DPG levels in RBC.

During the course of our previous studies on phosphate metabolism (5) and phosphate permeability (6) of human RBC we became particularly interested in special problems of 2,3-DPG metabolism (7-10). The recent results of these investigations may contribute to a better understanding of those processes responsible for the

[*] Supported in part by a grant from the Deutsche Forschungsgemeinschaft.

regulation of 2,3-DPG concentration and for adaptive
concentration changes of this compound subsequent to
oxygen deficiency.

The first part of this paper deals with in vitro
studies regarding the influence of inorganic sulfur compounds on 2,3-DPG metabolism and glycolysis as well as
with the role of ADP in the regulation of the rate of
2,3-DPG synthesis. In the second part most recent findings are presented concerning the concentration changes
of 2,3-DPG in rat RBC in vivo due to hypoxia and anemia
as well as the influence of the oxygenation state of
hemoglobin on the rates of synthesis and decomposition
of 2,3-DPG in human RBC in vitro.

Before reporting our results the pathways of 2,3-DPG
metabolism shall be recapitulated (Fig.1): 2,3-DPG is
formed from 1,3-DPG and decomposed to 3-PG. As was first
shown by RAPOPORT and LUEBERING the formation of 2,3-DPG
is catalyzed by DPG mutase, the decomposition by 2,3-DPG
phosphatase (11). It was only during recent years that
evidence was obtained to finally settle the question,
whether in RBC 1,3-DPG is mainly converted directly to
3-PG, or mainly via 2,3-DPG. As was demonstrated by
different authors (7,9,12,13) only about 20% of the total
glycolytic flux passes through the 2,3-DPG pool under
physiological conditions. Therefore we know now for certain that in RBC as in other tissues the main pathway of
glycolysis involves the phosphoglycerate kinase reaction.

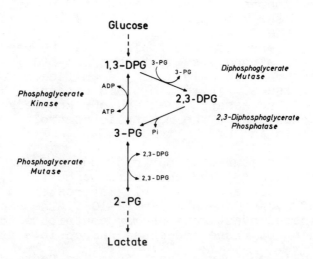

Fig.1. Pathways of 2,3-DPG metabolism in mammalian RBC

I. a) Effects of Inorganic Sulfur Compounds on 2,3-DPG
       Metabolism and Glycolysis in Human Red Blood
                     Cells in vitro

        When human RBC are incubated for several hours at
37°C and at a physiological pH in their own plasma containing an excess of glucose, the concentration of 2,3-DPG
decreases continuously at a rate of 0.17 μMol/ml RBC per
hour. The mechanism of this decrease which was also observed by other authors (14), is not yet understood. As
is shown in Fig.2 the spontaneous diminution of 2,3-DPG
becomes considerably enhanced in the presence of dithionite, sulfite and disulfite (5 mM), a finding, in agreement with early observations of MÁNIAY and VÁRADY (15)
and more recent results of other authors (16,17).

        In testing other inorganic sulfur compounds we made
the observation that tetrathionate, thiosulfate and
sulfate (5 mM) abolish almost completely the decrease of
2,3-DPG concentration. Corresponding effects of the different sulfur compounds were found to occur also in RBC
incubated without glucose in which no 2,3-DPG is synthesized.

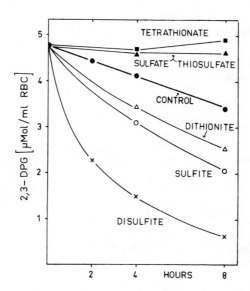

Fig.2. Effect of inorganic sulfur compounds (5 mM) on
the rate of 2,3-DPG decomposition in human RBC. Experimental conditions: Incubation of washed RBC in plasma,
37°C, pH 7.34, hematocrit 40%, glucose 15 mM. Analytical
procedures as described elsewhere (5,9). Each point is
the mean value of 3-7 experiments.

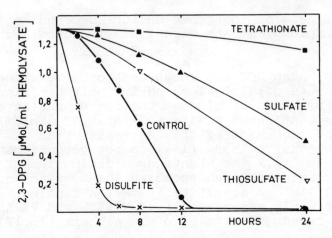

Fig.3. Effect of inorganic sulfur compounds (5 mM) on the rate of 2,3-DPG decomposition in hemolysates from human RBC. Incubation of hemolysates (2 parts of distilled water + 1 part of washed RBC (v/v), ghosts removed by centrifugation) at 37°C, pH 7.2, no glucose added. Each point is the mean value from 3 experiments.

In Fig.3 results are summarized concerning the effects of the different sulfur compounds on the rate of 2,3-DPG decomposition in hemolysates which were prepared from glucose-depleted RBC and incubated without any added substrates. Here too the decrease of 2,3-DPG is accelerated by disulfite, whereas it is inhibited by thiosulfate, sulfate and tetrathionate, the latter compound being again the most effective inhibitor.

From all these findings we have drawn the conclusion that the sulfur compounds under study act directly on the 2,3-DPG phosphatase (10). This view is further supported by experiments in which we could exclude the possibility that concentration changes of 3-PG, known to be a strong inhibitor of the 2,3-DPG phosphatase, mediates the effects of sulfur compounds on the metabolism of 2,3-DPG. Thus the sulfur compounds can be listed according to their action on the 2,3-DPG phosphatase (Table 1). It is interesting to note that very recently HARKNESS and ROTH demonstrated the activation by sulfite and dithionite of a highly purified 2,3-DPG phosphatase from human RBC (18).

Our data on the inhibitory action of sulfate provide a possible explanation of a special clinical observation: Patients with renal insufficiency or uremia exhibit

Table 1: <u>Classification of inorganic sulfur compounds</u>
<u>according to their influence on 2,3-DPG phosphatase</u>

Inhibitors:	Activators:
Tetrathionate $(S_4O_6^=)$	Disulfite $(S_2O_5^=)$
Sulfate $(SO_4^=)$	Sulfite $(SO_3^=)$
Thiosulfate $(S_2O_3^=)$	Dithionite $(S_2O_4^=)$

increased levels of 2,3-DPG in their RBC (19). Plasma
sulfate concentration in these patients is generally
found to be elevated to 5-8 mM (normally about 0.5 mM)
(20). Since according to our results 2,3-DPG phosphatase
is influenced by sulfate in the same range of concentration, it seems most likely that the high 2,3-DPG levels
in RBC of these patients result from a sulfate induced
inhibition of 2,3-DPG phosphatase.

Taking into account that the various sulfur compounds
have opposite effects on the 2,3-DPG phosphatase, our
results concerning their influence on glycolysis are
rather surprising: As we could demonstrate, all sulfur
compounds studied have in common that they increase the
glycolytic rate. This statement is supported by the
experimental data summarized in Table 2. As can be seen,
glucose consumption and lactate production of human RBC
are generally increased. However, in all cases glucose
consumption exceeds considerably lactate production; thus
the ratios Δlactate/2xΔglucose are always below the control value. Without going into further details it shall
be mentioned, that in the presence of the inhibitors of
2,3-DPG phosphatase the concentration of ATP decreases,
whereas under the influence of the activators ATP levels
remain constant (10).

From the difference between glucose consumption and
lactate production one would expect certain glycolytic
intermediates to accumulate. That this actually happens
is illustrated in Fig.4. The most remarkable changes
occur in fructose-1,6-diphosphate and the triosephosphates (DAP + GA-3-P), the concentrations of which increase
tremendously. In contrast the concentration changes of
3-PG and PEP are small.

Table 2: Influence of inorganic sulfur compounds (5mM) on glycolysis and ATP levels in human RBC [*]

	Glucose Consumption (% of Control)	Lactate Production (% of Control)	$\dfrac{\triangle \text{Lactate}}{2 \triangle \text{Glucose}}$	ATP (μMol/ml RBC)
Control	100	100	0.93	1.29
Inhibitors of 2,3-DPG Phosphatase:				
Tetrathionate	203	130	0.60	0.73
Sulfate	192	155	0.75	0.98
Thiosulfate	207	166	0.75	1.03
Activators of 2,3-DPG Phosphatase:				
Disulfite	221	192	0.81	1.31
Sulfite	165	154	0.88	1.34
Dithionite	198	176	0.86	1.25

[*] Incubation time: 4 hours. Mean values from 3 - 6 experiments. For experimental details see legend to Fig. 2

The action of the sulfur compounds on RBC glycolysis may be explained to result from an activation of phosphofructokinase (PFK). This interpretation seems most probable, since the observed changes closely resemble those occuring after the activation of PFK due to an increase in pH or an elevation of inorganic phosphate (21,22). Moreover it has been demonstrated that sulfate does activate PFK in hemolysates (23).

I. b) Control of 2,3-DPG Synthesis by ADP

According to findings of RAPOPORT (24) and SCHRÖTER (25) the rate of synthesis of 2,3-DPG in hemolysates is markedly influenced by the concentration of ADP. Until very recently there was no possibility to prove experimentally whether the extent of 2,3-DPG synthesis in intact RBC is also related to the level of ADP.

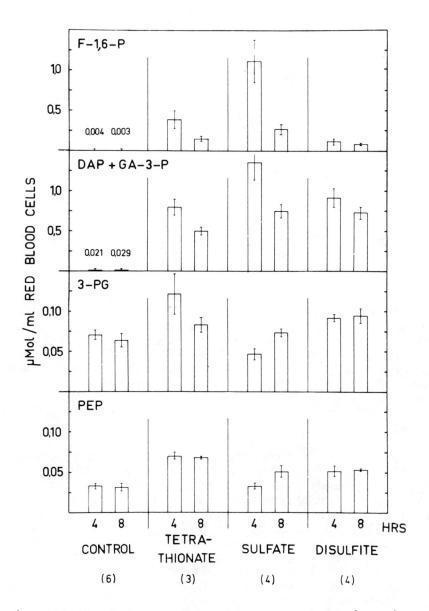

Fig.4. Effect of inorganic sulfur compounds (5 mM) on the concentrations of various glycolytic intermediates in human RBC. Mean values (± SEM) from number of experiments indicated.

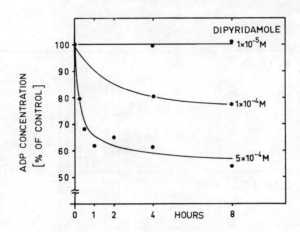

Fig.5. Influence of dipyridamole on the ADP concentration of human RBC. Experimental conditions see legend to Fig.2. Each point is the mean value of 5 experiments.

More or less accidentally we observed that dipyridamole* and some of its derivatives (6,26), which all strongly reduce phosphate permeability of RBC, induce a fall in the concentration of ADP and a stabilization of 2,3-DPG levels in these cells without causing detectable changes of glycolytic intermediates (9). On the basis of these findings it seemed therefore possible to use dipyridamole as a tool to establish that the concentration of ADP influences the rate of 2,3-DPG synthesis in intact RBC also.

The concentration changes of ADP brought about by dipyridamole in RBC incubated for 8 hours are given in Fig.5. While dipyridamole at 1 x 10^{-5} M is still ineffective, higher concentrations of this compound cause a rather rapid fall in ADP levels, which are reduced, respectively, to about 80 and 55% of the control values.

In Fig.6 results of experiments are summarized in which the influence of dipyridamole on 2,3-DPG metabolism was studied under various conditions. As can be seen, dipyridamole prevents the spontaneous diminution of 2,3-DPG in RBC incubated in the presence of glucose. In the absence of glucose, in IAA treated cells as well as in hemolysates it proved to be ineffective. In this

---

* 2,6-bis(diethanolamino)-4,8-dipiperidino-pyrimido-
  (5,4-d)pyrimidine = Persantin®

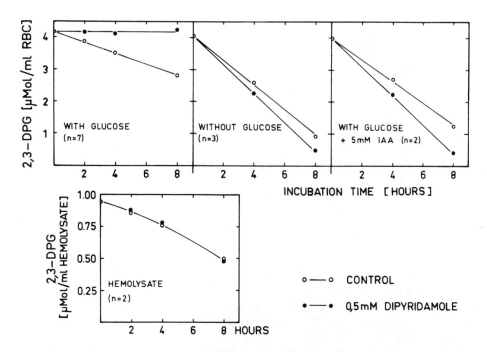

<u>Fig.6.</u> Influence of dipyridamole on 2,3-DPG decomposition in human RBC and in hemolysates. For experimental details see legends to Fig.2,3 and 14.

respect dipyridamole differs from those sulfate compounds which inhibit 2,3-DPG phosphatase.

Therefore one can conclude that dipyridamole maintains constant levels of 2,3-DPG in glycolyzing RBC not by inhibiting 2,3-DPG phosphatase, but by stimulating the synthesis of 2,3-DPG. This stimulatory effect, however, must be an indirect one, since in additional experiments on hemolysates an activation of DPG mutase by dipyridamole was excluded (9).

Such an indirect effect of dipyridamole on the formation of 2,3-DPG most probably results from the diminution of ADP (Fig.5): ADP and 1,3-DPG as well as ATP and 3-PG are the reactants in the phosphoglycerate kinase reaction which is at or near at equilibrium in RBC (27):

$$\frac{1.3\text{-DPG} \times \text{ADP}}{3\text{-PG} \times \text{ATP}} = K \; ; \quad K = 3.1 \times 10^{-4} \; (28).$$

Changes in ADP concentration must therefore result in inverse changes of 1,3-DPG, provided that the concentrations of 3-PG and ATP remain constant. Since this

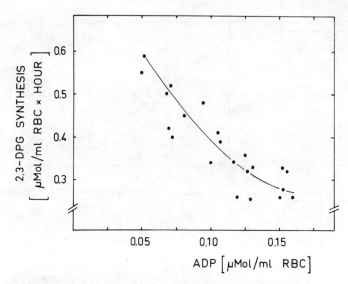

Fig.7. Relationship between the concentration of ADP and the rate of 2,3-DPG synthesis. The rates of synthesis were calculated as the difference between a constant rate of 2,3-DPG decomposition and the rate of changes of 2,3-DPG concentration at different levels of ADP induced by dipyridamole. The rate of 2,3-DPG decomposition (0.55 µMol/ml RBC per hour) was determined in RBC incubated without glucose. Experimental conditions as given in legend to Fig.2. For further details see (7,9).

actually happens under the influence of dipyridamole (9), the selective reduction of ADP will cause a rise of 1,3-DPG. Due to this elevation of 1,3-DPG the formation of 2,3-DPG increases.

Taking into account these considerations and the fact that dipyridamole does not inhibit 2,3-DPG phosphatase, the experimental results of our studies enable one to relate quantitatively the ADP concentration to the rates of 2,3-DPG synthesis. As can be seen from Fig.7 at very low concentrations of ADP the rate of 2,3-DPG synthesis is highest and diminishes progressively when ADP concentration increases. From all these findings it becomes evident that in the glycolyzing erythrocyte, as in hemolysates, synthesis of 2,3-DPG is indirectly controlled by the level of ADP.

II. a) Effect of Hypoxia and Anemia on the Concentration
         of 2,3-DPG in Rat Erythrocytes in vivo

According to the findings of LENFANT et al. (29) the
shift of the oxygen dissociation curve in man exposed to
high altitude is accompanied by an increase in the concentration of 2,3-DPG in RBC. Both phenomena seem to be
causally related. Nevertheless, the mechanism responsible for the elevation of 2,3-DPG content of RBC is not
fully understood. In order to contribute to the further
elucidation of this problem, experiments have been performed, in which the influence of hypoxia and anemia on
red cell 2,3-DPG and ATP levels were studied in vivo.

Sprague-Dawley rats of an average body weight of
200 g were placed in a 14 L glass chamber and exposed for
various periods of time to continuously flowing (7 L/min)
gas mixtures of O_2 and N_2. CO_2 and H_2O produced by the
animals were absorbed in an appropriate manner. From
each animal blood (0.7 ml) was taken by puncturing the
tongue vein during slight ether anesthesia at the beginning and after different periods of exposure. In a special series of experiments the animals were made anemic
by repeated bleeding within 8 hours (4 times 2-3 ml).
Polycythemia was produced within 5 days by three intra-
peritoneal injections of 4 ml of washed rat erythrocytes.

When rats are exposed to a gas mixture containing
11 Vol% O_2 and 89 Vol% N_2, the concentration of 2,3-DPG
in the RBC increases rapidly (Fig.8). Five hours after
the onset of hypoxia the 2,3-DPG level was already significantly elevated by about 2 µMol/ml RBC. At the end
of the first day 2,3-DPG reached a maximal value. After
3 and 6 days, respectively, the concentration was found
to be lower but still considerably above the initial
level. Compared with the changes of 2,3-DPG the alterations of ATP are delayed. Most likely they are due to
an increased count of reticulocytes.

Concomitant with the increase in 2,3-DPG and ATP
levels, changes of hemoglobin content and hematocrit were
observed. As can be seen from the data in Table 3, hematocrit and total hemoglobin were elevated after 6 days,
whereas RBC hemoglobin content was diminished. The inverse changes within the first day are most probably
caused by the repeated withdrawal of blood.

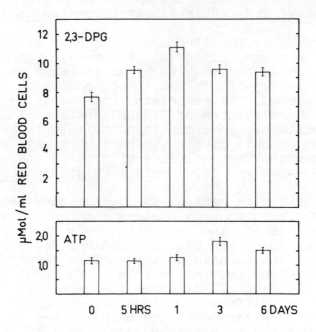

Fig.8. Influence of hypoxia on 2,3-DPG and ATP levels in RBC of rats. Experimental conditions: Exposure of rats to a gas mixture containing 11 Vol% of oxygen and 89 Vol% of nitrogen. Mean values ($\pm$ SD) from 4 animals after exposure times indicated.

Table 3: Hematological values during exposure
of rats to 11 Vol% O_2 *)

	Initial	5 h	1 d	3 d	6 d
Hematocrit %	44.8	43.0	40.7	44.5	52.6
Hemoglobin (µMol/ml Blood)	2.31	2.24	2.15	2.21	2.55
Hemoglobin (µMol/ml RBC)	5.15	5.20	5.28	4.98	4.85

*) Mean values from 4 and 8 experiments, respectively

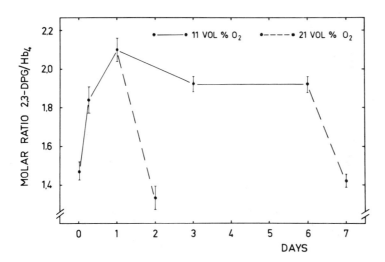

Fig.9. Influence of hypoxia (11 Vol% O₂) and of return
to normoxic conditions on the molar ratio of 2,3-DPG to
hemoglobin. Mean values (± SD) from 4 and 8 experiments,
respectively.

    In Fig.9 molar ratios of 2,3-DPG to hemoglobin are
plotted against time of exposure. In this kind of presentation the changes are more pronounced. As is further
shown the levels of 2,3-DPG decrease steeply when the
animals are exposed to normal air after a preceding period of hypoxia of either 1 day or 6 days. Within 24 hours
the molar ratio of 2,3-DPG to hemoglobin reaches the
range of the initial value.

    In order to evaluate the influence of different de-
grees of hypoxia on 2,3-DPG levels, rats were exposed for
24 hours to gas mixtures containing oxygen in various
concentrations. The results of these studies are summarized in Fig.10. For reasons of comparison a meter scale
is given below the abscissa, which allows the oxygen
content of the applied gas mixture to be related to altitude. From the data it is evident that a reduction of
oxygen to 18% - corresponding to an altitude of about
1500 m - is almost without effect on the concentration
of 2,3-DPG in RBC. However, between 17 and 7% of oxygen
a steep and nearly linear increase in 2,3-DPG levels
occurs. The absolute rise in 2,3-DPG at an oxygen concentration of 7% - corresponding to an altitude of about
7700 m - amounts to more than 60% of the normal value.
This severe hypoxia was only tolerated for 24 hours by
about half of our animals.

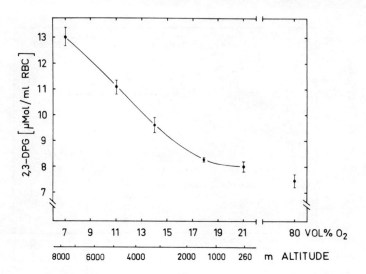

Fig.10. 2,3-DPG levels in rat RBC after 24 hours of exposure of the animals to gas mixtures of different oxygen
content. Mean values (± SD) from 4 and 8 experiments,
respectively.

        In contrast to the strong effects of hypoxia, hyper-
oxia due to an increase in the oxygen content of the gas
mixture to 80% causes only a small, but significant decrease of 2,3-DPG concentration (Fig.10). This finding
might explain the shift of the oxyhemoglobin dissociation
curve to the left observed during exposure of man to a
pressure of 2 atm. (30).

        Having thus demonstrated that rats principally re-
spond to lack of oxygen like man with an elevation of red
cell 2,3-DPG levels, it seemed of particular interest to
investigate whether an inverse correlation between
2,3-DPG concentration and whole blood hemoglobin (31-33)
can be shown also to exist in these animals. To clarify
this problem experiments were performed using anemic and
polycythemic rats. Fig.11 illustrates that a diminution
of whole blood hemoglobin due to repeated bleeding leads
generally within 24 hours to a pronounced increase of
2,3-DPG in RBC. As is evident from the lines connecting
the values for each animal, this effect occurred in all
the 8 animals studied.

        Inverse changes of the 2,3-DPG concentration were
found in rats which had been made polycythemic. The analytical data from this set of experiments as well as

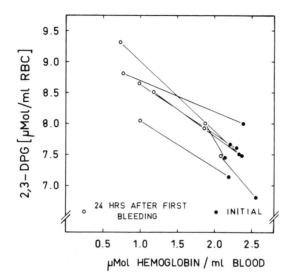

Fig.11. Increase in 2,3-DPG levels of rat RBC within 24 hours after reduction of whole blood hemoglobin by repeated bleedings.

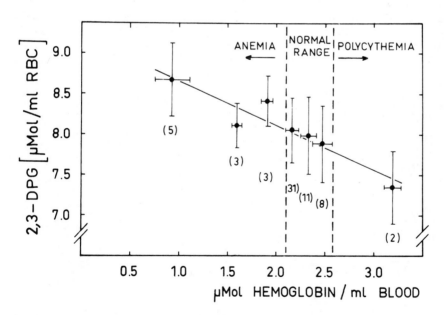

Fig.12. Relation between whole blood hemoglobin and 2,3-DPG concentration in rat RBC. For details see text.

those from anemic and control animals are compiled in
Fig.12. Obviously the levels of 2,3-DPG are negatively
correlated to whole blood hemoglobin concentration over
a wide range. Since in our experiments the concentrations of 2,3-DPG change subsequent to the shift in hemoglobin, it may be concluded that the concentration of
hemoglobin and/or its average saturation with oxygen is
somehow involved in the regulation of 2,3-DPG metabolism.

All our results reported so far as well as the findings of most other investigators who studied the changes
in 2,3-DPG do not explain the primary metabolic mechanism
which induces the shift in 2,3-DPG levels. An attempt was
therefore made to characterize in special experiments
those factors which may be of significance with respect
to the elevation of red cell 2,3-DPG in hypoxia.

Two factors have to be considered which may participate in the hypoxia induced changes of 2,3-DPG metabolism:
1. The transient increase in blood pH due to hyperventilation;
2. the diminution of the saturation of hemoglobin with
   oxygen.
The importance of the shift in blood pH was studied in
rats exposed for 24 hours to gas mixtures of low oxygen
content, to which 5% CO_2 was added in order to prevent
alkalosis. As is evident from the results summarized in
Fig.13, the rise in 2,3-DPG concentration occurring
within 24 hours of oxygen deficiency is abolished in the

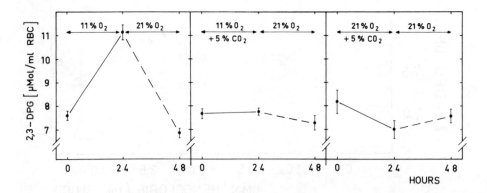

Fig.13. 2,3-DPG levels in RBC of rats exposed to 11 or
21 Vol% O_2 in presence or absence of 5 Vol% CO_2. Each
point is the mean (± SD) of 4 experiments.

presence of 5% CO_2. On the other hand, when the animals are exposed to gas mixtures containing normal amounts of oxygen and in addition 5% CO_2, the concentration of 2,3-DPG decreases moderately. All the changes are reversed within 24 hours when the animals are returned to normal conditions.

Although we did not measure blood pH in these animals, our findings indicate that an increase in pH contributes to the elevation of red cell 2,3-DPG levels in hypoxia, at least in the initial phase we have studied. In principle, this could be already expected from older observations of RAPOPORT and GUEST (34). These authors found in dogs with pyloric obstruction that an increase in blood pH of 0.1 unit causes within 24 hours a 50% rise in the 2,3-DPG content of RBC.

II. b) Effects of the Oxygenation State of Hemoglobin on the Metabolism of 2,3-DPG in Human Erythrocytes in vitro

The changes in blood pH of hypoxic animals cannot be the only reason for the elevation of 2,3-DPG, since it is well known that after a certain time of persistent hypoxia the blood pH returns to normal. Therefore we started investigations regarding the direct influence of the oxygenation state of hemoglobin on the metabolism of 2,3-DPG in human RBC in vitro. Since these studies are not yet completed only some preliminary results can be presented concerning the effects of deoxygenation of hemoglobin on the rate of decomposition of 2,3-DPG and on the rate of ^{32}P incorporation into 2,3-DPG and other organophosphates.

As was described above in RBC incubated in the absence of glucose for several hours the 2,3-DPG concentration diminishes at a constant high rate. According to the results given in Fig.14, this decrease proved to be independent of whether the cells are incubated aerobically or anaerobically. If greater amounts of 2,3-DPG are actually bound to deoxygenated than to oxygenated hemoglobin, as several authors have suggested (3,35), one can conclude from our results that the differences in the binding of 2,3-DPG do not affect the rate of its decomposition. In view of the very low Km value of 2,3-DPG phosphatase recently measured by HARKNESS and ROTH (18) this conclusion seems quite reasonable.

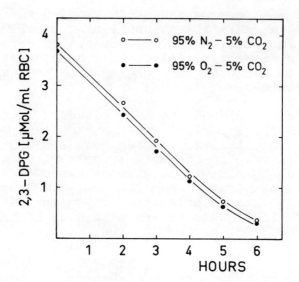

Fig.14. Decomposition of 2,3-DPG in human RBC incubated aerobically or anaerobically in glucose-free Locke solution.

Table 4: <u>Rate of glycolysis and incorporation of ^{32}P into</u>
<u>ATP, F-1,6-P and 2,3-DPG of human RBC</u>
Aerobic incubation: 95% O_2 - 5% CO_2
Anaerobic incubation: 95% N_2 - 5% CO_2

	Glucose Consumption (μMol/ml RBC per hour)	Lactate Production	Incorporation of ^{32}P x) ATP	F-1,6-P	2,3-DPG
Aerobic	1.44	2.66	599	67	15.5
Anaerobic	1.83	3.31	749	86	30.7
Change	+27%	+24%	+25%	+28%	+98%

x) Radioactivities in percent x 10^3 of the specific activity of the extracellular orthophosphate. Incubation of RBC in presence of ^{32}P: 5 min. Further experimental details see legend to Fig. 2

        In Table 4 data are summarized regarding the glycolytic rates and the incorporation of ^{32}P into ATP, F-1,6-P and 2,3-DPG both, in oxygenated and in deoxygenated human RBC. By comparing the figures it becomes evident that the rate of glycolysis as well as ^{32}P

incorporation is distinctly higher in the deoxygenated
cells than it is in the oxygenated erythrocytes. While
the percentage increase in glucose consumption and lactate production corresponds closely to the percentage
acceleration of ^{32}P incorporation into ATP and F-1,6-P
this is not true for 2,3-DPG. The percentage change of
^{32}P incorporation into this compound is much higher.

Though certain reservations are necessary with respect to the interpretation of these tracer experiments,
they nevertheless indicate that 2,3-DPG synthesis proceeds faster in the absence than in the presence of
oxygen. Detailed and convincing evidence, however, concerning the primary reason for the increased formation
of 2,3-DPG in deoxygenated RBC is not available as yet.
Some hypotheses have been put forward by different authors, but these have still to be proved experimentally
and therefore shall not be discussed. To further clarify
the interrelationship between the oxygenation state of
hemoglobin and 2,3-DPG metabolism appropriate in vitro
and in vivo experiments are presently in progress in our
laboratory.

REFERENCES

1) GREENWALD,I.: J. Biol. Chem. 63, 339 (1925)
2) CHANUTIN,A., and R.R.CURNISH: Proc. Soc. Exp. Biol.
   Med. 120, 291 (1965)
3) BENESCH,R., and R.E.BENESCH: Biochem. Biophys. Res.
   Commun. 26, 162 (1967)
4) CHANUTIN,A., and R.R.CURNISH: Arch. Biochem. Biophys.
   121, 96 (1967)
5) GERLACH,E., A.FLECKENSTEIN, and E.GROSS: Pflügers
   Arch. ges. Physiol. 266, 528 (1958)
6) GERLACH,E., B.DEUTICKE, and J.DUHM: Pflügers Arch.
   ges. Physiol. 280, 243 (1964)
7) DUHM,J., B.DEUTICKE, and E.GERLACH: In: Metabolism
   and Membrane Permeability of Erythrocytes and Thrombocytes, p. 69. Ed.: E.DEUTSCH, E.GERLACH, and K.
   MOSER. Stuttgart: G. Thieme 1968
8) DUHM,J., B.DEUTICKE, and E.GERLACH: Biochim. Biophys.
   Acta (Amst.) 170, 452 (1968)
9) DUHM,J., B.DEUTICKE, and E.GERLACH: Pflügers Arch.
   ges. Physiol. 306, 329 (1969)
10) DUHM,J., B.DEUTICKE, and E.GERLACH: Z. Physiol.
    Chem. 350, 1008 (1969)
11) RAPOPORT,S., and J.LUEBERING: J. Biol. Chem. 183,
    507 (1950)
12) SCHRÖTER,W.: In: Metabolism and Membrane Permeability

of Erythrocytes and Thrombocytes, p. 50. Ed.: E.
DEUTSCH, E.GERLACH, and K.MOSER. Stuttgart: G. Thieme
1968

13) RAPOPORT,S.: In: Essays in Biochemistry, Vol. 4,
p. 69. Ed.: P.N. CAMPBELL, and G.D.GEVILLE. London
and New York: Academic Press 1968

14) WHITTAM,R.: J. Physiol. 140, 479 (1958)

15) MÁNIAY,S., and Z.VÁRADY: Biochim. Biophys. Acta
(Amst.) 20, 594 (1956)

16) GÁRDOS,G.: Acta Biochim. Biophys. Acad. Sci. Hung.
1, 139 (1966)

17) PARKER,J.C.: J. Clin. Invest. 48, 117 (1969)

18) HARKNESS,D.R., and S.ROTH: Biochem. Biophys. Res.
Commun. 34, 849 (1969)

19) HURT,G.A., and A.CHANUTIN: J. Lab. Clin. Med. 64,
675 (1964)

20) HÄNZE,S.: Klin. Wschr. 44, 1247 (1966)

21) MINAKAMI,S., T.SAITO, C.SUZUKI, and H.YOSHIKAWA:
Biochem. Biophys. Res. Commun. 17, 748 (1964)

22) ROSE,I.A., and J.V.B.WARMS: J. Biol. Chem. 241,
4848 (1966)

23) RIZZO,S.C., and R.E.ECKEL: Am. J. Physiol. 211,
429 (1966)

24) RAPOPORT,S., F.DIETZE, and G.SAUER: Acta Biol. Med.
German. 13, 693 (1964)

25) SCHRÖTER,W., and H.v.HEYDEN: Biochem. Z. 341, 387
(1965)

26) GERLACH,E., B.DEUTICKE, and F.W.KOSS: Arzneim.
Forsch. 15, 558 (1965)

27) MINAKAMI,S., and H.YOSHIKAWA: Biochem. Biophys.
Res. Commun. 18, 345 (1965)

28) BÜCHER,TH.: Biochim. Biophys. Acta (Amst.) 1, 292
(1947)

29) LENFANT,C., J.TORRANCE, E.ENGLISH, C.A.FINCH, C.
REYNAFARJE, J.RAMOS, and J.FAURA: J. Clin. Invest.
47, 2652 (1968)

30) ASTRUP,P., M.RÖRTH, K.MELLEMGARD, C.LUNDGREN, and
R.O.MULHAUSEN: Lancet II, 732 (1968)

31) EATON,J.W., and G.J.BREWER: Proc. Nat. Acad. Sci.
61, 756 (1968)

32) EATON,J.W., G.J.BREWER, and R.F.GROVER: J. Lab. Clin.
Med. 73, 603 (1969)

33) SHOJANIA,A.M., L.G.ISRAELS, and A.ZIPURSKY: J. Lab.
Clin. Med. 71, 41 (1968)

34) RAPOPORT,S., and G.M.GUEST: J. Biol. Chem. 131, 675
(1939)

35) GARBY,L., G.GERBER, and C.-H.de VERDIER: In: Meta-
bolism and Membrane Permeability of Erythrocytes and
Thrombocytes, p. 66. Ed.: E.DEUTSCH, E.GERLACH, and
K.MOSER. Stuttgart: G. Thieme 1968

III

INTERACTION OF THE CARDIAC, PULMONARY, AND ERYTHROCYTE
SYSTEMS IN RESPIRATORY HOMEOSTASIS

SESSION 4 - R. Grover, Chairman

THE RESPIRATORY FUNCTION OF THE BLOOD

Giles F. Filley, M.D.

University of Colorado Medical Center; Webb-Waring

Institute for Medical Research, Denver, Colorado

Study of the physiological mechanisms of oxygen transport makes particularly clear the distinction between the pressure of oxygen (or its chemical potential - an intensity factor) and the amount of oxygen (or, per unit volume, its concentration - a quantity factor). This distinction is more recognized in thermodynamics than in physiological chemistry; it is especially important in considering systems capable of dissociating (1,2,7).

Figs. 1-4 illustrate the difference between quantity and intensity factors in oxygen transport. In Fig. 1 the coordinate system is the one usually used for the normal oxyhemoglobin dissociation curve with oxygen pressure as the intensity factor on the abscissa and oxygen saturation as the quantity factor on the ordinate. Only when total hemoglobin concentration is normal can this ordinate scale fairly represent oxygen quantity since its units are dimensionless. In Fig. 2 the normal dissociation curve (dotted line) is reproduced; it is identical to that in Fig. 1 when 200 ml O_2/L (the normal "O_2-capacity" of blood) is substituted for 100% saturation. Fig. 2 also shows the advantage of this ordinate scale: the dilutional effect of anemia is to lower the curve without changing its shape. (Other factors, including 2-3 DPG, change its shape.) The venous point in Fig. 2 is shown displaced vertically from its initial position in Fig. 1 but its final position is, of course, determined not only by the size and shape of the curve but by the arterio-venous O_2 concentration difference, i.e. the ratio of oxygen consumption to cardiac output.

Fig. 3 shows a pure change in the O_2 intensity factor, i.e. a lowering of Po_2 for a given O_2 quantity, or what could be called

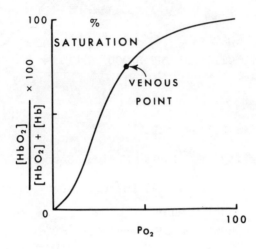

Fig. 1.   The normal human oxyhemoglobin dissociation curve at pH 7.4.

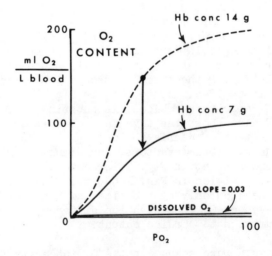

Fig. 2.   The "shape" of the curve is not affected by anemia per se.

EFFECT OF CO
ON O₂ INTENSITY

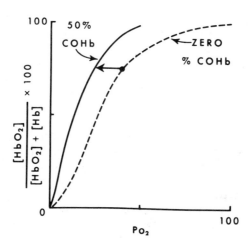

Fig. 3. CO lowers the O_2 unloading tendency (or the oxygen intensity) of oxyhemoglobin.

EFFECT OF CO
ON BOTH

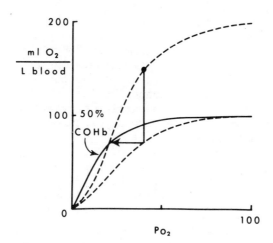

Fig. 4. The appropriate intensity-quantity coordinate system clarifies the double effect of CO on oxygen transport by hemoglobin.

a low oxygen intensity* of oxyhemoglobin. As is seen, carbon monoxide interferes with the ability of oxyhemoglobin to unload its
oxygen and therefore the curve is shifted to the left. The tradi-
tional units of % oxygen saturation on the ordinate are suitable
for displaying such an intensity change but, as is seen in Fig. 4,
when oxygen quantity is involved, O_2 concentration units should be
substituted for % saturation to show changes in both quantity and
intensity.

Oxygen uptake by the lungs and the level of oxygenation of
the mixed arterial blood leaving the lungs are affected by the
shape of the O_2-dissociation curve, especially in pulmonary disease.
This results from the fact that different portions of the lungs
have different O_2 intensity-quantity relationships, usually called
ventilation-perfusion relationships. Thus the Po_2 of blood leaving
a pulmonary capillary bed will be high if it flows thru a highly
ventilated portion of lung but the quantity of oxygen delivered to
the mixed arterial blood will depend on the O_2-capacity of the
blood and how much flows thru this highly ventilated portion.
These concepts can be clarified by a study of Figs. 5-7.

In Fig. 5, the left hand alveolus represents a "perfect" lung
in that the gas phase Po_2 of 100 mmHg is attained by the blood
which leaves the alveolus. (A normal lung is not perfect in this
sense; at rest the arterial blood Po_2 is about 90 mmHg, so that an
alveolar-arterial Po_2 difference of 10 mmHg is usually found.) The
right hand alveolus shows the effect of pure hypoventilation. The
narrow airway, by producing obstruction to airflow, has interfered
with ventilation of the alveolus so that a Po_2 of only 80 is developed and the blood which leaves the alveolus only contains oxygen at a concentration determined by the position of the dissociation curve at a Po_2 of 80.

In Fig. 6 are depicted two pulmonary "physiological lesions"
which interfere with arterial oxygenation. On the left a pure
shunt allows venous blood to bypass the gas phase completely and
the mixed arterial Po_2 and O_2 concentration will be low on this account. On the right a diffusion barrier prevents the blood from
achieving equilibrium with the oxygen pressure in the gas phase and
arterial hypoxemia therefore results.

In patients these pure lesions are unusual. In the commonest
pulmonary diseases causing arterial hypoxemia, a mixture of these
lesions exist along with disturbances of gas and blood distribution or ventilation-perfusion (V/Q) ratios. Fig. 7 shows how these

---

*The change can also be described as an increased affinity of
hemoglobin for oxygen - a term whose potential for obstructing the
process of understanding oxygen transport is insufficiently appreciated.

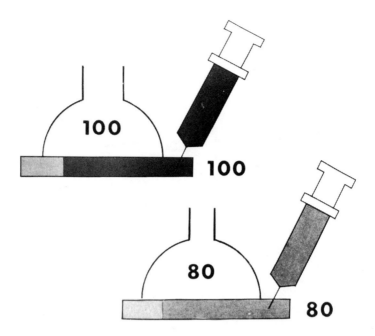

Fig. 5. The one alveolus model of a perfect lung (left) and of a hypoventilated lung (right). The latter has a narrow airway and therefore develops only a low oxygen pressure in alveolar gas and therefore in arterial blood.

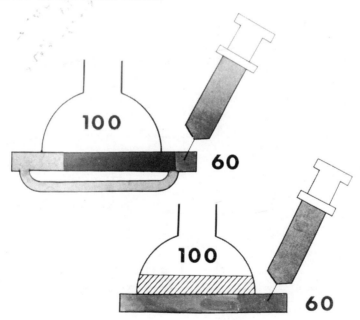

Fig. 6. The two classical physiological causes of arterial hypoxemia with normal ventilation.

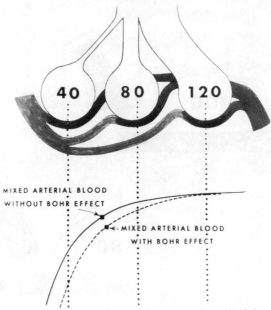

Fig. 7.   Disturbed ventilation-perfusion (V/Q) ratios. Equal quantities of blood are assumed to flow to three portions of lung - hypoventilated, normal and hyperventilated portions.

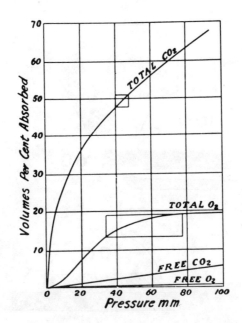

Fig. 8. CO_2 and O_2 dissociation curves "on the same figure and on the same scale" ((3), p. 77).

disturbances lower arterial oxygen concentration and emphasizes how
the normal shape of oxyhemoglobin dissociation curve is a disadvantage at this step in the oxygen transport process. This comes
about as follows. The obstructed and hence underventilated alveolus on the left delivers so small a quantity of oxygen to the blood
leaving it that the overventilated alveolus (with an intensity
factor just as much above the average as the obstructed alveolus'
Po_2 is below the average) cannot compensate. Obviously this effect
results from the fact that an increase in O_2 pressure above the
average in the gas phase does not lead to enough of an increase in
O_2 concentration in the blood to compensate for the decrease in
concentration caused by the low Po_2 developed in the underventilated alveolus.

It is interesting that the Bohr effect, though of great advantage in the tissues (especially in actively metabolizing, CO_2-
producing and pH-lowering tissues), is a disadvantage in pulmonary
disease so far as delivering a quantity of oxygen to arterial blood
is concerned. For the underventilated alveolus with a Po_2 of 40
must have a high Pco_2 and hence the blood leaving it must have a
low pH. This, of course, shifts the curve to the right, further
aggravating the arterial O_2 quantity effect of V/Q disturbances -
an aggravation which cannot be appreciated without considering CO_2
transport.

Indeed oxygen transport cannot be understood apart from CO_2
transport. The first complete analysis of these two transport
systems was carried out by L. J. Henderson in 1928 (3). Fig. 8,
reproduced from his book, clearly shows certain contrasts between
the physical chemistry of these systems. In addition to the im-
pressive height of the CO_2 curve and its steepness (reflecting,
respectively, the ability of blood to carry large quantities of CO_2
with little change in the intensity factors Pco_2 and pH), the CO_2
curve is nearly straight in the physiological range. This contrasts with the S-shape of the O_2 curve and explains why pulmonary
disease so seldom interferes with the transport of CO_2 from blood
to alveolar gas.

The explanation for both O_2 and CO_2 effects of disturbed V/Q
ratios is given in Fig. 9. For O_2 transport it is clear, as we
have shown, that hyperventilation of one portion of lung (high
V/Q) cannot make up for hypoventilation in another portion. This
is not true for CO_2 transport. Here, a high V/Q can make up in
CO_2 quantity transported (i.e. change on the ordinate) for a deficit caused by a low V/Q because the quantity-intensity ratio is
nearly constant between venous and arterial points (i.e. CO_2 dissociation curve is nearly straight).

The importance of even subtle changes in the shape of the O_2

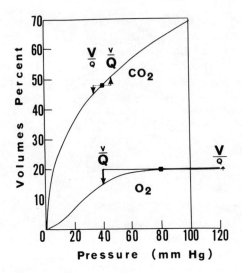

Fig. 9. The physicochemical reason why V/Q disturbances affect arterial oxygenation but scarcely affect CO_2 transport is reflected by the shape of the two dissociation curves.

TWO ALVEOLI LUNG MODEL

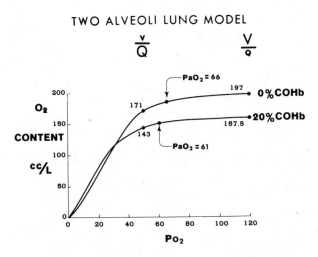

Fig. 10. Without CO, blood leaving the low V/Q region has a
Po_2 of 50 mmHg which corresponds to a saturation of 85.4%; thus
half the arterial blood contains .854 x 200 = 171 ml O_2/L blood.
This is mixed with blood at a Po_2 of 120 mmHg containing 197 ml
O_2/L, yielding a mixed concentration of 184 ml O_2/L at a Po_2 of 66.
With 20% COHb the mixed concentration is (143 + 157.5)/2 = 150.3
ml O_2/L at a Po_2 of 61 mmHg. (These calculations are those of
Brody (5)).

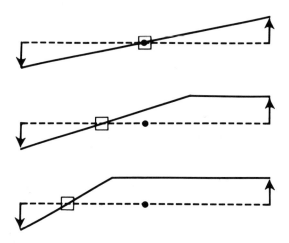

Fig. 11.   Linearizing the O_2 dissociation curve (top) eliminates the effect of a V/Q disturbance on mixed arterial blood since
the curve intersects the quantity level (dotted line) at an intensity level (open square) which would be reached if all alveoli had
the same V/Q.

The normal O_2 curve (middle) has a Po_2 to the left of center
because of the position of its major bend.

The O_2 curve in CO-poisoning (bottom) has a Po_2 further to the
left for the same % O_2 saturation because its major bend is shifted
to the left.

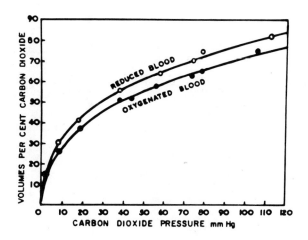

Fig. 12.   At any Pco_2 reduced (venous) blood contains a larger
quantity of CO_2 (mostly as bicarbonate) than arterial. At any CO_2
concentration, oxygenated blood has a greater CO_2 unloading tendency than reduced blood.

dissociation curve is indicated by the fact that a _left_-shifted curve can aggravate arterial hypoxemia in V/Q disturbances as recently shown by Brewer _et al_. (4) and by Brody and Coburn (5) - depending on the location of the major bend in the upper part of the curve.

The finding that the arterial Po_2 is reduced in patients inhaling carbon monoxide is depicted in Fig. 10. The arithmetic explaining how arterial Po_2 becomes lowered in such circumstances is given in the legend. The visualization of how the lowering occurs is shown in Fig. 11. In words the argument is as follows. A _linear_ O_2 dissociation curve would allow hyperventilation to correct for hypoventilation because intensity and quantity changes are proportional to each other. This beneficial effect of a linear O_2 dissociation curve in V/Q disturbances has recently been quantified by West (6). The normal O_2 dissociation curve has major bend in its upper portion such that a moderate drop in arterial Po_2 results from V/Q disturbances. In CO poisoning, the major bend in the O_2 curve is to the left of normal; hence the intersection of an ordinate value of quantity with an abscissa value of intensity is also to the left of normal. Hence arterial Po_2 is reduced in CO poisoning.

The _in vivo_ role of 2-3 DPG in oxygen transport is yet to be understood in terms of its behavior in intact red cells in flowing blood exchanging CO_2 and O_2. The behavior of this intracellular phosphate is linked with intracellular proton transfers (also yet to be understood, (7,8,9)) responsible for both the Christiansen-Douglas-Haldane effect (Fig. 12) and the Bohr effect in true plasma and in whole blood respectively. As a means of bringing concepts which have classically been thought to apply _in vivo_ into relation with gains in the chemistry of hemoglobin _solutions_, the following short review of the status of red cell pH is offered.

The Bohr effect in whole blood is usually studied in relation to the pH of plasma. Until the change in pH, ΔpH, inside the red cells as hemoglobin changes reversibly between Hb and O_2 Hb, even the Bohr effect is incompletely known. (The discrepancy between this ΔpH as estimated by workers in different laboratories (2,8) is of the order of 100%.) Hence how or even whether 2-3 DPG "affects the Bohr effect" are questions which must be carefully asked.

Perhaps the easiest way of changing the pH inside a cell is to change its Pco_2 (10). While venous blood is becoming arterialized in the lungs, its Pco_2 falls and the pH of _plasma_ rises - only about 0.03. What is the rise in the pH of the _red_ cells? Considerably greater than 0.03 if classical concepts are right (Fig. 13) but not if recent work on hemoglobin solutions is assumed to apply in intact red cells (8).

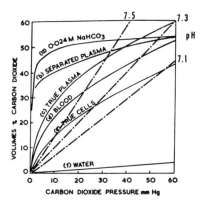

Fig. 13. As seen by the flatness of the top curve, the pro-
tein-free bicarbonate solution is the least well buffered at physiologic ranges of Pco_2. Plasma separated from cells is better buffered because it contains protein. The curve of plasma in contact
with cells (true plasma) is the steepest of all at $Pco_2 = 40$.
(Adapted from Roughton (12).)

For a given change in Pco_2 the pH inside true red cells apparently changes more than in true plasma because the curve for
true cells is less steep and lower than for true plasma.

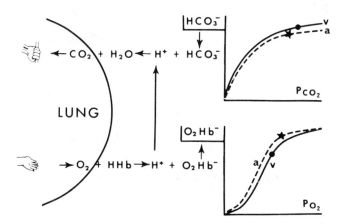

Fig. 14. As CO_2 leaves the blood and enters lung gas (upper
left) its unloading is facilitated by the donation of protons from
the fairly strong acid O_2HHb because these protons destroy bicarbonate. Thus pulmonary capillary blood bicarbonate, high in venous
blood (solid circle, upper right) becomes lowered and Pco_2 falls as
the blood becomes arterialized (star). The path followed is between the circle and the star - the physiological CO_2 dissociation
curve. This process is as important as the Bohr effect shown below since the two processes are reciprocally linked via a proton
shuttle.

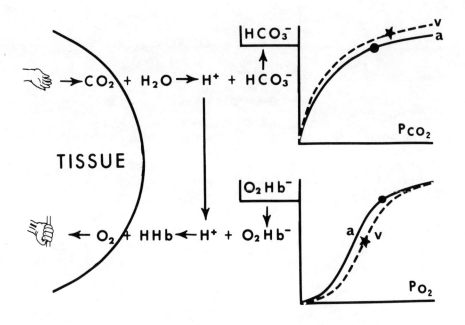

Fig. 15. As O_2 enters the tissues from the blood (lower left), reduced hemoglobin groups with a high pK (and hence proton-avid) either acquire protons or have protons thrust upon them from the Pco_2 bicarbonate system. The pH of plasma falls but slightly as blood moves along the physiological O_2 dissociation curve (solid circle to star). The unloading of oxygen could obviously be facilitated if within the red cell the pH were to fall more than in plasma - a possibility depending on the magnitude of the increase of the pK of conjugate bases. This is 6.2 in oxy- and 7.7 in deoxy-hemoglobin (9), but might be modified by 2-3 DPG.

Now although students of molecular structure (9) consider the physiological function of the Bohr effect "to be the neutralization of hydrogen ions released on the uptake of CO_2 by the blood," it seems more likely that this effect is but part of more general mechanism. As Henderson (3) emphasized (p. 82),

> "In studying the interaction between oxygen and carbonic acid, it is of the first importance not to regard the change in one substance as cause and the change in the other as effect. If we think of our terms mathematically as variables and functions, the difficulty does not arise."

Wyman (7) echoes these words and underlines the necessity to study the exchange system in its intact as well as its dissassembled state:

> "It is now possible to see, in a general way, how the α- and β-chains [of the hemoglobin molecule] move in relation to one another as oxygen enters and leaves and the Bohr protons leave and enter, the whole structure behaving like a miniature reciprocating engine which mimics us, at a molecular level, as we breathe....Until now those who have been trying to understand the mechanism of the hemoglobin molecule by taking off and putting on pieces and looking for what happens are still but as children playing with a watch."

In view of the foregoing it may be that 2-3 DPG, rather than displacing oxygen from hemoglobin by being bound to the deoxy form (11), simply facilitates proton transfer by changing the pKs of proton donating and accepting groups of the hemoglobin molecule. Exactly how 2-3 DPG will be fitted into the scheme presented in Figs. 14 and 15 must await further investigation.

Summary

1. Intensity and quantity factors in physiology should be clearly conceived and conveniently named.

2. The shape of the oxyhemoglobin dissociation curve, long known to be important with respect to O_2 unloading in the body tissues, is also important in affecting oxygen loading in the lungs if these are abnormal.

3. How important 2-3 DPG is in oxygen transport can be appreciated by considering how CO_2 and O_2 transport are linked via a proton transfer mechanism operating in the red cell.

References

(1) Clark, W.M.: The Determination of Hydrogen Ions. Baltimore,
     Williams and Wilkins Co., 3rd Ed., 1928, pp xiii,35,36.

(2) Wyman, J.,Jr.: Heme Proteins in Advances in Protein Chemistry.
     Ed. by M.L. Anson and J.T. Edsall, New York, Acad. Press, p
     436, 1948.

(3) Henderson, L.J.: Blood. A Study in General Physiology. New
     Haven, Yale Univ. Press, 1928.

(4) Brewer, G.J., J.W. Eaton, J. Weil, and R.F. Grover: Red cell
     metabolism in health and disease: Studies of red cell glycoly-
     sis and interactions with carbon monoxide, smoking and alti-
     tude. This symposium.

(5) Brody, J.S., and R.F. Coburn: Carbon monoxide-induced arte-
     rial hypoxemia. Science, 164, 1297, 1969.

(6) West, J.B.: Ventilation-perfusion inequality and overall gas
     exchange in computer models of the lung. Respiration Physiol-
     ogy, 7, 88, 1969.

(7) Wyman, J.,Jr.: Linked functions and reciprocal effects in
     hemoglobin: A second look. Advances in Protein Chemistry, 19,
     223, 1964.

(8) Rossi-Bernardi, L., and F.J.W. Roughton: The specific influ-
     ence of carbon dioxide and carbamate compounds on the buffer
     power of hemoglobin and Bohr effects in human hemoglobin solu-
     tions. J. Physiol., 189, 1, 1967.

(9) Perutz, M.F., H. Muirhead, L. Mazzarella, R.A. Crowther, J.
     Greer, and J.V. Kilmartin: Identification of residues respon-
     sible for the alkaline Bohr effect in hemoglobin. Nature, 222,
     1240, 1969.

(10) Waddell, W.J., and R.G. Bates: Intracellular pH. Physiologi-
     cal Reviews, 49, 285, 1969.

(11) Benesch, R., R.E. Benesch, and C.I. Yu. Reciprocal binding
     of oxygen and diphosphoglycerate. Proc. N.A.S., 59, 526, 1968.

(12) Roughton, F.J.W.: Handbook of Physiology, Sec. 3, Vol. I, p
     814, American Physiol. Soc., Washington, D.C., 1964.

SYSTEMIC OXYGEN TRANSPORT

Robert F. Grover, M.D., Ph.D. and John V. Weil, M. D.

Cardiovascular Pulmonary Research Laboratory, Division of Cardiology, Department of Medicine, University of Colorado Medical Center, Denver, Colorado.

Normal tissue metabolism is intimately dependent upon an adequate supply of oxygen and it is the primary function of the oxygen transport system to supply this oxygen to the tissues. In a simple single-cell organism such as the amoeba transport of oxygen is accomplished by simple diffusion into the cell from the surrounding aqueous medium. Even insects are sustained by simple diffusion of oxygen from the surrounding atmosphere with the aid of a system of air ducts penetrating the body. However, when organisms are larger and more complex simple diffusion is no longer adequate to maintain oxygenation and a specific system must be introduced to transport oxygen from the surrounding environment to the cells of the body. The basic requirement for this system is to bring adequate quantities of oxygen to the tissues at sufficient partial pressure to permit rapid diffusion of oxygen in sufficient quantity from the blood to the tissue. The intracellular oxygen tension must be adequate to maintain metabolic processes. As long as these basic requirements are met, the oxygen transport system is a success. We will discuss two topics relating to this oxygen transport system. The first is the relationship between oxygen transport and the regulation of red cell production and the second considers the comparative physiology of oxygen transport in several animal species.

A simple diagramatic representation of the mammalian oxygen transport system is shown in figure 1. The system begins with the lung which, given the partial pressure of oxygen in the atmosphere, determines the tension of oxygen in the blood within the pulmonary capillaries and systemic arteries. Each of the rectangles represents a container for oxygen and these containers in turn repre-

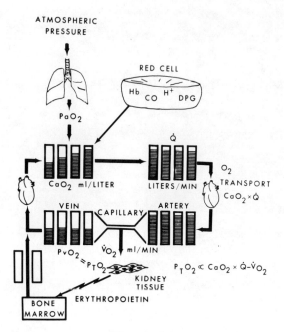

Figure 1

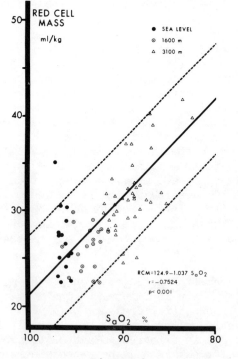

Figure 2

sent quantities of red cells. The affinity of the hemoglobin for oxygen in these red cells is influenced by such things as 2,3 DPG, pH and temperature of the plasma and in smokers the concentration of carbon monoxide as well. Hence these are the major factors which determine the oxygen saturation at a given oxygen partial pressure. The arterial oxygen content is the actual volume of oxygen carried by a given volume of blood and is determined by the amount of the hemoglobin in the container and by the arterial oxygen saturation. Oxygen transport is simply the product of the oxygen content and the rate of blood flow. This may be defined for a specific organ e.g. oxygen transport to the kidney = renal blood flow x arterial oxygen content or for the whole body (systemic oxygen transport = cardiac output x arterial oxygen content). In either case oxygen transport defines an upper limit for the total quantity of oxygen available to tissue.

At the arterial end of the systemic capillary the oxygen tension gradient favors diffusion of oxygen out of the blood and into the tissues. As blood flows along the capillary this process of diffusion continues until the oxygen tension of the blood is reduced to a value equal to that in the tissue. Tissue oxygen tension is determined by a dynamic balance between oxygen transport or delivery on the one hand and the amount of oxygen consumed by the tissue on the other. The difference between these two quantities ultimately determines the concentration of free oxygen molecules in tissue fluid and hence the tissue oxygen tension. It is generally believed that venous oxygen tension is a reasonably close reflection of the oxygen tension of the surrounding tissue (1).

There are several feedback interactions between tissue oxygen tension and oxygen transport. One important example is the regulation of erythropoiesis. There is now substantial evidence that erythropoietin release is regulated in accordance with renal tissue oxygen tension such that a decreased oxygen tension results ultimately in increased erythropoietin release with stimulation of red cell production (2). The consequent rise in hemoglobin concentration produces an augmentation of arterial oxygen content. Under certain conditions this results in increased oxygen transport unless the polycythemia becomes so severe as to depress blood flow due to increased viscosity. The increased quantity of oxygen delivered to the tissues can restore depressed tissue oxygen tension even in the face of decreased arterial oxygen tension. In other words an increase in quantity of oxygen (oxygen content) can compensate for a decrease in partial pressure of oxygen.

The control of erythropoiesis was examined in studies aimed at elucidating the relationship between blood oxygenation and the total red cell mass (3). Red cell mass was measured by tagging red cells with radioactive chromium. A range of arterial oxygen

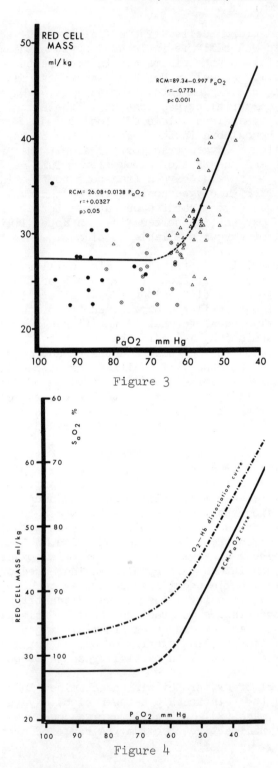

Figure 3

Figure 4

saturations was achieved by studying normal men living at 3 altitudes sea level, Denver, Colorado (1600 m) and Leadville, Colorado
(3100 m). In figure 2 it is evident that there is a strong linear
relationship between arterial oxygen saturation and red cell mass.
In contrast when red cell mass is viewed in relation to oxygen tension (figure 3) the relationship is considerably more complex, in
fact there is no correlation at the higher range of oxygen tensions
and it is only below a tension of about 60 mmHg that a strong correlation exists between red cell mass and oxygen tension.

We were struck by the resemblance of this latter curve to the
oxygen-hemoglobin dissociation curve, and that comparison is shown
in figure 4. The dissociation curve has been inverted so that both
curves take the form of classical stimulus response curves, the
stimulus being a decreased oxygen tension. The important thing
about this comparison is not the apparent similarity of the slopes
of the various portions of these curves because that can be
achieved by adjustment of the relative scale factors on the
ordinate. The important feature is that both of these curves bend
over the same range of oxygen tensions which means that only those
oxygen tensions which lower oxygen saturation cause an increase in
red cell production. This suggests that arterial oxygen saturation
is a more important determinant of red cell mass than arterial
oxygen tension. This is probably a reflection of the fact that
arterial oxygen saturation is closely related to oxygen content
and hence is a more direct determinant of tissue oxygen tension
than is arterial oxygen tension. We believe this is the basis for
the linear correlation between red cell mass and arterial oxygen
saturation rather than oxygen tension.

The position of the oxygen-hemoglobin dissociation curve is
another factor influencing tissue oxygenation. Several investigators have pointed out that shifting the curve to the right would
permit the unloading of oxygen at a higher oxygen tension. However,
oxygen transport, i. e. the quantity of oxygen brought to the
tissues, is also of major importance in determining tissue oxygenation. Therefore, we have examined the way in which oxygen transport is actually accomplished in three animal species with marked
differences in the position of the dissociation curve; these
species are man, sheep, and llama. Sheep hemoglobin has an unusually low affinity for oxygen, whereas the hemoglobin of the llama
has an extremely high affinity for oxygen. Oxygen transport in
the llama is or particular interest because this animal, being
native to high altitude in the Andes, could be considered the
prototype of adaptation to hypoxia.

For purposes of this comparative analysis, we have examined
the oxygenation of arterial and mixed venous blood (a-v difference).
Arterial oxygenation relates to oxygen brought to the tissues, and

OXYGEN-HEMOGLOBIN
DISSOCIATION CURVES

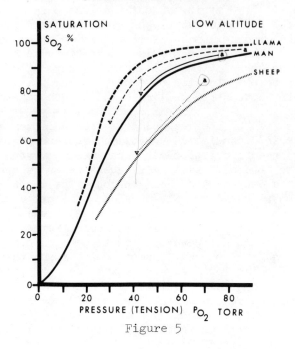

Figure 5

OXYGEN-HEMOGLOBIN
DISSOCIATION CURVES

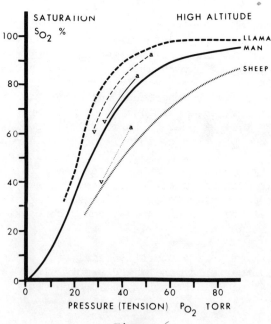

Figure 6

the resulting tissue oxygenation is reflected by the oxygen remaining in venous blood. The a-v difference was determined at
both low and high altitude, the latter indicating the response of
the oxygen transport system to the stress of arterial hypoxemia.

Studies from our laboratory are among the few with direct
measurements of mixed venous as well as arterial blood in the same
individuals at two different altitudes. The human data were
obtained by Dr. John Vogel and his associates (4) on four young
men in Denver at 1600 m at during 48 hours at 4300 m on the summit
of Mt. Evans. Drs. Banchero, Grover, and Will (5) studied three
young llamas born at sea level, first at low altitude (Madison,
Wis.) and then after 5 and 10 weeks at 3400 m (Climax, Colorado).
Twelve lambs 3-4 months old were studied by Reeves, Grover, and
Grover (6) at Denver, 1600 m, and after 2, 4 and 6 weeks at 3900 m
on Mt. Evans; the presence of hemoglobin type A or B was not determined in these lambs.

In each individual studied, arterial and mixed venous blood
were sampled simultaneously, the latter by means of a catheter
floated into the pulmonary artery. Promptly, pH, PCO_2, and PO_2
were measured at the individual's body temperature, 37.5° C for
men, and $39\text{-}40^{\circ}$ C for sheep and llamas. Blood oxygen capacity was
determined by Van Slyke analysis in all studies. For the sheep
and llamas, oxygen content was also measured and from this, saturation calculated. In the human studies, saturation was calculated from PO_2 and pH, and using the measured capacity, oxygen content was calculated.

Figures 5 and 6 present for reference average oxygen-hemoglo-
bin dissociation curves for llama at 39.0° C (8), man at 37.5° C
(7), and sheep at 39.4° C (hemoglobin type B) (8); all are at pH
7.40. Against this background we have plotted the values of
arterial and mixed venous oxygen tension and saturation actually
observed in vivo; these data have not been "corrected" for pH or
temperature.

At low altitude (Fig. 5), the llama with his dissociation
curve farthest to the left has the lowest $P_{\bar{v}}O_2$ (30 torr). In a
sense, this could be looked upon as a handicap for the llama at
sea level because it implies that he is "obliged" to function with
a lower tissue PO_2 than other species. The sheep with a dissociation curve well to the right of man does not have a higher $P_{\bar{v}}O_2$
than man. Apparently oxygen transport is regulated in both sheep
and man to maintain virtually identical values of $P_{\bar{v}}O_2$ (42-43
torr). The lower value of PaO_2 in sheep results from a higher
$PaCO_2$ (40 torr) and a higher water vapor pressure (57 torr at
39° C), both of which lower alveolar PO_2.

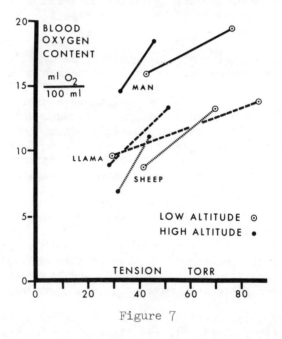

Figure 7

At high altitude, the reduction in atmospheric pressure lowers PaO_2. When man and sheep are compared at the same low value of PaO_2 (45 torr) in Fig. 6 they again have identical values for $P_{\bar{v}}O_2$ (32 torr) despite the difference in position of their dissociation curves. This implies similar adjustments in oxygen transport to maintain tissue oxygenation. In this lower range of oxygen tensions, the two dissociation curves are more nearly parallel, so that for the same decrease in PO_2 (45 to 32 torr) there is a comparable fall in saturation. The llamas were studied at a less high altitude and consequently had a somewhat higher PaO_2 of 52 torr. Nevertheless, his leftward dissociation curve requires him to unload oxygen at a lower $P_{\bar{v}}O_2$ (28 torr). Apparently, at all altitudes, the llama has lower values of $P_{\bar{v}}O_2$ than other species. This appears paradoxical for an animal so well adapted to life in an hypoxic environment.

Examination of the oxygen-hemoglobin dissociation curves in Figures 5 and 6 indicates how well tissue oxygen tension (i.e. $P_{\bar{v}}O_2$) is maintained, but the saturation data do not indicate the quantity of oxygen delivered. For this, we must examine blood oxygen content. (Figure 7). Numerous studies have concluded that under normal resting conditions, blood flow (cardiac output) is regulated so that from each 100 ml. of blood, 3.5-4.5 ml of oxygen is extracted (a-v difference of 3.5-4.5 volumes percent) (9). At low and high altitude respectively, the a-v differences are: llama 4.2 and 4.5, man 3.4 and 3.8, sheep 4.6 and 4.1. These data indicate that in all three species, tissue blood flow relative to tissue oxygen consumption at rest is maintained within the normal range.

Two factors operate to minimize the decrease in $P_{\bar{v}}O_2$ with little change in blood flow (a-v difference) at high altitude. First is the shape of the dissociation curve. By increasing in steepness at the lower range of PO_2, a given decrease in saturation can occur with a smaller change in PO_2. Secondly, the increase in hemoglobin concentration in response to altitude increases the oxygen carrying capacity of the blood. Consequently, there is less decrease in arterial oxygen content with the decrease in SaO_2 at altitude. Further, the greater capacity permits a normal decrease in blood oxygen content (a-v difference) with less reduction in saturation and hence less reduction in PO_2.

In comparing sheep with man, the theoretical advantage of the sheep's rightward curve in raising $P_{\bar{v}}O_2$ is not observed in normal animals. At the same time, the lower affinity of sheep's hemoglobin for oxygen has a significant effect on arterial oxygenation; at altitude, the PaO_2 of 45 torr gives an SaO_2 of only 63% compared with 84% in man. In other words, one third of the sheep's oxygen carrying capacity cannot be utilized as a consequence of the position of the dissociation curve. While this does not appear to be a handicap at rest, this should become a disadvantage when exercise increases the demands for oxygen transport.

In summary, a successful oxygen transport system supplies tissues with adequate quantities of oxygen through a combination of blood flow and arterial oxygen content, the latter being determined by the concentration of hemoglobin and its affinity for oxygen, i.e. saturation. Further, tissue oxygen pressure must be sufficiently high to maintain aerobic metabolism. Otis (10) found that the venous blood draining dog skeletal muscle must have a PO_2 of 30 torr at rest and 10 torr during exercise to maintain oxygen uptake. Donald et al (11), studying humans during leg exercise found the femoral venous saturation to be 14-24%, and the corresponding PO_2 would be in the range of 10-20 torr. Mixed venous PO_2 would be higher than the PO_2 of venous blood draining only muscle. Man, sheep, and llama all accomplish oxygen transport successfully even though they exibit a wide range in the position of the oxygen-hemoglobin dissociation curve are major factors in maintaining tissue oxygenation.

REFERENCES

1. Tenney, S. M. and Lamb, T. W.: Physiological consequences. of hypoventilation and hyperventilation. In Handbook of Respiration, W. O. Fenn and Rahn editors. 1965. Amer. Physiol. Soc. Vol. II, p. 982.

2. Stohlman, F.: Erythropoiesis. New England J. Med. 26:342,1967.

3. Weil, J. V., Jamieson, G., Brown, D. W., and Grover, R. F.: The red cell mass-arterial oxygen relationship in normal man. J. Clin. Invest. 47: 1627-1639, 1968.

4. Vogel, J. H. K., Goss, J. E., Mori, M., and Brammell, H. L.: Pulmonary circulation in normal man with acute exposure to high altitude (14,260 feet). Circulation 34:III-233, 1966.

5. Banchero, N., Will, J. A., and Grover, R. F.: Oxygen transport in the llama. Physiologist 12:166, 1969.

6. Reeves, J. T., Grover, E. B., and Grover, R. F.: Pulmonary circulation and oxygen transport in lambs at high altitude. J. Appl. Physiol. 18:560-566, 1963.

7. Lambertsen, C. J., Bunce, P. L., Drabkin, D. L., and Schmidt, C. F.: Relationship of oxygen tension to hemoglobin oxygen saturation in the arterial blood of normal men. J. Appl. Physiol. 4:873-885, 1952.

8. Blood O_2 dissociation curves: mammals. *In* Handbook of Respi-
    ration, D. S. Dittmer and R. M. Grebe editors. 1958,
    Philadelphia, Saunders, pp. 80.

9. Reeves, J. T., Grover, R. F., Filley, G. F., and Blount, S. G.,
    Jr.: Cardiac output in normal resting man. J. Appl. Physiol.
    16:276-278, 1961.

10. Otis, A. B.: The control of respiratory gas exchange between
    blood and tissues. *In* The regulation of human respiration,
    D. J. C. Cunningham and B. B. Lloyd editors, 1963. Oxford,
    Blackwell, pp. 111-119.

11. Donald, K. W., Wormald, P. N., Taylor, S. H., and Bishop, J. M.:
    Changes in the oxygen content of femoral venous blood and leg
    blood flow during leg exercise in relation to cardiac output
    response. Clin. Sci. 16:567-591, 1957.

ADAPTATION TO HYPOXIA (1)

C. Lenfant, J.D. Torrance, R. Woodson, and C.A. Finch

Departments of Medicine and of Physiology and Biophysics

University of Washington, Seattle, Washington 98105, USA

Hypoxia occurs if the oxygen requirement of the tissues is greater than the oxygen supply. In man at rest the basal requirement is fixed and if supply does not match this demand, normal function is interrupted.

The supply of oxygen is set by its availability in the environment and by the efficiency with which it can be transported from the environment to the mitochondria. This occurs in four distinct steps:

(a) Pulmonary ventilation, by which gas molecules are actively transferred from the environment to the alveoli.

(b) Pulmonary gas exchange, in which oxygen diffuses from alveolar air into the capillary blood.

(c) Circulation, in which the oxygen is carried in the blood to the tissue capillaries.

(d) Passive diffusion from the capillaries into the cells composing the tissues.

A decrease in oxygen availability or a dysfunction of any of these transport mechanisms would produce hypoxia if it were not for corrective compensation by one or more of the other factors. Some of these however have limited compensatory power--for instance, increased ventilation would do little to compensate for either a lack of oxygen in the environment or circulatory failure. Similarly passive diffusion, whether in the lungs or at the tissue level, cannot respond to improve a deficient oxygen supply. Thus the only mechanism by which impaired oxygen supply can be effectively and rapidly corrected is improved delivery of oxygen from the lung to tissue capillaries.

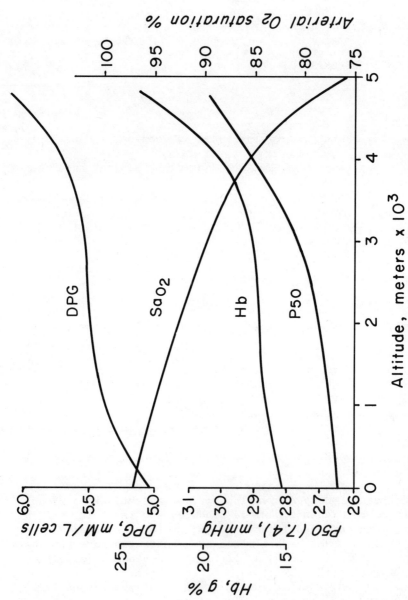

Figure 1: Average DPG concentration, Hb concentration and P50 (7.4) in residents at sea level and at altitudes ranging from 1000 to 4840 meters. The average arterial O₂ saturation is also shown. Lines shown are the best fitted lines.

This improvement can occur in two ways: (a) improved oxygen transport; (b) alteration in the oxygen affinity of hemoglobin.

(a) <u>Improved oxygen transport</u>.

An improvement in oxygen transport can be produced by an increase in the hemoglobin level which increases the oxygen capacity. Such a change however occurs slowly because an increase in the hemoglobin level can only be induced via erythropoietin stimulation of the marrow. Alternatively the transport can be improved by an increase in the cardiac output--this is able to compensate for a decreased oxygen tension or a lowered transport capacity due to anemia. The advantage of compensation by increased cardiac output is that it can occur immediately. It has however the considerable disadvantage that it increases significantly the basal oxygen requirement; this offsets the advantage.

(b) <u>Changes in the oxygen affinity of hemoglobin</u>.

Another mechanism available to the organism for promoting the supply of oxygen to the tissues is by decreasing the blood affinity for oxygen. This change, which results in a rightwards displacement of the oxygen dissociation curve, improves oxygenation because more oxygen can be delivered at the same or higher oxygen tension. Also, the increased PO_2 at the capillary would facilitate the final step of diffusion into the tissues.

This adaptive mechanism was investigated in conditions which in its absence would result in a decrease in O_2 supply. These conditions were: life at high altitude, low blood flow due to cardiac impairment and low O_2 carrying capacity due to anemia. These conditions are often referred to as hypoxic hypoxia, stagnant hypoxia and anemic hypoxia, respectively (Barcroft, 1920).

People living at high altitude are continually exposed to an environment with a low oxygen pressure. Figure 1 shows the composite changes from studies we have carried out at different altitudes. With increasing altitude there is a decreased hemoglobin affinity for oxygen as shown by an increase in P_{50}. This increase, however, is not proportional to the altitude but is rather a mirror view of the decrease in arterial oxygen saturation. It is small, below 3000 m, but at higher altitudes there is a rapid increase. It is of interest that in these residents oxygen delivery is further assisted by an increased hemoglobin level, which also increased more rapidly with increasing height above 3000 m. Figure 1 also shows that above this altitude the arterial O_2 saturation begins to decrease more sharply.

Similar adaptive changes in P_{50} have been described in both cardiac (Morse et al., 1950; Metcalfe et al., 1969; Lenfant et al., 1969) and anemic patients (Kennedy and Valtis 1954; Rodman et al., 1960; Mulhausen et al., 1967; Edwards et al., 1968). Our own studies have also demonstrated such changes and in addition have

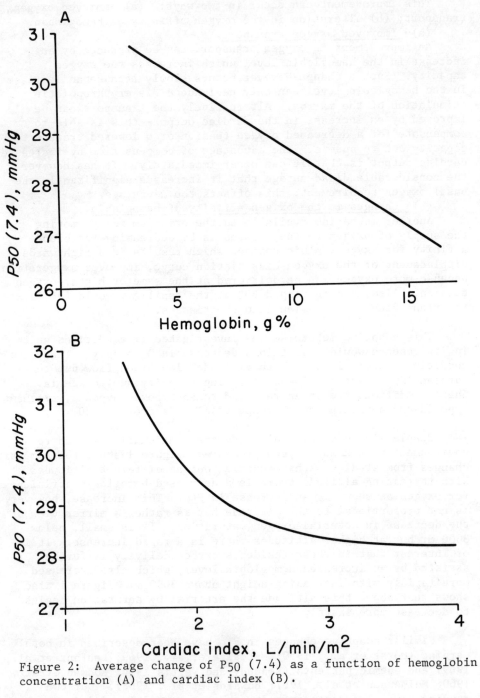

Figure 2: Average change of P_{50} (7.4) as a function of hemoglobin
concentration (A) and cardiac index (B).

established a relationship between the reduction in cardiac output
and the change in hemoglobin affinity (Fig. 2A). Likewise, there
is an increasing P50 associated with increasing severity of the
anemia (Fig. 2B). Thus in all three situations where the individual
has been exposed to hypoxia, changes occur in hemoglobin affinity
for oxygen which act to increase oxygen supply to body tissues.

Although changes in O_2 dissociation with hypoxia have been
established for many years, only recently has the mechanism been
disclosed by which this change is effected. In this respect, the
recent pioneering work of Chanutin (1967) and Benesch et al. (1967,
1968) constitutes a milestone. These investigators have convincing-
ly shown in vitro that intraerythrocytic organic phosphate compounds
are powerful modifiers of oxygen affinity of hemoglobin. The two
compounds, 2,3 diphosphoglycerate and adenosine triphosphate which
comprise 88% of the cell's organic phosphate were found most
effective. This observation was particularly interesting in view
of the large accumulation of 2,3 DPG in erythrocytes. To evaluate
the influences of these compounds on the oxygen dissociation curve
in vivo, their concentration was measured in individuals at high
altitude (Lenfant et al. 1968) and in patients with cardiac failure
(Woodson et al., 1969) and anemia, (Torrance et al., in preparation).
In all three, there was an increase in 2,3 DPG and ATP. The increase
in DPG concentration as a function of altitude is shown in figure 1.
Relationship between the severity of the cardiac or hematologic
abnormality and the change in DPG is shown in Figures 3A and 3B.
When the cardiac index fell below $2.5 L/min/m^2$ there was a marked
increase in DPG. The increase in DPG with decreasing hemoglobin
levels in anemia appeared more linear. This relationship between
erythrocyte DPG concentration and hemoglobin (within the normal
range of hemoglobin concentration) has also been found by Eaton
et al (1968) in healthy subjects.

In all groups of patients, there was an excellent correlation
between P50 and DPG; the calculated regression lines are given in
Table 1. The anemic patients are divided into 2 groups according
to the altitude at which they were studied.

Table 1.

Relationship between P50 and 2,3 DPG

Subjects	n	Regression equation	r*
Cardiac	36	P50 = 1.80 DPG + 17.86	0.866
Anemic Seattle (sea level) Medellin (1500 m)	119 52	P50 = 1.25 DPG + 21.09 P50 = 1.07 DPG + 21.01	0.723 0.803

* In all cases, P value of r was smaller than .001

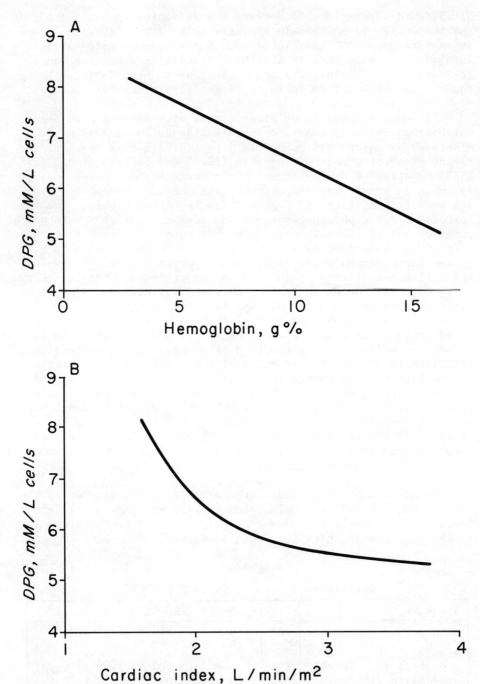

Figure 3: Average change of intracellular DPG as a function of
hemoglobin concentration (A) and cardiac index (B).

The shift in the oxygen dissociation curve which is a constant
occurrence in situations where oxygen delivery would be
otherwise impaired, is therefore associated with a predictable
increase in organic phosphate. On the basis of in vitro data,
it may be assumed that the change in organic phosphate is the
primary determinant of the change in oxygen affinity.

Scattering of the data in the patients studied raised the
question as to whether mechanisms other than DPG influence the
oxygen dissociation curve. An important variable is the effect of
the arterial pH on the in vivo position of the oxygen dissociation
curve. This is illustrated by two sets of observations.

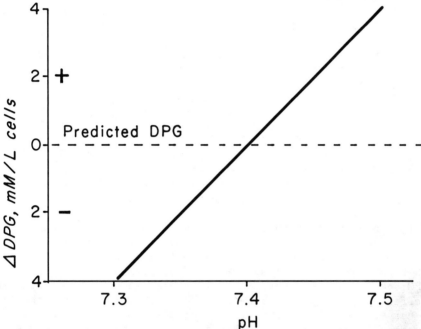

Figure 4: Average deviation of measured DPG from calculated DPG
(using the regression line DPG = -.194 Hb + 8.89) as a function of
arterial pH. Data obtained from a group of anemic patients at
Medellin (Colombia).

The arterial pH was measured in a group of anemic subjects to
see if it influenced either the P_{50} or the DPG level. The data
suggested that as the in vivo pH decreased the 2,3-DPG level fell.
An analogous fall in P_{50} occurred. The effect of in vivo pH on
the 2,3-DPG level was examined by plotting the difference between
the measured DPG and the mean predicted value of DPG deduced from
the hemoglobin level (using the regression equation DPG= -.194 Hb
+ 8.89) against the arterial pH (Figure 4). This shows that at

normal pH, predicted and actual DPG are the same but at acid pH
the 2,3-DPG concentration is less than the predicted value and at
alkaline pH it is more. Thus in an alkalotic subject whose in
vivo oxygen dissociation curve is displaced to the left (Bohr
effect) the increase in 2,3-DPG level is greater than at a normal
arterial pH of 7.4. The opposite effects occur in acidosis.
It would therefore seem that changes in pH appear to negate
their direct effect on the hemoglobin oxygen affinity by changes
which they produce in 2,3-DPG concentration.

Further insight into the role of pH in the adaptive mechanism
was obtained from the sudden exposure of normal subjects to an
altitude of 4350 m.

Normally, after arriving at high altitude there is a rapid
increase in both 2,3-DPG and P_{50} (Lenfant et al., 1968). The
DPG level reaches 1/2 its maximum value in about 6 hours and the
change in P_{50} is parallel. At the same time a marked alkalosis
due to hypocapnia of hyperventilation occurs (7.48 at 4350 m).
By 24 hours the 2,3-DPG and P_{50} changes are maximal and no further
change occurs. The pH on the other hand starts declining and
reaches 7.42 - 7.43 by the second day.

Upon returning to sea level, the pH falls to normal or slightly
acid levels and the DPG and P_{50} decrease to normal levels over a
five-day period. Readjustment to sea level values occurs at a
much slower rate than the response to hypoxia.

If, in order to maintain an acidotic pH, Diamox is taken
before going to high altitude and during the stay there, the
pattern of change is entirely different. Indeed, in this case
neither DPG nor P_{50} increase, probably because of the pH effect
on DPG concentration. Yet, in terms of oxygen unloading capacity
the effect is the same as previously because the shift of the in
vivo curve, due to the Bohr effect, equals that resulting from a
decreased affinity due to DPG binding. It seems, then, that a
fall in pH replaces an increase in 2,3-DPG level as an adaptation
to arterial hypoxia. It is significant that the alkalosis
occurring in untreated subjects shifts the in vivo oxygen dissociation curve to the left which aggravates the anoxia already
present. This may act as a trigger for the rapid formation of
2,3-DPG observed at high altitude which then shifts the curve
back to the right.

Conclusion

These studies show that an important adaptation to hypoxia
is a decrease in the hemoglobin oxygen affinity. This change is
mediated in vivo by changes in the intracellular concentration
of 2,3-DPG. An in vivo shift of the oxygen dissociation curve

can however also occur by means of the Bohr effect. Because of the interrelationship between DPG concentration and pH it is quite possible that the changes in pH occurring at the onset of hypoxia may have an enhancing effect on other adaptive mechanisms.

(1) This work was supported by grants HE-06242 and HE-12174 from the National Heart Institute and by the Boeing Employees' Medical Research Fund.

REFERENCES

Barcroft, J. (1920). Anoxaemia - Presidential Address. Lancet 199: 485-489.

Benesch, R., and Benesch, R.E. (1967). The effect of organic phosphates from the human erythrocyte on the allosteric properties of hemoglobin. Biochem. Biophys. Res. Commun. 26: 162-167.

Benesch, R., Benesch, R.E. and Yu, C.I. (1968). Reciprocal binding of oxygen and diphosphoglycerate by human hemoglobin. Proc. Natl. Acad. Sci. U.S. 59: 526-532.

Chanutin, A., and Curnish, R.R. (1967). Effect of organic and inorganic phosphates on the oxygen equilibrium of human erythrocytes. Arch. Biochem. Biophys. 121: 96-102.

Eaton, J.W., and Brewer, G.J. (1968). The relationship between red cell 2,3-diphosphoglycerate and levels of hemoglobin in the human. Proc. Natl. Acad. Sci. U.S. 61: 756-760.

Edwards, M.J., Novy, M.J., Walters, C.L., and Metcalfe, J. (1968). Improved oxygen release: an adaptation of mature red cells to hypoxia. J. Clin. Invest. 47: 1851-1857.

Kennedy, A.C., and Valtis, D.J. (1954). The oxygen dissociation curve in anemia of various types. J. Clin. Invest. 33: 1372-1381.

Lenfant, C., Torrance, J., English, E., Finch, C.A., Reynafarje, C., Ramos, J., and Faura, J. (1968). Effect of altitude on oxygen binding by hemoglobin and on organic phosphate levels. J. Clin. Invest. 47: 2652-2656.

Lenfant, C., Ways, P., Aucutt, C., and Cruz, J. (1969). Effect of chronic hypoxic hypoxia on the O_2-Hb dissociation curve and respiratory gas transport in man. Respir. Physiol. 7: 7-29.

Metcalfe, J., Dhindsa, D.G., Edwards, M.J., and Mourdjinis, A.
    (1969). Decreased affinity of blood for oxygen in patients
    with low-output heart failure. Circulation Research 25:
    47-51.

Morse, M., Cassels, D.E., and Holder, M. (1950). The position of
    the oxygen dissociation curve of the blood in cyanotic
    congenital heart disease. J. Clin. Invest. 29: 1098-1103.

Mulhausen, R., Astrup, P., and Kjeldsen, K. (1967). Oxygen
    affinity of hemoglobin in patients with cardiovascular
    diseases, anemia, and cirrhosis of the liver. Scand.
    J. Clin. Lab. Invest. 19: 291-297.

Rodman, T., Close, H.P., and Purcell, M.K. (1960). Oxyhemoglobin
    dissociation curve in anemia. Ann. Intern. Med. 52: 295-309.

Torrance, J.D., Jacobs, P., Restrepo, A., Eschbach, J.,
    Lenfant, C. and Finch, C.A. (in preparation).
    Intraerythrocytic adaptation to anemia.

Woodson, R.D., Torrance, J.D., and Lenfant, C. (1969). Oxygen
    transport in low cardiac output hypoxia. Physiologist
    12: 399.

ADAPTATION OF THE RED BLOOD CELL TO MUSCULAR EXERCISE

John A. Faulkner, George J. Brewer, and John W. Eaton

Departments of Physiology, Medicine (Simpson Memorial

Institute) and Human Genetics, The University of

Michigan Medical School, Ann Arbor

The shift to the right in the oxygen dissociation curve of vigorously exercising subjects beyond that attributable to the decrease in blood pH and/or the increase in blood temperature has been noted by several investigators (Mitchell et al., 1958; Rowell et al., 1964; Sproule and Archer, 1959). The right shift is more pronounced in venous than arterial blood because of the greater decrease in pH (Sproule et al., 1960) and the slight increase in temperature (Sproule and Archer, 1959) of the venous compared to the arterial blood. Mitchell et al., (1958) recognized the potential of the right shift in the oxygen dissociation curve to maintain an adequate tissue oxygen gradient or to increase oxygen unloading at a given tension. However, they concluded that the mechanism was unknown.

Rowell et al., (1964) observed that the arterial oxygen desaturation of athletes was greater than that of normal subjects when both groups were exercising strenuously. The greater desaturation of the athletes could not be accounted for by pH or temperature changes. They proposed that following athletic training, 3 mechanisms might operate separately or in unison to increase the arterial oxygen desaturation: a) a greater A-a oxygen gradient because the large cardiac outputs of athletes result in high flow rates in pulmonary capillaries and transit time is not sufficient for gas equilibration; b) the opening of more A-V shunts, and c) greater changes in the shape of the oxygen dissociation curve because athletes exert greater physical effort.

The right shifted oxygen dissociation curve can now be reassessed in terms of the known negative relationship between

213

2,3 - diphosphoglycerate   (DPG) and the oxygen affinity of hemoglobin (Benesch and Benesch, 1967; Chanutin and Curnish, 1967).
The red blood cell concentration of DPG increases in response to
hypoxia (Brewer and Eaton, 1969; Eaton et al., 1968; Lenfant et al.,
1967) and the increased DPG accounts for the right shift of the
oxygen dissociation curve of high altitude natives compared to that
of sea level residents (Aste - Altazar and Hurtado, 1944). Because
of the displacement of the oxygen dissociation curve to the right,
the transition from arterial to venous blood occurs on the steeper
portion of the oxygen dissociation curve (Figure 1). Therefore,
with a constant oxygen consumption the arterial to venous oxygen
gradient is smaller or with a given oxygen tension more oxygen is
released to the tissues. We have recently reported an increase in
the concentration of red blood cell DPG after 60 min of strenuous
exercise (Eaton et al., 1969b). In the following paper, the cardiovascular response of man during acute exposures and chronic
exposures (training) to maximum exercise will be discussed and the
possible role of an increased red blood cell DPG will be interpreted in relation to the factors that limit maximum physical work
capacity in trained and untrained subjects.

Red, Intermediate, and White Skeletal Muscle Cells. The
immediate event in the contraction of skeletal muscle is the
hydrolysis of adenosine triphosphate (ATP). In vivo, ATP is rapidly phosphorylated by coupling to the breakdown of creatine phosphate. Skeletal muscle concentrations of 2 mM of ATP/100 g and
7 mM creatine phosphate/100 g dry weight (Hultman et al., 1967)
provide anaerobic sources of energy for muscle contraction. Creatine phosphate may be rephosphorylated from ATP produced by anaerobic glycolysis or by oxidative phosphorylation.

In man, most skeletal muscles are composed of different proportions of red, intermediate, and white skeletal muscle cells
that have very different structural and functional characteristics
(Henneman and Olson, 1965; Romanul, 1965). Motor units composed
of red skeletal muscle cells have a low stimulus threshold and are
recruited frequently for low tension, repetitive movements. The
red fibers have many capillaries, have a high mitochondrial density, oxidize pyruvate rapidly, have a low ATPase activity, and
are slow to fatigue. Motor units composed of white skeletal muscle
cells have a high stimulus threshold and are recruited infrequently
for rapid, powerful movements. White fibers have few capillaries, few mitochondria, high concentrations of glycolytic enzymes, a high ATPase activity, and fatigue rapidly (for review see
Faulkner, 1970). During contraction, red skeletal muscle cells
rephosphorylate ATP primarily by oxidative phosphorylation while
white skeletal muscle cells rephosphorylate ATP by anaerobic glycolysis. In recovery periods between contractions, white fibers
likely utilize their very limited capacity for pyruvate oxidation
to rephosphorylate ATP aerobically.

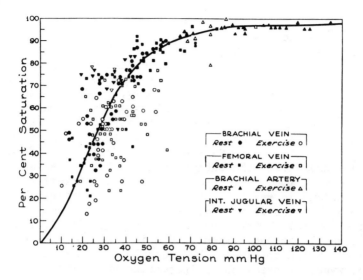

Fig. 1. The % oxygen saturation plotted against oxygen tension for
normal subjects at rest and during exercise (from Sproule et al.,
1960 with permission).

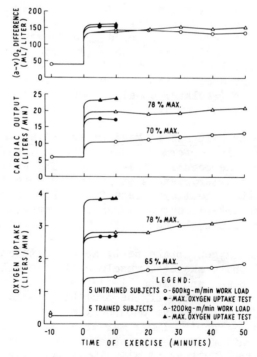

Fig. 2. The arteriovenous oxygen difference, cardiac output, and
oxygen uptake of trained and untrained men during 50 min of heavy
work and during a maximum oxygen uptake test of 10 min duration.

The Maximum Oxygen Uptake Test. The most objective measure of man's maximum physical work capacity or his physical fitness is the maximum oxygen uptake test (Astrand and Saltin, 1961a; Mitchell et al., 1958; Taylor et al., 1955). The maximum utilization of oxygen per unit time is specific to the task performed (Astrand and Saltin, 1961b; Christensen and Hogberg, 1950; Hermansen and Saltin, 1969); however, reasonable estimates of maximum oxygen uptake may be obtained for most subjects during either a treadmill run (Mitchell et al., 1958; Taylor et al., 1955) or a bicycle ergometer ride (Astrand and Saltin, 1961a; Hermansen and Saltin, 1969). In either test, the subject begins at a submaximum work load and the work load is increased in regular increments until voluntary fatigue is reached. The work periods are usually from $2\frac{1}{2}$ to 10 min duration with 10 min rest periods between each bout of exercise. Oxygen uptake increases linearly with increasing work loads until maximum oxygen uptake is reached. The criterion that maximum oxygen uptake has been attained is a plateau or decrement in oxygen uptake with an increasing work load as voluntary fatigue is reached. If the approximate physical work capacity of the subject is known, a single work load with an energy requirement above the maximum oxygen uptake may be used after a 5 min warm-up. The work load should be selected to exhaust the subject in from 5 to 10 min. With a single supra-maximum work load, the criterion for maximum oxygen uptake is a plateau in oxygen uptake for several minutes, usually followed by a decrease in oxygen uptake as voluntary fatigue is reached (Astrand and Saltin, 1961a). In a study that involved 14 track athletes, a clear plateau or a plateau followed by a decrement was observed in 175 of 180 maximum oxygen uptake tests (Faulkner et al., 1968). The maximum oxygen uptake is extremely reproducible (r = +0.95, Taylor et al., 1955).

Cardiovascular Response to Maximum Exercise. When a maximum oxygen uptake test is performed after a warm-up, the transition to maximum oxygen uptake occurs within 2 min. The oxygen uptake, cardiac output and arteriovenous oxygen difference during a 10 min maximum oxygen uptake test are presented in Figure 2. Heart rate, stroke volume and arteriovenous oxygen difference all reach asymptotes at maximum values throughout the middle portion of the run.

In a maximum oxygen uptake test, motor units composed of red, intermediate and white skeletal muscle cells are all recruited continuously (Henneman and Olson, 1965) and the hydrolysis of ATP greatly exceeds the capacity of the skeletal muscle cells to rephosphorylate ATP by oxidative phosphorylation, by anaerobic glycolysis, or both (Margaria, 1967; Margaria et al., 1969). Muscle glycogen concentration (Hermansen et al., 1967) and creatin phosphate concentration (Hultman et al., 1967; Margaria et al., 1964) decrease and eventually the ability of skeletal muscle cells to develop tension is impaired (Merton, 1956). With the onset of

fatigue, arteriovenous oxygen difference remains at maximum levels
and oxygen uptake decreases because of a decrease in cardiac output
(Mitchell et al., 1958). Under these circumstances, blood lactates
reach maximum concentration of from 135 to 175 mg/100 ml (Astrand
and Saltin, 1961a).

Maximum oxygen uptake can be sustained continuously for about
5 to 10 min (Astrand and Saltin, 1961a; Faulkner et al., 1968).
In prolonged exercise only a percentage of maximum oxygen uptake
can be maintained. The percentage is inversely related to work
duration and directly related to the maximum oxygen uptake of the
subject. Runners, for example, maintain 75% of their maximum
oxygen uptake for approximately $2\frac{1}{2}$ hours in the 26 mile marathon
(Costill, 1969). Data are presented in Figure 2 for 5 trained
subjects pedalling at 1200 kg-m/min and 5 untrained subjects pedalling at 600 kg-m/min. The subjects maintained these work loads
for 50 min. The arteriovenous oxygen difference is fairly stable
throughout the work period but subjects displayed a steadily increasing cardiac output and oxygen uptake. The gradual increase
in oxygen uptake in heavy work of long duration has been reported
previously (Saltin and Stenberg, 1964).

At work intensities of this magnitude (55 to 90% of maximum)
red fiber motor units are continuously active and white fiber motor
units are cycling at a rate necessary to develop the tension required in the work task. If the white fiber recruitment cycle
allows sufficient recovery time between contractions for the creatine phosphate concentrations to be restored to resting levels
aerobically, lactate will not be formed. Such work loads, usually
less than 50% of maximum, may be carried out for an eight hour
work day without undue fatigue (Astrand, 1960) and blood lactates
do not change from resting levels (Strydom et al., 1962). More
rapid cycling of white fibers results in a decrease in the creatine phosphate concentration which stimulates glycolysis. Lactate
production increases as more pyruvate is formed than can be oxidized (Margaria et al., 1964). The factors that limit maximum
performance differ in work of different durations (Astrand et al.,
1963). In work of up to 2 min duration, the speed and power of
muscle contractions depend on the rate at which ATP can be hydrolyzed and the resting concentration of creatine phosphate. When
maximum work must be sustained for from 2 to 12 min, physical work
capacity is limited by the resting concentrations of creatine
phosphate and glycogen and by the amount of ATP that can be phosphorylated by oxidative phosphorylation and glycolysis. In prolonged work, physical work capacity is related to the muscle
glycogen concentration (Hermansen et al., 1967), but the most significant relationship is between physical work capacity and maximum
oxygen uptake (Balke, 1963). The hemoconcentration that occurs in
severe exercise has been observed in many studies over the past 35

years (Dill et al., 1935; Mitchell et al., 1958; Saltin and
Stenberg, 1964). The increase in hemoglobin concentration from
14.9 g/100 ml to 16.4 g/100 ml (Mitchell et al., 1958) results in
an increased oxygen carrying capacity even with the lower arterial
oxygen saturation that occurs in maximum exercise (Figure 3). The
exact magnitude of the decrease in arterial oxygen tension
varies from an estimated oxygen tension of 65 mm Hg (Rowell et
al., 1964), to measured values of 88 and 89 mm Hg (Mitchell et al.,
1958; Holmgren and Linderholm, 1958).

Increased Red Blood Cell DPG during Muscular Exercise. We
first observed a significant increase (p< 0.01) in red blood cell
DPG (18% above resting) in 10 subjects immediately after 60 min of
competitive basketball (Eaton et al., 1969b). A 50 min bicycle
ergometer ride was then used to provide a more controlled physiological stress. Five untrained subjects pedalled at a work load
of 600 kg-m/min and 5 trained subjects pedalled at 1200 kg-m/min.
These work loads required an energy expenditure of approximately
70% of maximum oxygen uptake with a range of from 55% to 90%.
Average cardiovascular responses to the ergometer ride are plotted
in Figure 2. Venous blood samples were drawn at 0, 30, and 50 min,
and extracts were prepared for DPG and lactate assays. The ana-
lytic methods for DPG (Eaton et al., 1969a) and lactate (Marbach
and Weil, 1967) have been reported previously.

No change was observed in red blood cell DPG concentrations
after 30 min of pedalling. However, after 50 min of work, 7 of
the 10 subjects had increased DPG concentrations (Table 1). Although blood lactate does not reveal the actual muscle lactate concentration (Astrand et al., 1963), the blood lactate has been used
on many occasions as a measure of physiological strain (Astrand et
al., 1963; Astrand and Saltin, 1961; Hermansen and Saltin, 1969;
Saltin and Stenberg, 1964). Since the half response time for lactate is about 5 min (Margaria et al., 1969), the best estimate of
the physiological stress throughout the 50 min test was taken as
the average of the 30 and 50 min lactate concentrations minus the
resting value. If blood lactate is a valid measure of physiological strain, the subjects who were stressed the most had the great-
est increases in DPG. Three subjects who had slight or negative
changes in blood lactate with exercise had no change or a slight
decrease in DPG. The coefficient of correlation between the delta
blood lactate and the delta DPG was +0.743 (Figure 3). A similar
relation was observed between the delta DPG and the percentage of
maximum oxygen uptake required to perform the work load.

The red blood cell DPG response does not appear to be stimulated or is not sustained by low intensity work of long duration.
The red blood cell DPG concentration of three subjects who trav-
ersed a 14 mile distance at the fastest possible speed (1 3/4, 2,
and 4 hours respectively) were the same as resting values.

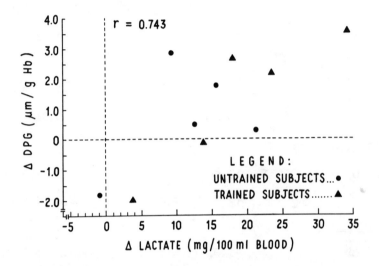

Fig. 3.   A scatter diagram showing the correlation between the
changes from resting levels in blood lactate and red cell DPG
during exercise on a bicycle ergometer.   DPG is expressed in μmoles
per gram hemoglobin and lactate in mg. per 100 ml. of whole blood.
Solid triangles = trained subjects, solid circles = untrained subjects.   Correlation coefficient = +0.743, p < 0.01.   (Modified from
Eaton et al., 1969c)

Table 1. Mean DPG and Blood Lactate Changes in Response to Exercise
in Two Groups of 10 Adult Males
(from Eaton et al., 1969c with Permission).

TIME (minutes)	DPG (μmoles per gram hemoglobin)	LACTATE (mg. per 100 ml. whole blood)
Basketball:		
0	11.14 ($\pm$ 1.53)	16.9 ($\pm$ 1.57)
60	13.12 ($\pm$ 1.90)	27.0 ($\pm$ 3.00)
Δ	+1.98 (t = 3.38, p < 0.01)	+10.1 (t = 2.99, p < 0.01)
Bicycle ergometer:		
0	12.84 ($\pm$ 2.17	9.3 ($\pm$ 4.84)
50	13.85 ($\pm$ 2.06)	24.4 ($\pm$ 8.47)*
Δ	+1.01 (t = 1.26, NS)	+15.1 (t = 3.29, p < 0.01)

*Average of the 30 and 50 minute lactate concentrations.

To determine the effect of short exhaustive work on the DPG
concentration in red blood cells, 3 untrained and 3 trained subjects warmed up for 5 min and then ran to voluntary fatigue in
from 8 to 12 min on a motor driven treadmill (maximum oxygen uptake test). The cardiovascular responses were approximately the
same as that plotted for the 5 untrained and 5 trained subjects in
Figure 2. Venous blood samples were taken immediately before the
warm-up and immediately after voluntary fatigue was reached. The
lapsed time between the resting and the immediate post-exercise
blood sample varied from 20 to 27 min with an average of 23 min.
The data for each subject are presented in Table 2.

Table 2. Blood Lactate and Red Blood Cell DPG Concentrations at Rest, and after Maximum Short Duration Exercise.

Subject	Oxygen Uptake (liters/min)	Blood Lactate (mg/100 ml)	DPG** (μM/g Hb)	Hb (g/100 ml)
JF*	Rest	5.8	15.9	14.9
	3.49	91.7	16.7	15.0
GH*	Rest	10.0	11.0	15.6
	4.98	91.5	10.1	17.3
RL*	Rest	9.5	11.1	14.6
	4.72	83.8	13.2	15.6
RD	Rest	13.8	8.4	15.6
	3.10	70.7	12.2	15.5
CK	Rest	11.6	11.7	15.3
	2.86	78.6	12.5	16.4
LM	Rest	7.8	12.3	13.6
	2.91	75.7	12.8	15.3
Mean	Rest	9.7	11.7	14.8
	Maximum	82.0	12.8	15.8

* The asterisk indicates the 3 trained subjects. The other 3 subjects were untrained.

**In our paper presented at the First International Conference on Red Cell Metabolism and Function, we reported preliminary data on 4 subjects following 10 min of exhaustive work who had DPG concentrations higher than the values reported here. The post-exercise DPG concentrations reported at the Conference now seem to have been high due to the appearance following maximum work of one or more substances in the plasma that resulted in additional color development in the chromatropic method.

The mean increase in red blood cell DPG after the 8 to 12 min exhaustive run was 10% compared to 13% after the 50 min bicycle

ergometer ride and 18% after 60 min of basketball. An increase in
DPG of from 0.5 to 3.8 μ moles/g Hb occurred in 5 of 6 subjects
during the 20 to 27 min between the beginning of the warm-up run
and the completion of the maximum voluntary effort. The increase
in red blood cell DPG after elapsed times of from 20 to 60 min
indicates a half response time during adaptation to heavy exercise
that is much more rapid than the 6 hour half response time observed
during adaptation to high altitude (Lenfant et al., 1968).

A relationship between blood lactate concentration and DPG
concentration was neither expected nor observed because the subjects reached voluntary fatigue after runs of different durations.
The blood samples were drawn immediately after work ceased and the
blood lactate concentrations would not be representative of the
maximum concentration that occurred. After maximum exercise of
from 8 to 12 min duration, lactate concentration in the brachial
vein may not reach a peak value until 5 min or more after work has
stopped (Astrand and Saltin, 1961a; and unpublished data). At
present, the time response of red blood cell DPG during and following maximum exercise is unknown.

The right shift in the oxygen dissociation curve in maximum
exercise appears to provide the same physiological advantage as
enjoyed by high altitude natives. The right shifted curve seems
to be of particular value in maintaining an adequate oxygen gradient between capillary blood and muscle cell mitochondria in
maximum work when a maximum arteriovenous oxygen difference makes
a major encroachment on end capillary oxygen tension. The slight
increase in DPG of 1 μ mole/g of Hb coupled with a .25 decrease in
pH (Mitchell et al., 1958) and the increase in venous blood temperature of 0.7 C (Sproule and Archer, 1959) is not sufficient to
account for the 10 to 15 mm Hg right shift previously observed in
the oxygen dissociation curve (Figure 1).

Training. The frequency, duration and intensity of chronic
exposures to muscular exercise necessary to produce significant
changes in cardiovascular variables and cell structure and function have not been resolved. The physiological status of the
individual is certainly a major determinant and sedentary men
(maximum oxygen uptake 38 ml/kg-min) increase their maximum oxygen
uptake 17% with 30 min of jogging twice a week for 20 weeks while
some college track men (maximum oxygen uptake 70 ml/kg-min) may
show no change in maximum oxygen uptake with 2 to 3 hours of running 5 days a week for 4 years (Faulkner, 1968).

The differences between the trained and the untrained state
are much more significant when trained endurance athletes are compared to subjects with normal physical activity than when changes
before and after training are compared in the same individual

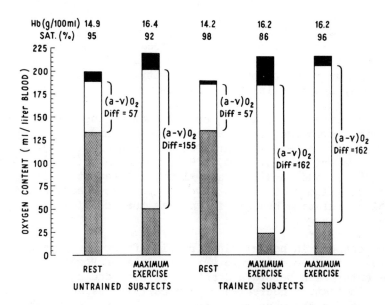

Fig. 4. The arteriovenous oxygen difference of trained and untrained men at rest and in maximum exercise. Oxygen capacity is
represented by the height of each bar graph. Black shading is
desaturated hemoglobin. Stipled area is mixed venous oxygen content. Data were compiled from Mitchell et al., 1958; Holmgren and
Linderholm, 1958; Reeves et al., 1967; Rowell et al., 1964; and
unpublished data University of Michigan.

(Ekblom et al., 1968). At rest, the most widely observed change with training is the decrease in heart rate (Holmgren et al., 1960) and the concomitant increase in stroke volume. However, equally significant changes occur in the red blood cell (Gollnick et al., 1965; Davis, 1939), in cardiac muscle cells (Hakkila, 1955), and skeletal muscle cells (Carrow, 1967; Gordon et al., 1966).

Data on the response of the red blood cell to regular muscular exercise are conflicting. Although an increased integrity of the human and dog red blood cell is described in the older literature, the more recent data of Gollnick et al. (1965) on rats supports the findings of Davis (1939) that regular training increases the fragility of red blood cells. The decrease in the integrity of the red blood cell wall with training is attributed to increases in circulatory rate, temperature, acidity, and compression of the cell (Davis, 1939; Gollnick et al., 1965).

On the effect of training on hemoglobin concentration and hematocrit, investigators have reported no change (Kjellberg et al., 1949), an increase (Knehr, Dill and Neufeld, 1942), and a decrease (Oscari et al., 1968). Holmgren et al. (1960), Kjellberg et al. (1949), and Oscari et al. (1968) all report an increase in total blood volume. The first two groups also observed an increase in total circulating hemoglobin whereas the Oscari group did not observe any change.

The changes in hemoglobin directly affect the oxygen carrying capacity of the blood (Figure 4). The data of Rowell et al. (1964) on 4 sedentary men before and after training and on 4 endurance athletes indicate a decreased oxygen carrying capacity at rest and in exercise for the physically trained subject. Although a decrease in oxygen transport capability with training appears incongruous, the decreased blood viscosity and the increased blood volume may contribute to the greatly enhanced cardiac output in maximum exercise (Ekblom et al., 1968). Controversy exists as to the amount of desaturation that occurs in arterial blood in exercise particularly in trained subjects (Figure 4). However, regardless of the arterial oxygen content, the trained subject can make a greater encroachment than the untrained subject on the mixed venous oxygen content and further widen the arteriovenous oxygen difference. The increased red blood cell DPG concentration may play a significant role in the preservation of an adequate capillary to mitochondrial oxygen tension gradient under these circumstances.

In summary, red blood cell DPG appears to have a much more rapid half response time than previously recognized. DPG concentration increases 18% in the red blood cells of human subjects following 60 minutes of exercise. The red blood cell DPG did not respond or was not sustained during long term work of 2 to 4 hours duration. An increase of 10% in the red blood cell DPG was observed following an 8 to 12 min exhaustive run on a treadmill. The increase in DPG, decrease in pH, and increase in venous blood temperature are not sufficient to account for the 10 to 15 mm Hg right shift in the oxygen dissociation curve that has been reported previously. Insufficient data and conflicting data make conclusions regarding the effect of training in muscular endurance on red blood cell metabolism and function very tenuous.

ACKNOWLEDGMENT

We thank Dinu Patel for his technical assistance with the DPG analyses and Donald Roberts and Robert Dixon for their aid in the administration of the exercise tests. The research was supported by USPHS training grant T01-GM-0071, USPHS research grant Am-09381, Career Development Award AM 07959 (GJB), Contract DADA17-69-9103 with the U.S. Army and Navy Medical Research and Development Commands and the Michigan Heart Association.

REFERENCES

Aste-Salazar, H. and Hurtado, A. (1944). Am. J. Physiol. 142:733.
Astrand, I. (1960). Acta Physiol. Scand. 49:Suppl. 169.
Astrand, P.-O., Hallback, I., Hedman, R., and Saltin, B. (1963). J. Appl. Physiol. 18:619.
Astrand, P.-O., and Saltin, B. (1961a). J. Appl. Physiol. 16:971.
Astrand, P.-O., and Saltin, B. (1961b). J. Appl. Physiol. 16:977.
Balke, B. (1963). Proceedings of First Canadian Fitness Seminar 1:5.
Benesch, R., and Benesch, R. E. (1967). Biochem. and Biophys. Res. Commun. 26:162.
Brewer, G. J. and Eaton, J. W. (1969). J. Clin. Invest. (abst.). 48:11a.
Carrow, R. E., Brown, R. E., and Van Huss, W. D. (1967). Anat. Record. 159:33.
Chanutin, A. and Curnish, R. R. (1967). Arch. Biochem. Biophys. 121:96.
Costill, D. L., and Fox, E. L. (1969). Med. Sci. Sports. 1:81.
Christensen, E. H., and Hogberg, P. (1950). Arbeits. 14:292.
Davis, J. E. (1939). J. Lab. Clin. Med. 23:786.
Dill, D. B., Edwards, H. T., and Talbot, J. H. (1935). J. Physiol. (Lond.). 69:267.
Eaton, J. W., Brewer, G. J., and Grover, R. F. (1969a). J. Lab. Clin. Med. 73:603.

Eaton, J. W., Faulkner, J. A., and Brewer, G. J. (1969b).
    Physiologist (abst.). 12:212.
Eaton, J. W., Faulkner, J. A., and Brewer, G. J. (1969c). Proc.
    Soc. Exp. Biol. (In Press).
Ekblom, B., Astrand, P.-O., Saltin, B., Stenberg, J., Wallstrom, B.
    (1968). J. Appl. Physiol. 24:518.
Faulkner, J. A. (1968). J. Am. Med. Assoc. 205:741.
Faulkner, J. A. (1970). In Physiology and Biochemistry of Muscle
    as a Food. Briskey, E. J., Cassens, R. G., Marsh, B. B., Eds.
    Univ. of Wisconsin Press. (In Press).
Faulkner, J. A., Kollias, J., Favour, C. B., Buskirk, E. R., and
    Balke, B. (1968). J. Appl. Physiol. 24:685.
Gollnick, P. D., Struck, P. J., Soule, R. G., and Heinrick, J. R.
    (1965), Arbeits. 21:169.
Gordon, E. E., Kowalski, K., and Fritts, M. (1967). Arch. Phys.
    Med. Rehab. 48:296.
Hakkila, J. E. (1955). Annales Med. Exper. Biol. Fenniae 33:Suppl.
    10.
Henneman, E., and Olson, C. B. (1965). J. Neurophysiol. 28:581.
Hermansen, L., Hultman, E., and Saltin, B. (1967). Acta Physiol.
    Scand. 71:129.
Hermansen, L., and Saltin, B. (1969). J. Appl. Physiol. 26:31.
Holmgren, A. and Linderholm, H. (1958). Acta Physiol. Scand. 44:
    203.
Holmgren, A., Mossfeldt, A. R., Sjostrand, T., and Strom, G. (1960)
    Acta. Physiol. Scand. 50:72.
Hultman, E., Bergstrom, J., and Anderson, N. McLennan (1967).
    Scand. J. Clin. Lab. Invest. 19:56.
Kjellberg, S. R., Rudle, U., and Sjostrand, T. (1949). Acta Physiol.
    Scand. 19:146.
Knehr, C. A., Dill, D. B., and Neufeld, W. (1942). Am. J. Physiol.
    136:148.
Lenfant, C., Torrance, J., English, E., Finch, C. A., Reynafarje,
    C., Ramos, J., and Fauru, J. (1968). J. Clin. Invest. 47:2652.
Marbach, E. P., and Weil, M. H. (1967). Clin. Chem. 13:314.
Margaria, R. (1967). In Exercise at Altitude. Margaria, R. Ed.
    Exerpta Medica Foundation, New York. p. 15.
Margaria, R., Cerretelli, P., and Mangili, E. (1964). J. Appl.
    Physiol. 19:623.
Margaria, R., Oliva, R. D., DiPrampero, P. E., and Cerretelli, P.
    (1969). J. Appl. Physiol. 26:752.
Merton, P. A. (1956). J. Physiol. 123:553.
Mitchell, J. H., Sproule, B. J., and Chapman, C. B. (1958). J.
    Clin. Invest. 37:538.
Oscari, L. B., Williams, B. T., and Hertig, B. A. (1968). J. Appl.
    Physiol. 24:622.
Pollard, M. L., Cureton, T. K., and Greninger, L. (1969). Med.
    Sci. Sports. 1:70.
Reeves, J. T., Grover, R. F., and Cohn, J. E. (1967). J. Appl.
    Physiol. 22:546.

Romanul, F. C. A. (1965). Arch. Neurol. 12:497.

Rowell, L. B., Taylor, H. L., Wang, Y., and Carlson, W. S. (1964). J. Appl. Physiol. 19:284.

Saltin, B. and Stenberg, J. (1964). J. Appl. Physiol. 19:833.

Sproule, B. J. and Archer, R. K. (1959). J. Appl. Physiol. 14:983.

Sproule, B. J., Mitchell, J. H., and Miller, W. F. (1960). J. Clin. Invest. 39:378.

Strydom, N. B., Wyndham, C. H., v. Radhenand, M., and Williams, C. G. (1962). Intern. Congr. Physiol. Sci., 22nd, Leiden. P.6.

Taylor, H. L., Buskirk, E. R., and Henschel, A. (1955). J. Appl. Physiol. 8:73.

A COMPARISON OF MECHANISMS OF OXYGEN TRANSPORT AMONG SEVERAL MAMMALIAN SPECIES

James Metcalfe and Dharam S. Dhindsa

Heart Research Laboratory, University of Oregon

Medical School, Portland, Oregon

INTRODUCTION

One important function of the circulation is to provide oxygen to the peripheral tissues in quantities adequate for their metabolic needs. Since the final link in the chain of oxygen supply depends upon diffusion from capillary blood to the mitochondria, and since cellular oxygen tensions seem to be of the order of a few millimeters of mercury (Chance et al., 1962), the rate of oxygen diffusion is governed over short periods of time by the oxygen tension of capillary blood and the intercapillary diffusion distances (Krogh, 1941). Therefore, the first sentence of this paragraph could read that one important function of the circulation is to maintain an oxygen tension in tissue capillary blood adequate to supply tissue demands by diffusion.

The oxygen tension in tissue capillary blood depends not only upon the quality of the circulating blood but also upon the rate of blood flow and its distribution with respect to oxygen consumption; therefore, knowledge of the respiratory characteristics of blood must be combined with hemodynamic data and knowledge of oxygen utilization before the role of the circulation in tissue oxygen supply can be defined.

METHODS

Figure 1 represents an attempt to illustrate and analyze

229

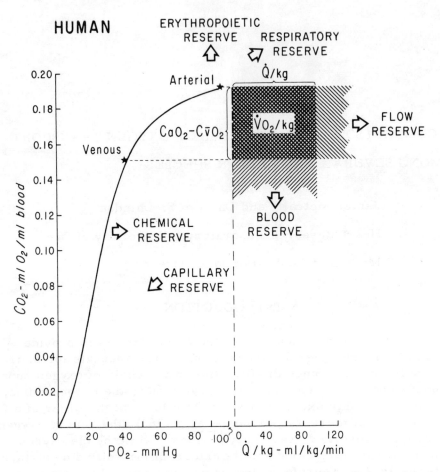

Figure 1. A representation of factors influencing O_2 tension in peripheral capillary blood. The abscissa is divided by the vertical dashed line. To the left is the O_2 dissociation curve for human blood at 37°C and pH 7.400. The ordinate has been converted from % saturation to O_2 concentration (C_{O_2}) assuming an O_2 capacity of 20 vol% (0.20 ml/ml). Average values for C_{O_2} and O_2 tension (P_{O_2}) in arterial and mixed venous blood are shown by stars; the vertical distance between them represents the arterio-venous O_2 concentration difference across the peripheral circulation (Ca_{O_2}-$C\overline{v}_{O_2}$); their horizontal span embraces the range of P_{O_2} in blood flowing through the "average peripheral capillary". To the right of the vertical dashed line the abscissa expresses the blood flow per kg of body weight ($\dot{Q}$/kg). The cross-hatched area is the product of $\dot{Q}$/kg and Ca_{O_2}-Cv_{O_2}, i.e. the rate of O_2 consumption per kg ($\dot{V}_{O_2}$/kg). The open arrows indicate the physiological reserves of O_2 transport and are discussed in the text.

graphically the factors which modify capillary oxygen tension.
Notice that the abscissa is fractured by the vertical dashed line.
To the left lies an oxygen dissociation curve whose ordinate has
been changed by knowledge of blood hemoglobin concentration;
the ordinate now expresses oxygen concentration in milliliters of
oxygen per milliliter of blood (Bartels, 1964). The curve is that
of human blood at 37°C and a pH of 7.40 (Severinghaus, 1961).
An arterial point located by both its oxygen concentration and
tension can be recorded; so can a venous point. The vertical
distance between them represents the difference in oxygen concentration between arterial and venous blood. Their horizontal span
embraces the oxygen tension in capillary blood as it passes from
artery to vein.

The right-hand section of the figure has the same dimensions on its ordinate (that is, blood oxygen concentration), but
uses blood flow per kilogram of tissue as its abscissa. The rec-
tangular shaded area represents the product of blood flow per
kilogram and the arteriovenous oxygen concentration difference;
that is, the rate of oxygen consumption per kilogram of tissue.
We can, therefore, express blood flow in relation to oxygen removal and since that relationship is also expressed by arteriovenous oxygen concentration difference, we can translate the
result into oxygen tension by knowing the respiratory characteristics of the blood of the individual or species.

For constructing these graphs we have used data obtained
from resting, unanesthetized individuals, and we have used data
from mixed venous blood to locate the "venous" point. It is
correct and appropriate to point out that mixed venous blood does
not represent any particular capillary, nor even any particular
tissue; the oxygen concentration and tension in coronary vein
blood is much lower than in renal vein blood and their differences
are undoubtedly important to our eventual concept of hemoglobin
function. However, simplifications are necessary at our stage of
sophistication and mixed venous blood represents a sample of
blood leaving all the peripheral capillaries with each tissue con-
tributing to the sample in proportion to its rate of blood flow.
Any conclusions that we reach must be limited by the knowledge
that they may not apply to any individual anatomical area or organ.
For the resting, unanesthetized human (Bartels et al., 1955) the
average oxygen consumption is 4.1 ml/kg/min and this is supplied
by a blood flow of 100 ml/kg/min and an arteriovenous oxygen
concentration difference of 4.1 ml/100 ml of blood, so that mixed

venous blood has an oxygen tension of 39 mm Hg.

Figure 1 also indicates some of the reserves in oxygen supply. The rate of oxygen transport by the circulation could be increased by increasing blood flow as represented by the arrow labeled "Flow Reserve". Oxygen availability in blood can also be increased a little by hyperventilation and a lot by breathing oxygen-rich or hyperbaric gases and this potential is represented by the diagonal arrow labeled "Respiratory Reserve". An increase in hemoglobin concentration expands the curve vertically as represented by the arrow labeled "Erythropoietic Reserve". Displacement of the blood oxygen dissociation curve to the right would increase the average oxygen tension and would permit a greater extraction of oxygen from blood; this arrow is labeled "Chemical Reserve" because the location of the blood oxygen dissociation curve depends upon hemoglobin's primary structure and the configurational changes induced by pH or intracellular phosphates. All of the reservoirs which I have listed so far can be tapped without lowering the oxygen tension of capillary blood. In contrast, the oxygen remaining in blood which is returning to the lungs can only be used at the expense of a fall in mean capillary oxygen tension and such a fall decreases the pressure gradient for oxygen diffusion; additional tissue capillaries must open or be developed for a new equilibrium to be achieved. These two interrelated reserves are labeled "Blood Reserve" and "Capillary Reserve".

RESULTS AND DISCUSSION

Comparisons Among Species

A major commitment of our laboratory is to explore the dimensions of these reserves of oxygen delivery and their integration. This commitment began a few years ago when we recognized that the dynamics of tissue oxygen supply are quite different in sheep as compared to human beings (Parer et al., 1967; Parer and Metcalfe, 1967). A summary of our data, arranged in the graphical form which I have just presented, is shown in Figure 2. To the left are the average data for resting, unanesthetized humans for which we owe thanks to Bartels and his colleagues (1955). To the right are the data for sheep, again at rest and unanesthetized. The oxygen consumption per kilogram is very similar in the two species as are also the dimensions of oxygen consumption, blood

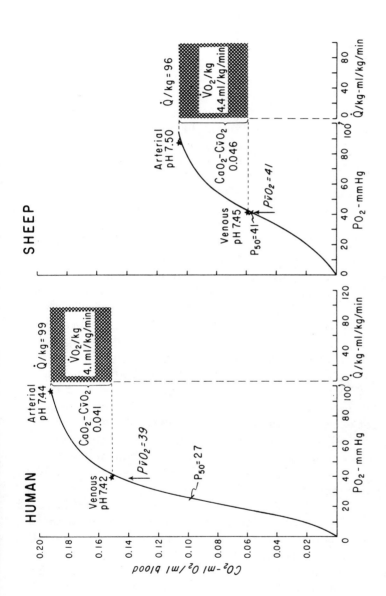

Figure 2. A comparison of blood O_2 transport in resting, unanesthetized sheep and humans. Despite a much lower blood O_2 capacity, sheep supply their peripheral tissues with O_2 at the same rate and over the same average range of O_2 tension as humans do; this is possible because sheep blood has a much lower O_2 affinity ($P_{50}=41$ mm Hg) than human blood ($P_{50}=27$ mm Hg). The O_2 tension in mixed venous blood ($P\bar{v}O_2$) is indicated.

flow and arteriovenous oxygen difference. However, the oxygen concentration in arterial blood of sheep is only half that found in the arterial blood of humans. Despite this natural ovine anemia, the mixed venous oxygen tensions are almost identical in the two species because the dissociation curve of the sheep is much farther to the right than is the human curve; the oxygen tension necessary to half-saturate blood's hemoglobin with oxygen (P_{50}) at a pH of 7.4 and the normal body temperature of each species is 27 mm Hg for the human and 41 mm Hg for our sheep. Because of rightward displacement of the sheep's blood oxygen dissociation curve, 50% of the oxygen in its arterial blood can be extracted at oxygen tensions above 40 mm Hg; in the human only 25% of the oxygen in arterial blood is removed before the oxygen tension falls to 40 mm Hg. Clearly, the sheep has a lower "Blood Reserve" than does the human, unless its tissue can extract oxygen at lower capillary oxygen tensions than human tissues can.

Animals of small body weight have high rates of oxygen consumption per kilogram and Figure 3 compares data for the rabbit with the human data. In this small animal with an average body weight of 1.9 kg, the rate of oxygen consumption is three-fold greater than those of the human and sheep (Korner and Darian Smith, 1954). However, this high oxygen need is again provided to the tissues over a range of capillary P_{O2} which is very similar to that in the two larger species; oxygen tension falls from 90 mm Hg in arterial blood to 38 mm Hg in mixed venous blood (we assumed the pH values shown, because we could find none in the literature). The arteriovenous oxygen concentration difference is 1-1/2 times that in the human and sheep; nevertheless, using blood with an oxygen affinity between the values for human and sheep blood ($P_{50} = 31$) and a blood oxygen capacity which is also intermediate, the same range of capillary oxygen tension is maintained despite a three-fold increase in oxygen delivery. This is accomplished by doubling the cardiac output relative to body size. It seems likely that the rabbit has less "Flow Reserve" than the other two species have, and a "Blood Reserve" which lies between the large one of the human and the small one of the sheep. But, does the sheep have a lower blood oxygen reserve than the human, or does it have, rather, a richer capillary supply? Will the rabbit's response to stress be limited by its high basal cardiac output?

Responses to Anemia

We don't know the answers to these questions, but we have

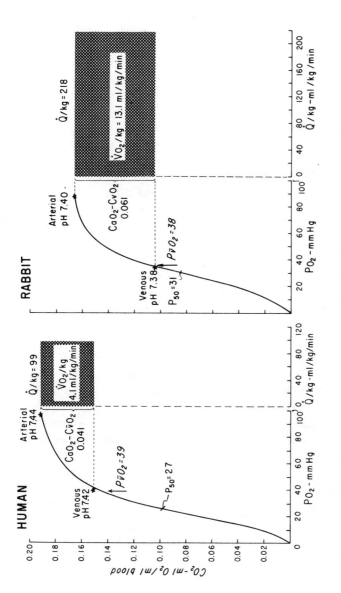

Figure 3. The parameters of blood O_2 transport in resting, unanesthetized humans and rabbits are compared. The rate of O_2 delivery is 3 times larger in rabbits than humans. By doubling the rate of blood flow (per kg of tissue) and increasing the O_2 extraction from blood with a lower O_2 affinity, the rabbit maintains the same range of O_2 tension in "average capillary" blood as do humans and sheep (see Figure 2).

begun to investigate the dimensions of each of the reservoirs of circulating oxygen which have been identified. Our technique, essentially, has been to upset the normal equilibrium by disturbing some component of the system and then to quantify the adjustments which occur in the other components of tissue oxygen supply. I would like to show you data from two species, dog and goat, which have different biochemical responses to anemia.

We chose anemia as the experimental stress because it is easily quantifiable and, to the best of our knowledge, reversible. Moreover, there is already a large literature on several pertinent physiological and biochemical responses of human beings to chronic anemia. Anemia was produced in these laboratory animals by bleeding, on two successive days, of amounts of blood calculated to reduce the circulating red cell mass to 50% or less of its control value; the plasma removed with each of those two initial bleedings was promptly restored to minimize hypovolemia and hypoproteinemia. On subsequent days the anemia was maintained by additional small bleedings. The data presented here reflect the response after days or weeks of sustained anemia without hypovolemia. This integrated response differs quantitatively in its component parts from the immediate response which, in some animals at least, is accompanied by transient acidosis, causing an immediate decrease in blood oxygen affinity.

Figure 4 shows the hemodynamic and hematologic responses which we identified during sustained normovolemic anemia in four of our eight dogs (Dhindsa et al., in preparation). They shifted their blood oxygen dissociation curves an average of 2-1/2 mm Hg to the right (as expressed by the P_{50} value), increased their cardiac outputs by 70%, and maintained the same rate of oxygen delivery to their tissues as before anemia despite a fall in the average mixed venous P_{O_2} of 9 mm Hg. Four other dogs, treated in the same way, did not shift their blood oxygen dissociation curves; their average cardiac output rose to the same degree as the dogs shown in the figure, but because their blood oxygen affinity did not change, their mixed venous oxygen tension fell to a mean of 27 mm Hg, 5 mm Hg lower than the animals shown here.

Unfortunately, organic phosphate concentrations in the erythrocytes of these animals were not measured because of our biochemical ignorance. However, since then we have been deeply impressed with the powers of 2, 3-DPG and are repeating these

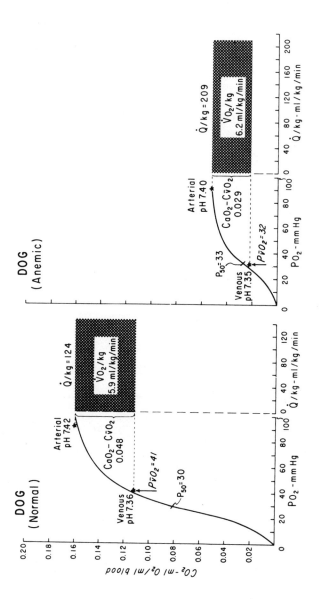

Figure 4. Changes in the dynamics of tissue oxygen supply in four dogs studied at rest and unanesthetized, before and about a week after the production of anemia by bleeding. The rate of oxygen delivery is maintained by an increase in blood flow in the anemic period. In these dogs the blood oxygen affinity fell during anemia (P50 rose from 30 to 33 mm Hg) and P$\bar{v}$O₂ fell to 32 mm Hg; in four other dogs with the same degree of anemia, blood oxygen affinity did not change and P$\bar{v}$O₂ fell to 27 mm Hg.

studies, combining them with simultaneous DPG analyses. But there are other fascinating questions raised by these results; for example, why did only half the dogs lower the oxygen affinity of their blood? Were the others unable to do so? These questions are also worthy of answers, but finding the answers may be difficult.

In learning about DPG we were fascinated by the finding (Harkness et al., 1969) that goat erythrocytes contain it in only minute amounts. Goats are one of our favorite experimental animals (Metcalfe et al., 1968). Furthermore, the protective potential of a lowered blood oxygen affinity in guarding against tissue hypoxia seems to us such an obvious survival advantage that its abandonment by higher animals was unlikely. So, this past summer, our colleague, Don Wodtli, studied their hemodynamic and hematologic responses to anemia produced by bleeding in the same manner as we have already described for dogs. Figure 5 shows a comparison of blood oxygen transport in one animal before anemia and two weeks after anemia was produced. The responses to anemia are qualitatively indistinguishable from those of dogs. However, only negligible concentrations of DPG were detectable in the goats' red cells both during the control period and after the curve had shifted in response to anemia. How, then, do goats accomplish the decrease in blood oxygen affinity which anemic humans seem to produce by increases in erythrocyte DPG concentration? The answer to that question is also being actively sought; but the careful systematic studies of Huisman have shown (Adams et al., 1968; Huisman, et al., 1967; Huisman et al., 1968) that goats shift their primary hemoglobin structure during anemic stress and this seems the likely explanation. The physiological point is that our Pygmy goats, when made anemic, lower their blood oxygen affinity and increase their cardiac output.

SUMMARY

In summary, several biochemical and physiological factors have been defined which modify mean capillary oxygen tension. These variables are used in different combinations by different species to maintain a range of oxygen tension in the "average tissue capillary" which is remarkably similar in several mammals, despite wide variations in their rate of oxygen consumption, blood hemoglobin concentration, and blood oxygen affinity. These generalizations can only be made for resting, unanesthetized individuals.

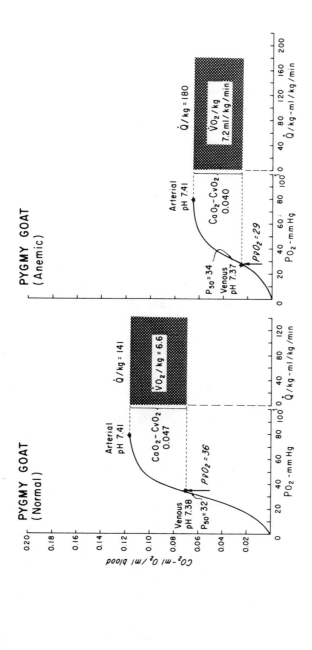

Figure 5. Changes in the dynamics of tissue oxygen supply in one Pygmy goat studied at rest and unanesthetized, before and after two weeks of anemia produced by bleeding.

We have studied the hemodynamic and hematologic responses of dogs and goats to anemia produced by bleeding. In both of these species, as in the human, a lowered blood oxygen affinity is one of the compensatory adjustments to the stress of anemic hypoxia.

ACKNOWLEDGMENT

The work reported in this paper was supported in part by USPHS Training Grant HE 05499 and Research Grant HE 06042 of the National Heart Institute, and by the Oregon Heart Association.

REFERENCES

Adams, H. R., Boyd, E. M., Wilson, J. B., Miller, A. and Huisman, T. H. J. (1968). Arch. Biochem. Biophysics 127: 398.

Bartels, H. (1964). The Lancet 2: 599.

Bartels, H., Beer, R., Fleischer, E., Hoffheinz, H. J., Krall, J., Rodewald, G., Wenner, J. and Witt, I. (1955). Pflügers Arch. Ges. Physiol. 261: 99.

Chance, B., Cohen, P., Jobsis, F. and Schoener, B. (1962). Science 137: 499.

Dhindsa, D. S., Hoversland, A. S., Neill, W. A. and Metcalfe, J. (In preparation).

Harkness, D. R., Ponce, J. and Grayson, V. (1969). Comp. Biochem. Physiol. 28: 129.

Huisman, T. H. J., Adams, H. R., Dimmock, M. O., Edwards, W. E. and Wilson, J. B. (1967). J. Biol. Chem. 242: 2534.

Huisman, T. H. J., Brandt, G. and Wilson, J. B. (1968). J. Biol. Chem. 243: 3675.

Korner, P. I. and Darian Smith, I. (1954). Austral. J. Exptl. Biol. 32: 499.

Krogh, A. (1941). The Comparative Physiology of Respiratory Mechanisms. Dover Publications, Inc., New York.

Metcalfe, J., Hoversland, A. S., Erickson, L. F., Rogers, A. L. and Clary, P. L. (1968). In: Animal Models for Biomedical Research. Publication #1594, National Academy of Science Washington, D. C., pp. 55-63.

Parer, J. T., Jones, W. D. and Metcalfe, J. (1967). Resp. Physiol. 2: 196.

Parer, J. T. and Metcalfe, J. (1967). Nature. 215: 653.

Severinghaus, J. W. (1961). In: Blood and Other Body Fluids., edited by P. L. Altman and D. S. Dittmer. Federation of American Societies for Experimental Biology, Washington, D. C., p. 165.

IV

ERYTHROCYTE FUNCTION AFTER BLOOD STORAGE

SESSION 5 - G. Bartlett, Chairman

PATTERNS OF PHOSPHATE COMPOUNDS IN RED BLOOD CELLS OF MAN AND
ANIMALS

Grant R. Bartlett

Laboratory for Comparative Biochemistry

San Diego, California

For several years the Laboratory for Comparative Biochemistry
has been studying the water-soluble phosphate compounds of the red
blood cells of man and of different animals. The spectrum of phosphates in the red cell has certain distinguishing features as compared to other tissue, but there are large species differences.

Figure 1 shows a fairly typical pattern of water-soluble phosphates present in the fresh normal human erythrocyte. This sample
of blood was collected in heparin at the San Diego Blood Bank,
cooled and processed within an hour. The process involves centrifugation, removal of plasma and white cells and extraction of the
red cells with trichloroacetic acid. The extract is passed through
a column of Dowex 1x8-formate and the adsorbed phosphate compounds
are eluted with a linear gradient increase in the concentration of
ammonium formate buffer, pH 3. The compounds present in the eluate
are detected by phosphorus assay and by their optical density in the
ultraviolet and they are identified by a variety of chemical and
enzymatic tests as well as by their elution position.

As can be seen in Figure 1 the predominating compound is 2,
3-diphosphoglycerate (DPG) which averages about 10 uM (as phosphorus) per ml of red cells. In the following discussion amounts
of compounds will be expressed in terms of their phosphorus content.
The concentration of ATP is relatively high in the human erythrocyte
averaging about 2.5 uM (P) per ml of cells. In this particular
sample of blood the monophosphoglycerate (MPG) is a little higher
than usual and the fructose diphosphate (FDP) a little less. You
will note that eluting between these two compounds is a fairly large
double peak which our Laboratory first identified as the glucose
and mannose 1,6-diphosphates (GDP and MDP). These two sugar diphos-

245

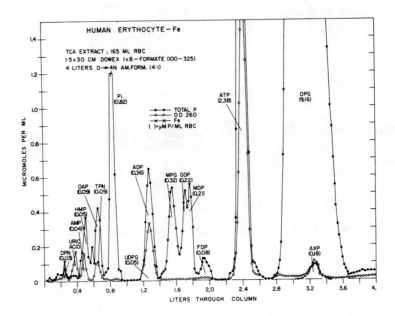

Figure 1

phates have been found to be present in all mammalian red cells so far examined. As far as is known they do not accumulate in such quantities in any other kind of tissue. Red cells in general are characterized by a high ratio of ATP to ADP and of ADP to AMP. They all have in addition only a very small pool of hexose monophosphates.

This recent chromatographic analysis was chosen for presentation here because it includes special information about a compound we call AXP. Although we have been showing this compound in charts of red cell phosphates for many years no progress has been made in its identification – other than the early findings that it contained adenine, ribose and phosphorus – until very recently when we discovered that it also contained iron. Assays for iron were carried out by the dipyridyl method on all fractions of the column eluate and reaction was found only in the AXP peak. The assay indicates that the AXP has close to one atom of ferric iron per mole of adenine. The AXP elutes between the ATP and DPG or sometimes, as in this case, with the DPG. AXP and DPG can be completely separated from each other by rechromatography with Dowex 1-formate at a lower pH. We have found the AXP to be present in all mammalian erythrocytes examined in a concentration ranging form 0.2 to 1.0 uM per ml of RBC.

The phosphate compounds of the human erythrocyte change greatly during the storage of blood in ACD in the cold under the usual blood-banking conditions as shown in the next chromatograph (Figure 2)

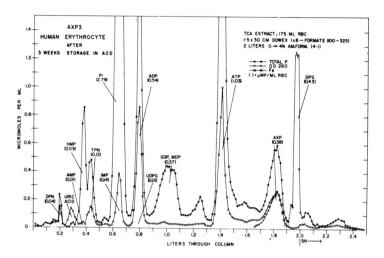

Figure 2

describing red cells stored for three weeks. There is a precipitous
fall in the concentration of DPG, in this particular case to about
5% of the original. The ATP drops during this period of storage to
from one half to one third of the level in the fresh cell. ADP does
not decrease and AMP is variably higher. No FDP is present, but GDP
and MDP remain unchanged. An interesting feature of the stored cells
at this stage is the rather marked elevation in the concentration of
the hexosemonophosphates. Inosinic acid (IMP) and inorganic phosphate (Pi), which elute together, are greatly increased.

This chromatographic assay was made a few days ago in order to
obtain more of the iron nucleotide for further structural study.
Analyses for iron were carried out on all eluate fractions and were
positive only in the peak indicated. The AXP does not decrease in
concentration during the first few weeks of storage of the human
red cell in ACD.

Figure 3 represents a chromatograph of red cells from human
blood which had been stored in ACD at 4° for four weeks. The ATP
is down to about 20% of the original, DPG has almost disappeared
and the pool of AXP is now larger than that of ATP.

Old stored human red cells can synthesize a large amount of organic phosphate if they are incubated with inosine and adenine as
shown in Figure 4. Red cells which had been stored in ACD for four
weeks were separated from plasma and preservative and incubated in
saline-phosphate containing inosine and adenine for 3 hours at 38°.
The TCA extract of the cells was chromatographed as usual. There
was a large accumulation of FDP and of the diphosphates of the 7
and 8-carbon keto-sugars, sedoheptulose (SDP) and octulose (ODP).

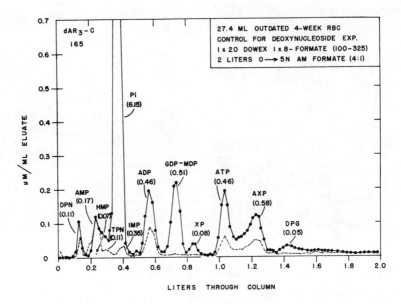

Figure 3

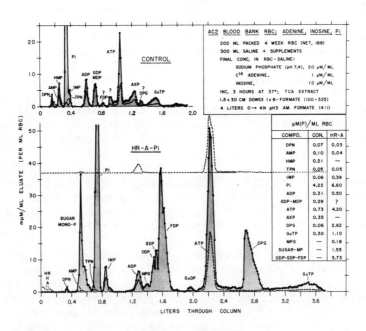

Figure 4

The sugar monophosphate elution area contained octulose, sedoheptulose, glucose, fructose, ribose, ribulose and xylulose monophosphates. There was a considerable resynthesis of DPG and, most striking, an increase of the ATP to a level exceeding that present in the fresh cell. When inosine alone was incubated with stored cells of the same age there was a similar snythesis of the various organic phosphates except for the ATP which increased only slightly due to phosphorylation of preexisting ADP. When adenine alone was used nothing happened.

As most of you know if adenine is present with ACD from the outset of the storage of human blood there is a delayed breakdown of total adenine nucleotide of the red cells with a resulting improvement in their viability.

We have isolated phosphate compounds by ion-exchange column chromatography from the red cells of several mammals and of a few non-mammalian vertebrates.

The phosphate pattern of the porpoise red cell was found to be more like the human than any of the other animals studied (Figure 5).

The erythrocytes of some animals were found to contain twice as much DPG as the human. The rabbit is one example (Figure 6). The rabbit red cell has the highest concentration of ATP we have seen in the mammals, about double that in man.

The red cells of the rat and mouse also have a very high level

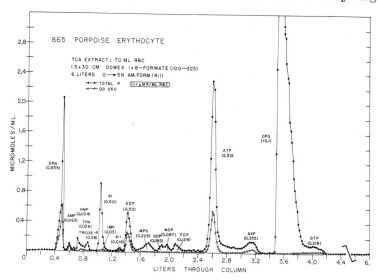

Figure 5

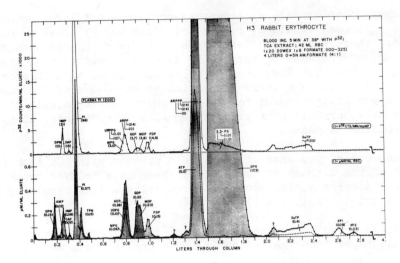

Figure 6

of DPG (Figure 7). These two rodents give very similar chromato-
grams except for a lower content of ATP in the rat. Both are characterized by their high concentration of fructose diphosphate and
triose phosphate.

The pig too has a very high concentration of DPG in it's red
cells and also large amounts of ATP (Figure 8). However the erythrocytes of this animal are peculiar in that they do not metabolize
glucose. The source of energy for maintaining a relatively high
turnover of ATP is not known. We have studied the pig red cell in

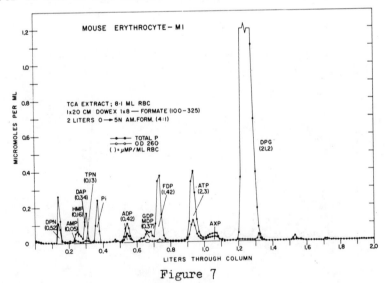

Figure 7

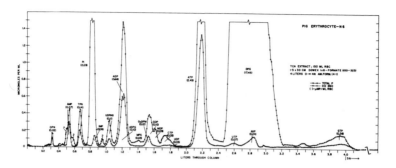

Figure 8

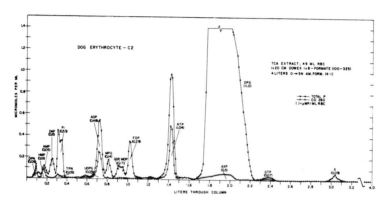

Figure 9

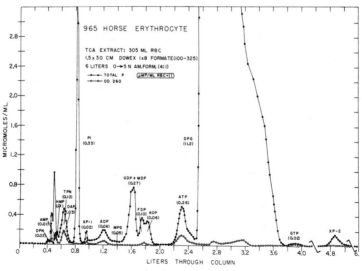

Figure 10

collaboration with Dr. Hyun-dju Kim, who has just completed his doc-
toral research on this subject with Dr. Thom McManus at Duke University. Red cells of the pecary and of the wild boar were compared
with the domestic hog and found to be very similar to each other.
Neonate pig red cells, which can utilize glucose, were found to contain low DPG, very high ATP, FDP and the hexose monophosphates. No
sugar phosphates (other than the GDP and MDP) were present in the
adult red cell.

The erythrocytes of dog and horse have about the same amount
of DPG as in man, but much less ATP (Figures 9 and 10). The horse
has only about 0.5 uM of ATP phosphorus per ml of RBC, one fifth of
that present in the human cell. The cats which we have examined
have had very low concentrations of both DPG and ATP in their red
cells (Figure 11).

The erythrocytes of the ruminants, cow and sheep, also had a
low concentration of both DPG and ATP (Figures 12 and 13). The
cow red cell is of special interest because of it's high concentration of uric acid riboside and ribotide, compounds not present in
any other species.

We have looked at the red blood cells of a few of the non-mammalian vertebrates by the same analytical techniques. These cells
are quite different histologically than in the mammals. They are,
in general, much larger, ovoid in shape rather than biconcave dis-
coid and possess a nucleus as well as other cellular organelles.

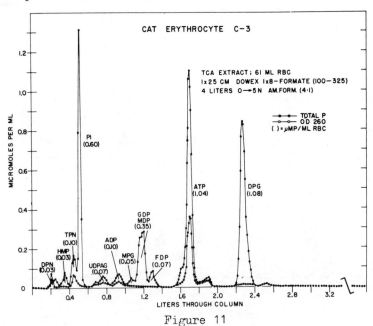

Figure 11

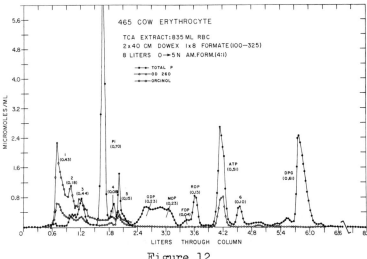

Figure 12

Erythrocytes from the pigeon, chicken and pelican proved to be remarkably alike in their patterns of water-soluble phosphates except for a lower concentration of ATP in the chicken. The chromatogram from the pigeon is shown as an example (Figure 14). There is a very high concentration of inositol hexaphosphate, a compound found to be characteristic of the bird red cell by Rapoport many years ago. Distinguishing features of the bird red cells, in addition to the inositol phosphate, were high ATP, low sugar phosphate, lack of DPG and substantial pools of UDPG, UDPAG, CTP, UTP, GTP and an unidentified guanine nucleotide.

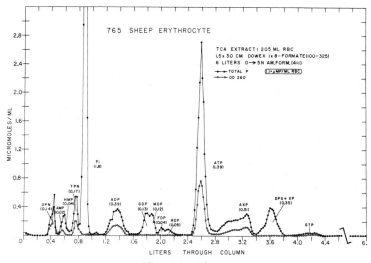

Figure 13

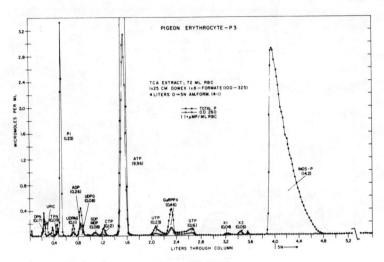

Figure 14

The frog was selected as the most readily available example of the amphibians (Figure 15). The frog red cells had a very high concentration of ATP and considerable pools of pyridine nucleotide, UDPG, UDPAG, UTP, CTP, and GTP. The sugar phosphates were very low, but there was a relatively large amount of DPG.

The red cells of the green sea turtle and of the snapping turtle were studied as examples of the reptilians (Figure 16). These

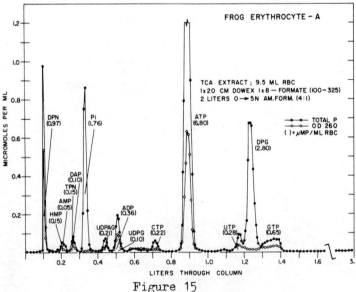

Figure 15

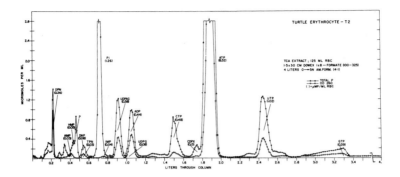

Figure 16

two were very similar to each other and much like the frog except that only a trace of DPG was found.

Figure 17 and 18 show how the concentrations of ATP and DPG varied in the red cells of man and the different animals studied. There appear to be no easily identifiable environmental or genetic factors which might determine the concentrations of these two substances in the red cell. For those of you who would like to relate the phosphate concentration of the red cell to it's oxygen transport capabilities, these figures should provide an interesting challenge.

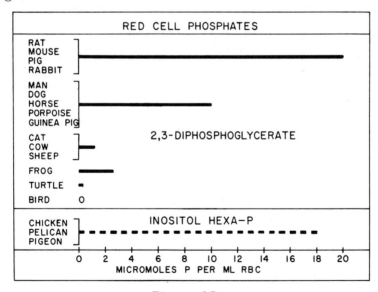

Figure 17

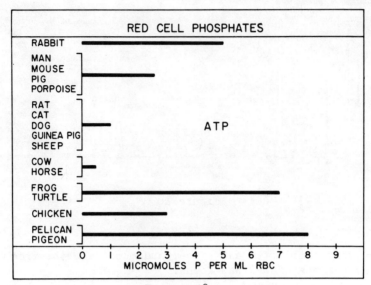

Figure 18

The following reference concerning ATP-iron complexes has recently come to our attention:

Konopke, K., Leyko, W., Gondko, R., Sidorczyk, Z., Fabjanowska, Z. and Swedowska, N.: Clin. Chim. Acta. 24,359, 1969.

BIOLOGICAL ALTERATIONS OCCURRING DURING RED CELL PRESERVATION

LTC Charles E. Shields, MC, Harold S. Kaplan, M.D.*
MAJ Roy B. Dawson, Jr., MC

Blood Transfusion Division, US Army Medical Research
Laboratory, Fort Knox, Kentucky 40121
*Washington University School of Medicine, St. Louis,
Missouri 63110

Removal of the red blood cell from the normal circulation drastically alters its external environment, depriving the cell of necessary nutrients as well as removing certain protective factors. To counter the loss of nutrient, various blood collecting solutions have been devised in which glucose is used to supply the cell with an energy source. At the same time, attempts are made to reduce cellular metabolism, hence cell demand for energy, usually by using solutions of low pH and/or mechanical factors, that of cooling the blood. The combination of a slower metabolism and a glucose supplement have permitted most storage of red cells in a useful state for perhaps 20-30 days (1,2,3).

Despite the practical value of these storage solutions, the removal and storage process combined with the natural loss of the oldest cells to the aging process lead to progressive decrease throughout storage in the number of red cells remaining in a functional state (1,2,3). The total breakdown of the cell is not necessarily apparent or immediate; however, certain changes can be detected as they increase with longer storage. The rate of the increase of these adverse changes can be altered in different collection solutions or under various storage conditions (1-6). Since the maintenance of intact red blood cells appeared to be the primary goal, measurements of the degree of red cell preservation have concentrated upon those reflecting the degree of hemolysis. Unfortunately, the measurement of hemolysis has not been found to correlate very well with the ability of the cell to remain in the circulation after transfusion (1-10).

257

Table 1.

Biochemical Changes in Stored Blood

	Days Stored						
	0	7	14	21	28	35	42
Hemoglobin mg/%	9.5 ± 3	21.7 ± 3	33.0 ± 4	73 ± 10	84 ± 29	144 ± 23	174 ± 28
Sodium mEq/L	145 ± 3	149 ± 4	154 ± 4	147 ± 4	151 ± 7	145 ± 6	146 ± 7
Potassium mEq/L	4 ± 1	9 ± 1	17 ± 1	23 ± 1	30 ± 2	37 ± 2	46 ± 3
Hematocrit %	44 ± 1	43 ± 1	43 ± 1	41 ± 1	41 ± 1	40 ± 2	38 ± 2
Os Fragility %	17 ± .5	16 ± .5	16 ± 1.0	14 ± 1.0	12 ± 1.5	12 ± 1.5	8 ± 2.0
Slope	.87 ± .05	.72 ± .08	.69 ± .08	.60 ± .08	.51 ± .12	.39 ± .07	.31 ± .10
pH units	6.89 ± .02	6.85 ± .03	6.80 ± .03	6.79 ± .03	6.64 ± .04	6.65 ± .04	6.61 ± .04
ATP mg/%	27.4 ± 1.5	20.3 ± 1.5	14.2 ± 1.7	15.2 ± 2.0	14.2 ± 2.0	12.3 ± 2.3	7.7 ± 2.5
2,3 DPG μM/ml	2.80 ± .1	1.25 ± .2	.26 ± .2	.09 ± .1	.10 ± .1	.10 ± .1	.10 ± .1
RBC cnts x 10^6	4.7 ± .1	4.3 ± .1	4.2 ± .1	4.1 ± .1	4.0 ± .2	3.8 ± .2	3.3 ± .3
MCV micron^3	97 ± 3	96 ± 3	101 ± 4	103 ± 5	101 ± 5	97 ± 5	101 ± 5
Cholesterol mg/%	270 ± 40	280 ± 40	250 ± 30	245 ± 40	270 ± 30	260 ± 20	240 ± 40
Bilirubin mg/%	.8 ± .2	.9 ± .2	1.0 ± .2	.9 ± .1	.8 ± .3	.9 ± .3	1.0 ± .3
G6PD units/gm hgb	4.97 ± 1.2	5.71 ± 1.5	6.66 ± 1.0	6.62 ± 1.5	5.74 ± 1.5	5.34 ± 1.2	4.76 ± 1.5
GSH mg/100 ml rbc	47.3 ± 5.0	45.1 ± 5.0	42.9 ± 7.5	46.0 ± 5.5	45.6 ± 6.7	41.0 ± 8.5	53.3 ± 10.5
ACHase units/mg hgb	134 ± 4	130 ± 3	127 ± 4	135 ± 4	130 ± 4	124 ± 5	122 ± 5
SGOT units/gm hgb	3478	3185	3084	3050	----	2610	2280
SGPT units/gm hgb	227	251	240	218	273	---	261
HKase units/gm hgb	40.0 ± 2	40 ± 2	46 ± 2	44 ± 3	28 ± 7	29 ± 7	23 ± 8
ATPase Δ O.D.	.151	.172	.162	.141	.130	.140	.095
ADase Δ O.D.	.172	.162	.155	.111	.115	.089	.121

The difficulty in assessing function by chemical means was further complicated after recent studies on biochemical changes during storage. In these experiments, alteration of storage conditions was employed to determine possible significant factors. Because of the importance of temperature control, particularly involving cellular metabolism, and because of problems in protecting blood against temperature variation during blood shipment, a series of experiments was set up in which blood was stored for selected time periods at various temperatures. Mechanical agitation was added as another variable commonly encountered in blood shipments. It was recognized that the mechanical buffeting occurring in the normal vascular system was not critically damaging to the normal red cell; however, the stored cell might be considered more vulnerable because of the absence of various defenses inherent in the *in vivo* circulation.

Methods and Materials

Throughout the experiments, blood was collected from healthy normal males in acid-citrate-dextrose (ACD). These units were stored for various periods up through 42 days. Samples were at weekly intervals when taken. The usual tests consisted of measuring free hemoglobin in the plasma, sodium, and potassium. Hematocrit and red cell osmotic fragility were obtained. In the final phase, red cell oxygen function and 2,3-diphosphoglycerate (2,3-DPG) levels were determined in addition.

The overall effect of the storage process was also examined in more detail on a series of nine units. These were sampled weekly over 42 days of storage. Tests included hematocrit, red blood cell count, and a calculated mean corpuscular volume. Chemical tests in addition to the above included: total cholesterol, bilirubin, glucose-6-phosphate dehydrogenase (G6PD), glutathione (GSH), acetylcholinesterase (ACHase), serum glutamic-oxaloacetic transaminase (SGOT), serum glutamic pyruvic transaminase (SGPT), hexokinase (HKase), adenosine triphosphate (ATP), and ATPase, aldolase (ADase), as well as electrophoretic mobility and pH.

In the study designed to determine the effects of warming the blood, temperatures were selected as follows: 4°C as control, with 10°C and 22°C as variables. One group was exposed to the 4° temperature throughout storage. The other groups were exposed to either temperature for periods of 1, 2, 14, 16, or 24 hours and then returned to 4° for subsequent storage. The exposures were also repeated at weekly intervals. The mechanical agitation consisted of one hour on a mechanical shaker at weekly intervals, with and without warming.

The final phase involved comparison between units that had

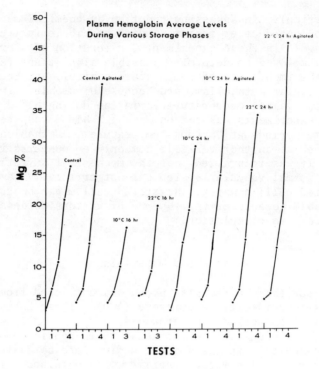

Figure 1

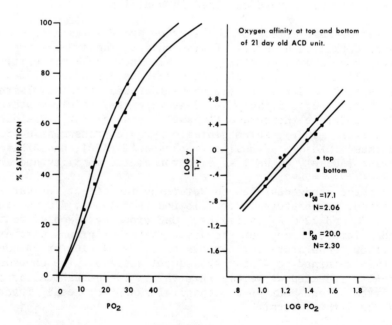

Figure 2

been stored undisturbed in a vertical position and units stored
and mixed. The units left undisturbed were sampled after the red
blood cells had settled. Each unit was sampled for red cell tests
in two areas, with one area being the red cells removed from the
layer at 2 cm above the bottom of the unit, and the second area
being red cells removed from a layer 2 cm down from the top of the
sedimented cell portion. These were then analyzed as the top and
bottom red cell portions of the unit. The controls for this group
were units that had been stored in either full units that were
mixed prior to sampling, or as units with most of the plasma removed. These control units were stored undisturbed between intervals of sampling, and mixed only prior to the sampling procedure.

Results

Long periods of storage at 4°C were associated with progressive loss of hemoglobin and potassium from the red blood cell,
along with decreased resistance of the cell to hypotonic saline.
Decrease in oxygen carrying function, as well as decreased levels
of 2,3-DPG, occurred during the storage periods.

The first tables indicate the changes in the multiple chemicals and enzymes analyzed in detail during 42 days of storage.
Despite the depth of analysis, the changes were seldom significant
except in the case of the pH, plasma hemoglobin, ATP, sodium, potassium, 2,3-DPG, osmotic fragility, and oxygen carrying capacity.
Because the demands of a blood bank for a screening test must include simplicity and usefulness within the range of technicians
and equipment available, subsequent studies concentrated on the
more obvious tests of hemolysis.

The rate of change in degree of hemolysis during early storage was similar in whole blood units or packed cell units exposed
to warmer temperatures or to mechanical agitation early in storage. However, by the third period of storage or over 21 days
since collection, most of the tests had levels higher than the
controls. The appearance of free hemoglobin was more obvious in
the units warmed to 22°C with and without mechanical agitation,
with significant differences being present after 28 days of storage (Fig. 1). Generally, exposure of less than 16 hours did not
lead to consistent changes in the rate of damage, but over 16 hours
of exposure did lead to increased damage. Comparison of the whole
units to the packed cell units was similar, though the packed cell
units (Table 2) had higher levels of free hemoglobin and potassium,
and had more susceptibility to osmotic lysis throughout the study.
The changes were greater than calculated from the dilution effect
of plasma suggesting that the plasma did have some protective effect.

Table 2.   Packed Cell Study

	Plasma Hemoglobin (mg/100 ml)				Hematocrit (%)		
	WB		PC		WB		PC
	Cont	Ag	Cont	Ag		Cont	Ag
Pre	3.0	4.1	316	1611	42	69	69
Day 21	5.1	6.5	580	3153	42	68	71
Day 28	10.8	13.7	856	4580	41	68	71

WB - whole blood
PC - packed erythrocytes
Cont - control
Ag - agitated

The settling of red cells during static storage was apparently involved in changing the external environment of the stored cell.   In Table 3 the differences in the electrolyte concentration of the upper and lower layers of settled red cells indicate significant alteration in concentration in the plasma and, by calculation, within the cell.   The increase of potassium in the supernatant plasma with longer storage follows the expected change with storage, but the ratio of the differences between the plasma and intracellular values between top and bottom layers is significantly different.   As seen in Table 3, the top layer has been able to maintain a definite gradient, while apparently the bottom layer is nearly in equilibrium with the external environment.   The capability to maintain a differential in salt concentration would imply that active metabolic processes are present with the bottom layer having less effective activity.   The lower concentration of glucose in the extracellular plasma from the bottom layer was significantly different from the top layer and may imply more metabolic requirement for an energy source.   Differences in blood urinary nitrogen were not marked and this metabolic system was apparently unaffected by the layering effect.   The differences in osmotic fragility were not as marked, however, though changes in the percent hemolysis were significant (Table 4).

Table 3.

Electrolyte Values of Stored Blood at Various Levels*

	Glucose mg% 21-22 da. n=10	BUN mEq/L	Sodium mEq/L		Potassium mEq/L		Ratio $\frac{Intra}{Extra}$ Na	Ratio $\frac{Extra}{Intra}$ K
			Fresh n=10	21-23 da. n=17	Fresh n=10	21-23 da. n=17		
Plasma Supernatant	344 ± 7 **	6.9 ± .3	165.6 ± .6	165.2 ± 2.2	3.3 ± .1 **	12.1 ± .4 **		
Extracell Top	270 ± 6 **	6.9 ± .3		150 ± 2.7 **		30 ± 1.1 **	15.9 ± 1.6	
Bottom	213 ± 6 **	6.8 ± .3		117 ± 1.1 **		60 ± 1.2 **	22.2 ± 1.2	
Intracell Mixed			9.2 ± .8		92.9 ± .5			
Top				25.6 ± 1.3		63 ± .9 **		49 ± 2.5
Bottom				26.1 ± .9		70 ± .8 **		85 ± 2.8

*Average ± standard deviation of mean

**Comparisons significant (p < .001)

Table 4

Spontaneous Hemolysis in Different
Regions of 21-23 Day Stored Blood

Location	% Hemolysis $\overline{X} \pm SDM$	Hematocrit $\overline{X} \pm SDM$
Top	0.74±0.07*	67%±1*
Bottom	0.38±0.03*	85%±.5*

*p<.001

Whether the cell was metabolically active enough to resist lysis
was not as critical as the detectable loss of ability of the top
layer cells to carry out oxygen function. The altered oxygen affinity or shift to the left was associated with lowered DPG levels
as well. These changes in oxygen curves have been shown graphically, both in the usual form and in a linear transformation using
log ratios (Fig. 2).

Discussion

Transfusion therapy with whole blood has the two major functions of replacing vascular volume and oxygen carrying capacity.
The latter function has been found to be dependent upon hemoglobin
activity. Hemoglobin in the red blood cell has been found to have
a relationship with the metabolic activity in two areas. First,
the red cell must maintain a satisfactory internal and cell wall
function, so as to retain the hemoglobin within the cell. Second,
more recently, the internal pathways involving particularly ATP
and 2,3-DPG have been found to relate to the ability of the hemoglobin to handle the oxygen (3,7,8).

Traditionally, blood bank personnel have used the red color
of the plasma caused by the escape of hemoglobin from the cell as
a sign of a damaged unit. As a simple screening test, it has some
value; however, some degree of hemolysis can be seen in many units
with some of these still able to be tolerated by the recipient
after a transfusion. Tests measuring other chemicals and red cell
function were devised to improve the detection of the borderline
or unusable unit. Many of these tests were found to be too complex for practical blood banking, and the tests did not necessarily correlate with tests devised to measure the function of the
stored cells in the recipient (1-6).

Despite these drawbacks, the present series of studies employed several tests to indicate damage during storage under various physical stresses. The experimental units were compared to controls and differences in rate of appearance of the changes previously associated with damage were considered signs that the experimental variable did have an adverse effect. Changes did occur under stress in many of the tests; however, the plasma hemoglobin remained the most sensitive of the purely chemical type tests.

The particular effect of heat on the red blood cell has been observed in several studies (9,10,11), indicating that exposure to temperatures in excess of 40°C can produce sufficient damage to result in sequesteration in the reticuloendothelial system of the recipient after transfusion. At the other extreme, exposure to cold sufficient to involve the internal cell water can lead to lysis of the cell wall. Storage in the cold between these two extremes has been helpful in blood banking. Cold storage can slow the metabolism which results in less energy demand and substrate expenditure. A secondary effect is the reduction in the rate of growth of bacteria accidentally included in the unit. Present mechanical refrigeration resources are sufficiently accurate to permit storage of the blood just above the critical freezing point and without excessive temperature variation. In contrast to the mechanical ability to maintain a temperature range between 3-6°C, blood being shipped by other means (such as wet ice) is exposed to more variability, and hence must have a wider temperature tolerance of 4-10°C. To add to the blood bank problems, the practical problem created in many hospitals, in which the physician asks that the unit be warmed prior to transfusion, must be considered. Warming to room temperature is still reasonably below the critically hot temperature, but if this is done frequently, or for long periods, it may have an adverse effect (9).

The present study, using blood in whole units and as packed red cells stored for periods through 28 days, used temperature and mechanical agitation as variables. During the course of storage, all units had signs of gradual damage, including the experimental units early in storage. However, after 15 days of storage, more marked effects were noted with the 22°C temperature when exposure to this temperature was 16 hours or longer. Mechanical agitation, though increasing the damage, had more effect in the packed units and later in storage.

Though the appearance of potassium and free hemoglobin in the plasma was considered a sign of cell damage, there did not seem to be any particular product present in the plasma that aggravated storage damage, though this has been considered possible in the earlier literature (1,3,4). The changes in the packed cell units were more marked at all stages compared to the full units, suggesting that the plasma did provide some protection during storage.

Further analysis of these differences was carried out in units left undisturbed. Samples taken from the top and bottom layers of the sedimented cells were found to have significant differences in various chemical concentrations. An electrolyte gradient was being maintained, implying that both layers did have active homeostatic mechanisms which required energy. Possibly the ability of the top layer to maintain a greater gradient than the bottom layer would indicate that the top layer was more active, hence requiring more energy, or that the cell population was in some way better able to handle the electrolyte gradient. In contrast, measurement of oxygen function showed that the top layer had a greater shift to the left of the oxygen dissociation curve. Perhaps the shift in the curve may reflect an energy pattern, in which the cell resources have been diverted to maintain one cell function at the expense of another. Hence, there is a possibility that oxygen function may be more complexly related to total metabolic function and/or the actual electrolyte concentration. In prior storage studies, a definite decrease in oxygen function has been observed in well-mixed units, and these changes have often been related to decreasing levels of 2,3-DPG (3,7,8,12). These findings tend to broaden the interrelationships of red cell function and metabolism and represent areas of concern in the development of satisfactory preservation of bank blood.

Summary

Chemical analysis of blood stored was studied under a variety of environmental stresses. These stresses accentuated changes resulting from storage. The changes occurred in units already in storage for at least two weeks, under stress of temperatures of 22°C, with and without mechanical agitation. Units of packed red cells had similar effects of a slightly greater magnitude.

Units left undisturbed and sampled from the top and bottom layers of the sedimented cells showed different electrolyte distribution. In addition, the layers had different oxygen carrying capacity, which may have been related to the changes in biochemical or electrolyte balance.

Acknowledgment

The studies presented represent joint efforts of several laboratories. We are grateful for the enzyme and biochemical data done in detail, which represents work done under Dr. Frank DeVenuto, and Dr. W. F. Kocholaty, Director of the Biochemistry Division.

References

1. Mollison, P.L.: Blood Transfusion in Clinical Medicine.
    Philadelphia, F.A. Davis Co., 4th ed., 1967.

2. Strumia, M.M., W. H. Crosby, J. G. Gibson, II, T. J.
    Greenwalt, and J. R. Krevans: General Principles of Blood
    Transfusion. From Transfusion, by National Academy of
    Science, 1963.

3. Bartlett, G. R.: Influence of glucose and nucleoside metab-
    olism on viability of erythrocytes during storage. Arch.
    Intern. Med. 106: 234, 1960.

4. Rapoport, S.: Dimensional, osmotic, and chemical changes of
    erythrocytes in stored blood. I. Blood preserved in sodium
    citrate, neutral, and acid-citrate-glucose (ACD) mixtures.
    J. Clin. Invest. 26: 591, 1947.

5. Strumia, M.M., A. D. Blake, Jr., and W. A. Wicks: The pre-
    servation of whole blood. J. Clin. Invest. 26: 667, 1947.

6. Shields, C.E.: Comparison studies of whole blood stored in
    ACD and CPD and with adenine. Transfusion, 8: 1, 1968.

7. Sugita, Y., and A. Chanutin: Electrophoretic studies of red
    cell hemolysates supplemented with phosphorylated carbohy-
    drate intermediates. Proc. Soc. Exp. Bio. 112: 72, 1963.

8. Chanutin, A., and R. R. Curnish: Factors influencing the
    electrophoretic patterns of red cell hemolysates analyzed
    in cacodylate buffers. Arch. Biochem. Biophys. 106: 433,
    1964.

9. Gibson, J. G., II, T. Sack, R. D. Evans, and W. C. Peacock:
    The effect of varying temperatures on the posttransfusion
    survival of whole blood during depot storage and after trans-
    portation by land and air. J. Clin. Invest. 26: 747, 1947.

10. Ham, T. H., S. C. Shen, E. M. Fleming, and W. B. Castle:
    Studies on the destruction of red blood cells. IV. Thermal
    injury: Action of heat in causing increased spheroidicity,
    osmotic and mechanical fragilities and hemolysis of erythro-
    cytes in dogs and in a patient with a fatal thermal burn.
    Blood, 3: 373, 1948.

11. Baar, S.: Osmotic resistance of heat-damaged erythrocytes.
    J. Clin. Path. 20: 239, 1967.

12. Dawson, R.B., Jr., W. F. Kocholaty, C. E. Shields, T. J.
     Ellis, and E. Bowles-Ledford: The hemoglobin function of
     blood stored at 4°C. USAMRL Lab. Rept., in press.

THE PREDICTION OF POSTSTORAGE RED CELL VIABILITY FROM ATP LEVELS *

Raymond J. Dern

Department of Medicine, Loyola University
Stritch School of Medicine, and the Department of
Hematology of the Hektoen Institute for Medical Research
Chicago, Illinois

Of the many chemical and physical changes that occur in blood
during storage, [1-5] the poststorage erythrocyte adenosine
triphosphate (ATP) level has the highest reported correlation with
poststorage erythrocyte red cell viability (R = 0.94).[6-8]
Although the correlation was great enough to be of predictive
value for the regression, it was obviously not applicable to the
estimation of expected cell viability from the ATP data for an
individual unit of stored blood. Furthermore, the study was
limited to blood which had been stored in acid-citrate-dextrose
(ACD) U.S.P. formula A, or in citrate-phosphate-dextrose (CPD)[8]
solutions for either 21 or 28 days. The studies reported herein
were undertaken for two primary reasons: (1) to expand the total
number of cases and the experimental conditions of blood storage,
and (2) to evaluate possible applications of the relationship.

MATERIALS AND METHODS

Using conventional blood bank techniques, 450 ml of blood
was withdrawn from each of 158 young, healthy, adult male
volunteers into plastic bags of the commercial type. The anticoagulants used were solutions of acid-citrate-dextrose (ACD)
U.S.P. formula A, citrate-phosphate-dextrose (CPD), or ACD-
adenine (ACD-Ad). ACD-Ad was prepared to provide 0.5 micromoles
of adenine per ml of blood. The duration of subsequent storage
at 4 ± 1°C is indicated by the number following the symbol

*Supported by Research Grant AM-09919, from the National Institute
of Arthritis and Metabolic Diseases.

indicating the anticoagulant, e.g., ACD-Ad-35 represents blood which had been stored for 35 days in ACD-adenine solution before testing.

Storage conditions were of two types. In the "standard" protocol, (136 cases) the blood was stored according to conventional blood bank techniques with the exception that, at the midpoint of the storage period, the blood was mixed and an aliquot removed for bacteriological study. After the storage period, the in vivo red cell viability was determined by reinfusion of a Cr-51 tagged aliquot of the stored blood into the donor. The numbers of tests, by type of bag, were: ACD-21, 55; CPD-21, 17; CPD-28, 42; ACD-Ad-35, 8; ACD-Ad-42, 14. In another group of 44 studies, a different protocol was followed ("experimental"), in which each unit of blood was divided into two subunits at the time of phlebotomy. Subsequently, one of the pair was stored motionless while the other was mixed from three to five times weekly for the duration of the storage period. The viability of the erythrocytes from each of the two subunits was measured in compatible recipients by Cr-51 tagged aliquots. The numbers of cases were: ACD-21, 8; CPD-28, 22 and ACD-Ad-42, 14.

Poststorage erythrocyte survivals were measured both by a modification of the blood volume method described by Button, Gibson, and Walter,[9] and by the extrapolation procedure, using the red cell activities of the 5, 15 and 25 minute postinfusion samples extrapolated to zero time as a measure of V_{100}.[10] Red cell survival is defined as the RBC Cr-51 activity remaining 24 hours after injection, expressed as a percentage of the infused RBC activity. Erythrocyte ATP levels (expressed as micromoles per gram hemoglobin) were determined by the firefly technique.[11] In all cases, the ATP concentration was measured immediately before injection of the Cr-51 tagged aliquot.

In order to estimate the technical error, the viability of red cells from each of 19 units of stored blood was measured simultaneously in 2 compatible recipients. The precision of ATP measurement was evaluated from duplicate determinations on 25 different samples of stored blood. A study was also made of the effects of the time at which the ATP level was measured; in 20 studies, estimation of ATP was made both immediately after removal of the blood from the 4°C refrigerator and again after 1 hour at room temperature (for Cr-51 tagging), immediately before the aliquot was injected into the recipient for in vivo red cell viability measurement.

The methods for data analysis have been described in detail in an earlier communication.[8] In summary, calculations were made with the appropriately programmed IBM 7094 computer. Curves of the quadratic form were fitted to the data by the method of least squares regression, and those of the exponential form, by the use of the BMD-06R program.[12] Prediction of variability and inter-comparison of the individual curves for different anticoagulants and durations of storage were based on methods utilizing orthogonal polynomials.[8,13] The 0.70 red cell viability point on the regression curve was arbitrarily selected for computation of confidence intervals in view of the practical significance of that region of the curve. A poststorage red cell survival of 70 percent is accepted as the minimal point for acceptance of stored blood for use in human transfusion.

RESULTS

The gross configuration of the data by graphic plot of poststorage ATP levels versus red cell viability resembled that previously reported,[8] except that the curve appeared somewhat flatter in the middle region. This was reflected by failure of attempts to fit an exponential curve to the data by the BMD-06R program, the coefficients failing to converge to an equation of the from $a + b \rho^{ATP}$. When a curve of the quadratic form was fitted, the equation yielded was:

Poststorage RBC viability = $0.131 + 0.389 (ATP) - 0.051 (ATP)^2$ where (ATP) is the red cell ATP level measured at the time when the blood was injected for the erythrocyte viability determination.

From the data of Table I, it is evident that the multiple correlation coefficients (R) are lower for the present data than reported previously, but the 0.95 confidence intervals were similar in both studies. This is probably due to an increase in the variance in ATP levels with the increased amount of data available at the extreme ends of the curve. When viability was measured by the extrapolation procedure, in contrast to 'the blood volume method, there was a trend toward higher correlation coefficients (Table I, method B vs. A), but the confidence intervals were similar for both techniques of viability measurement.

Individual curves for different anticoagulants and experimental conditions were tested against the hypothesis that all curves are the same. The hypothesis was accepted ($p > 0.10$) for ACD-21 vs. ACD-28, for CPD-21 vs. CPD-28, for ACD-Ad-35 vs. ACD-Ad-42, and for standard vs. experimental protocols. However, it was rejected ($p < .02$) for the comparison of ACD vs. CPD, ACD vs. ACD-Ad, and CPD vs. ACD-Ad. With respect to the different anticoagulants, this indicates that the curve for the pooled data is a composite of the three separate curves. It should be noted, however, that consideration of the curves individually does not

Table I. Multiple correlation coefficients and 0.95 confidence intervals for quadratic regression of poststorage ATP levels on poststorage red cell viability.

	No. of cases	Multiple correlation coef. R	Multiple correlation coef. R^2	0.95 confidence interval at 0.70 (70% RBC viability) for regression	0.95 confidence interval at 0.70 (70% RBC viability) for individual
Previous data[7]	37	0.93	0.86	± 0.03	± 0.10
Current data					
Method A					
Standard	126	0.83	0.69	± 0.013	± 0.09
Experimental	44	0.84	0.71	± 0.021	± 0.12
Pooled	170	0.82	0.69	± 0.011	± 0.11
Method B					
Standard	136	0.90	0.81	± 0.012	± 0.12
Experimental	44	0.82	0.68	± 0.017	± 0.15
Pooled	180	0.87	0.76	± 0.021	± 0.13
Subsets (standard)					
ACD-21	55	0.79	0.63	± 0.018	± 0.10
CPD-21,28	59	0.92	0.84	± 0.015	± 0.13
ACD-Ad-35,42	22	0.93	0.87	± 0.012	± 0.08

The red cell viability, in almost all cases, was measured both by the independent blood volume method (A) and by the extrapolation procedure (B).

result in narrower confidence intervals (Table I, subsets), and accordingly, there is no gain in considering the curves individually rather than as a composite.

In the comparison of the results of duplicate estimates of cell viability from 19 different units of stored blood, the variance of the difference was 8.22×10^{-4}. This accounts for approximately 20 to 25 percent of the residual error after fitting the regression equation. Technical errors in measurement of ATP levels account for an additional 1 percent (approx.) of the residual error. The mean increase in ATP level, during the one hour preinjection incubation period, was 0.16 micromoles ATP per gram hemoglobin (range 0.03 to 0.37); the magnitude of the rise appeared to be independent of the initial (4°C) level.

DISCUSSION

The results of this series of experiments confirm earlier observations that there is a significant correlation between erythrocyte poststorage ATP levels and viability. The relationship appears to be valid for all three anticoagulants tested and for storage periods up to 42 days. In addition, the marked deleterious effect on ATP levels produced by non-mixing of blood during prolonged storage[14] also affects the red cell viability to the extent predicted by the regression line for standard storage conditions. However, in spite of the wide range of conditions over which the relationship holds, it cannot be accepted as valid for every set of experimental conditions. For example, cell washing can affect ATP levels and viability independently; when stored red cells are washed in solutions containing phosphate and glucose, there is some increase in ATP level which is not accompanied by a change in red cell viability. Therefore, use of the relationship as the basis for an in vitro test for accurate determination of the effectiveness of proposed new anticoagulants, plastics, storage techniques, etc., cannot be recommended. However, in our experience, marked deviation from the curve has not been observed, and it is believed that the test is very useful as a screening procedure. Its judicious use can serve to reduce the number of confirmatory in vivo tests required to guide further work on proposed storage materials.

In view of the marked variation among donors with respect to their poststorage erythrocyte viability,[15] various approaches were considered which might permit the prestorage prediction of the true acceptable storage period for a given donors blood. Prestorage ATP levels appeared to be of no use since the correlation between such data and poststorage viability was low.[8] Evidence has also been presented which suggests that ATP levels may be regulated by at least two hereditary mechanisms, one which determines an individual's prestorage or inherent ATP level, and a second which regulates the rate of fall of ATP concentration during storage.[16] Biochemical tests to permit prestorage prediction of the ATP decline rate have been unsuccessful to date. In view of the precision limitations noted below, further pursuit of this approach does not appear promising.

From the data of Table I, it is obvious that the correlation coefficients and confidence intervals are quite similar for all data sets. Attempts to increase precision by considering the curves individually, by technical modification, or by estimating ATP levels at different preinjection times were not successful. While the correlation is great enough to be of predictive value for the regression curve, the confidence interval (individual) is too great to permit prediction of cell viability from the ATP level of a given bag. Therefore, the relationship does not appear useful for identifying those units of blood which remain acceptable for human transfusion beyond the automatic outdating period of 21 days. How much of the unaccounted for residual variation is due to biological, and how much to technical elements is unknown, but the former is believed to contribute a large fraction. If so, it is possible that the necessary level of precision for individual predictions of cell viability from ATP data may not be attainable.

REFERENCES

1. Rapoport, S.: Dimensional, osmotic, and chemical changes of erythrocytes in stored blood. I. Blood preserved in sodium citrate, neutral, and acid-citrate-glucose (ACD) mixtures, J. Clin. Invest. 26: 591, 1947.

2. Schechter, D. C., and Swan, H.: Biochemical alterations of preserved blood, Arch. Surg. 84: 269, 1962.

3. Gabrio, B. W., and Huennekens, F. M.: The role of nucleoside phosphorylase in erythrocyte preservation, Biochim. et biophys. acta 18: 585, 1955.

4. DeVerdier, C. H., Garby, L., Hjelm, M., and Hogman, C.: Adenine in blood preservation: Posttransfusion viability and biochemical changes, Transfusion 4: 331, 1964.

5. Valeri, C. R., Mercado-Lugo, R., and Danon, D.: Relationship between osmotic fragility and in vivo survival of autologous deglycerolized resuspended red blood cells, Transfusion 5: 267, 1965.

6. Brewer, G. J., and Powell, R. D.: The adenosine triphosphate
    content of glucose-6-phosphate dehydrogenase-deficient and
    normal erythrocytes, including studies of a glucose-6-
    phosphate dehydrogenase-deficient man with "elevated
    erythrocytic ATP," J. Lab. & Clin. Med. 67: 726, 1966.

7. Nakao, K., Wada, T., Kamiyama, T., Nakao, M., and Nagano, K.:
    A direct relationship between adenosine triphosphate level
    and in vivo viability of erythrocytes, Nature 194: 877, 1962.

8. Dern, R. J., Brewer, George J., and Wiorkowski, J. J.:
    Studies on the preservation of human blood. II. The
    relationship of erythrocyte adenosine triphosphate levels and
    other in vitro measures to red cell storageability, J. Lab.
    & Clin. Med. 69: 968, 1967.

9. Button, L. N., Gibson, J. G. II, and Walter, C. W.:
    Simultaneous determination of the volume of red cells and
    plasma for survival of stored blood, Transfusion 5: 143,
    1965.

10. Dern, R. J.: Studies on the preservation of human blood. III.
    The posttransfusion survival of stored and damaged erythro-
    cytes in healthy donors and patients with severe trauma,
    J. Lab. & Clin. Med. 71: 254, 1968.

11. Beutler, E., and Baluda, M. C.: Simplified determination of
    blood adenosine triphosphate using the firefly system,
    Blood 23: 688, 1964.

12. Dixon, W. J., editor: Biomedical computer programs, Health
    Sciences Computing Facilities, Department of Preventive
    Medicine and Public Health, School of Medicine, University
    of California, Los Angeles, 1964.

13. Kendall, M. G., and Stuart, A.: Advanced theory of
    statistics, ed. 3, New York, 1960, Hafner Publishing
    Company, Inc., vol. 2, p. 356.

14. Dern, R. J., Matsuda, T., and Wiorkowski, J. J.: Studies
    on the preservation of human blood. V. The effect of
    mixing of blood during storage on postinfusion red cell
    survival. (In press J. Lab. & Clin. Med.)

15. Dern, R. J., Gwinn, R. P., and Wiorkowski, J. J.: Studies on
    the preservation of human blood. I. Variability in
    erythrocyte storage characteristics among healthy donors,
    J. Lab. & Clin. Med. 67: 955, 1966.

16. Dern, R. J. and Wiorkowski, J. J.: Studies on the
     preservation of human blood. IV. The hereditary component
     of pre-and poststorage erythrocyte adenosine triphosphate
     levels, J. Lab. & Clin. Med. 73: 1019, 1969.

APPLICATION OF A MECHANISED METHOD FOR THE DETERMINATION OF DIFFERENT

GLYCOLYTIC INTERMEDIATES IN THE ROUTINE QUALITY CONTROL OF RED CELLS

J.A.Loos, Ph.D and H.K.Prins, Ph.D., with the technical
assistance of Miss B.M.T.Scholte

Central Laboratory of the Netherlands Red Cross Blood
Transfusion Service, P.O.B. 9190, Amsterdam

INTRODUCTION

For the routine quality control of red cells methods are required by which glycolytic intermediates, especially energy-rich
phosphates and 2,3-diphosphoglycerate, can easily be determined in
large series of blood samples.

In the course of a study on the carbohydrate metabolism of human
lymphocytes specific and sensitive methods were developed or adopted
by using enzymatic systems, based on principles as outlined by Glock
and McLean, Biochem. J. 61:381, 1955, Passonneau et al., J.Biol.Chem.
244:902, 1969, and Owens and Belcher, Biochem. J. 94:705, 1965; in
those systems reaction velocities are proportional to the concentrations of the compounds to be assayed. As it was possible to use
systems in which $NADH_2$, resp. $NADPH_2$ are formed or consumed,
fluorimetry offered a way to further refinement.

Fluorimetric determination of reaction rates requires a clean
system as well as highly reproducible pipetting, mixing and incubation. Therefore the use of a continuous flow system (AutoAnalyzer)
proved to be of great advantage in adapting the methods for the
performance of large series of determinations.

The high sensitivity of the methods allows the performance of
determinations in 900 to 27,000 fold dilutions of blood in 1 mM
ammonia, which are prepared with a simple semi-automatic diluting
device (Autodiluter), instead of extracts prepared with laborious
deproteinisation and neutralisation procedures.

With the continuous flow system one determination per minute can be carried out, which means about 300 determinations per day, including preparation of standards and reagents. The capacity may be increased by making a multichannel system, in which different determinations are performed simultaneously.

The sensitivity of the system enables us to determine ATP + ADP, glucose-1,6-diphosphate (GDP), 2,3-diphosphoglycerate (DPG), glycerol + glycerol-1-phosphate, L-lactate and pyruvate in 0.1 ml of blood or 3.10^6 human lymphocytes.

Apart from applications in the study of lymphocyte carbohydrate metabolism the mechanised system is being intensively used in the search for optimal conditions for the collection and transport of blood by our mobile teams and furthermore in the study of biochemical properties of packed cells and washed cell suspensions during preparation and storage. A number of examples are presented here.

MATERIALS AND METHODS

Principles of the Methods

In the determination of ATP + ADP the velocity of the conversion of 3-P-glycerate to 1,3-diP-glycerate with ATP and phosphoglycerate kinase is measured. All ADP, already present or newly formed is converted immediately to ATP by phosphoenolpyruvate and pyruvate kinase. The formation of 1,3-diP-glycerate is measured by converting it immediately after formation into 3-P-glyceraldehyde with $NADH_2$ and phosphoglyceraldehyde dehydrogenase. Pyruvate and 3-P-glyceraldehyde are trapped as hydrazones. The conditions are chosen so that reaction velocity is proportional to the concentration of ATP + ADP.

2,3-Diphosphoglycerate is determined by measuring the velocity of the conversion of 3-P-glycerate into 2-P-glycerate with 2,3-diP-glycerate and phosphoglyceromutase. The conditions are chosen so that the reaction velocity is proportional to the concentration of 2,3-diP-glycerate, according to Krimsky, Methoden der enzymatischen Analyse (H.U.Bergmeyer, Ed., Verlag Chemie Weinheim), 253, 1962. The formation of 2-P-glycerate is measured by converting it immediately after formation into lactate with enolase, pyruvate kinase + ADP, and lactate dehydrogenase and $NADH_2$.

Glucose-1,6-diphosphate is measured according to Passonneau et al., J. Biol. Chem. 244:902, 1969, by measuring the rate of conversion of glucose-1-P into glucose-6-P by phosphoglucomutase and glucose-1,6-diP. The conditions are chosen so, that the reaction velocity is proportional to the concentration of glucose-1,6-diP. The formation of glucose-6-P is measured by converting it immediately after formation to 6-P-gluconate with glucose-6-P dehydrogenase and NADP.

L-lactate is determined according to Hohorst, Biochem. Z. 328:509, 1957, by measuring the total increase of $NADH_2$ concentration in a system, containing lactate dehydrogenase, NAD, and hydrazine.

Pyruvate is measured according to Bücher et al., Methoden der enzymatischen Analyse, p. 253, 1962, by measuring the total decrease of $NADH_2$ concentration in a system containing lactate dehydrogenase and $NADH_2$.

Glycerol + glycerol-1-phosphate is determined according to Wieland, Methoden der enzymatischen Analyse p. 211, 1962, with the aid of glycerol kinase, glycerol-1-P dehydrogenase, NAD and hydrazine.

In the six systems $NADH_2$, resp. $NADPH_2$ is measured fluorimetrically after a fixed incubation time (appr. 14 minutes) at $37^{\circ}C$. Mixing of samples with reagents, incubation and recording of fluorescence is performed with the AutoAnalyzer system.

Reagents

All enzymes and biochemicals are obtained from Boehringer. The used 3-P-glycerate preparation contained approximately 1 percent of 2,3-diP-glycerate, and the glucose-1-P preparation was contaminated with traces of glucose-1,6-diP. For the determination of 2,3-diP-glycerate, resp. glucose-1,6-diP the preparations had to be purified. Purification was achieved by column chromatography on Dowex-1 formate, using a linear gradient of formate, according to Bartlett, Biochim. Biophys. Acta 156:221, 1968.

The composition of the reagents is represented in Table I; all enzyme concentrations were found experimentally as the minimum concentrations required to obtain optimal standard calibration curves.

Preparation of Samples and Standards

Red cell lysates are used as samples: whole blood or red cell suspensions of approximately the same hematocrit are submitted to three subsequent 30 fold dilution steps with 1 mM ammonia. The 900 fold dilution is most appropriate for the determination of ATP + ADP, lactate and pyruvate; the 27,000 fold dilution is used for the determination of DPG and GDP. Which dilution is to be used for the glycerol determination depends entirely on the stage of deglycerolisation. The dilution, as carried out with a Hook and Tucker Autodiluter Mk II, takes about 30 seconds per blood sample. The diluted samples are stable for at least one day at $0-4^{\circ}C$; for longer periods

Table I - Composition of reagent solutions.

Reagent		Composition
ATP + ADP	I	0.025 M tris(hydroxymethyl)aminomethane-HCl buffer pH 7.4, containing 50 μM $NADH_2$.
	II	0.025 M "tris"buffer pH 7.4, containing 0.008 M P-enolpyruvate, 0.04 M 3-P-glycerate (non-purif.), 1.0 M KCl, 0.3M $MgSO_4$ and 0.4 M hydrazine.
	III	0.4 vol of a suspension of P-glyceraldehyde dehydrogenase (20 mg/ml) + 0.15 vol of P-glycerate kinase suspension (10 mg/ml) + 0.15 vol of pyruvate kinase suspension (10 mg/ml) + 0.5 vol of 20% albumin solution + 1 vol of 2.4 M $(NH_4)_2SO_4$ + 1 vol of 0.04 M $Na_4P_2O_7$ + 22 vol 0.025 M "tris"buffer pH 7.4.
2,3-diP-glycerate	I	0.025 M "tris"buffer pH 7.4, containing 150 μM $NADH_2$.
	II	0.025 M "tris"buffer pH 7.4, containing 0.007 M ADP, 0.006 M 3-P-glycerate (purified), 1.0 M KCl and 0.3 M $MgSO_4$.
	III	0.08 vol of lactate dehydrogenase suspension (5 mg/ml, BOEHRINGER code: 15371 ELAC) + 0.04 vol pyruvate kinase suspension (10 mg/ml) + 0.04 vol enolase suspension (10 mg/ml) + 0.13 vol P-glyceromutase suspension (5 mg/ml) + 1 vol 20% albumin solution + 24 vol 0.025 M "tris"buffer pH 7.4.
Glucose-1,6-diP	I	0.05 M iminazole-HCl buffer pH 7.0, containing 0.1 mM EDTA.
	II	0.05 M iminazole-HCl buffer pH 7.0, containing 0.006 M glucose-1-P (purified), 0.03 M $MgSO_4$ and 0.0015 M NADP.
	III	0.005 vol of P-glucomutase suspension (2 mg/ml) + 0.06 vol of glucose-6-P dehydrogenase suspension (5 mg/ml) + 0.20 vol 20% albumin solution + 10 vol of 0.025 M "tris"buffer pH 7.4.
L-lactate	I	A solution of 0.33 M glycine and 0.13 M hydrazine; pH 9.5.
	II	0.025 M "tris"buffer pH 7.4, containing 0.007 M NAD
	III	0.85 vol of lactate dehydrogenase suspension (5mg/m BOEHRINGER code 15371 ELAC) + 1.0 vol 20% albumin + 24 vol of 0.025 M "tris"buffer pH 7.4.

Table I - Continued

Reagent		Composition
Glycerol + glycerol-1-P	I	A solution of 0.33 M glycine, 0.13 M hydrazine and 0.0017 M EDTA; pH 9.5.
	II	0.025 M "tris"buffer pH 7.4, containing 0.007 M ATP, 0.007 M NAD and 0.3 M $MgSO_4$.
	III	0.15 vol of glycerokinase suspension (1 mg/ml) + 0.08 vol of glycerol-1-P dehydrogenase suspension (2 mg/ml) + 0.2 vol of 20% albumin + 9.6 vol of 0.025 M "tris"buffer pH 7.4.
Pyruvate	I	0.025 M "tris"buffer pH 7.4, containing 5 μM $NADH_2$.
	II	water
	III	0.034 vol of lactate dehydrogenase suspension (5 mg/ml, BOEHRINGER code 15371 ELAC) + 0.4 vol of 20% albumin solution + 9.6 vol of 0.025 M "tris"buffer pH 7.4.

N.B. All reagent solutions are prepared with deionized water containing 1 drop of LEVOR IV per liter. The solutions are sufficiently stable for one week, when kept at 0-4°C free from light and air.

------

of storage they are kept at -15°C. The standards are prepared from stock solutions in the appropriate range and then diluted in exactly the same way as the samples.

Equipment and Procedure

The flow scheme is represented in Fig. 1. Details of equipment and operation were presented elsewhere, Prins and Loos, Advances in Automated Analysis, Mediad, New York, 1969 (in press).

As standards and samples are diluted in exactly the same way, concentrations are calculated by comparing peak heights of samples and standards; the concentrations thus obtained are divided by the hematocrit, giving the concentration per ml of red cells.

Table II - Range and Reproducibility of the Different Determinations.

	ATP+ADP	2,3-DPG	Glucose-1,6-diP	Lactate	Pyruvate	Glycerol +glyc-1-P
Range	50-1000nM	5-50nM	1-10nM	5-50μM	1.5-7.5μM	3-12μM
Reproducibility	4-10nM	1-2.5nM	0.1nM	0.6-1μM	60-80nM	0.1-0.2μM

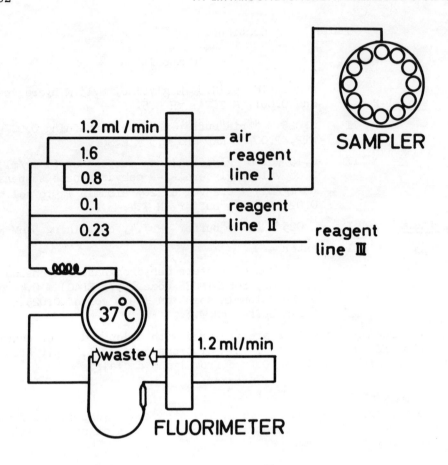

Fig. 1 - Flow diagram of the mechanised system.
Reagents I, II, and III are specified in Table I.

RESULTS

Decrease of 2,3-DPG in Blood after Collection

Fig. 2 illustrates the temperature-dependence of DPG loss in
ACD blood. A rapid loss of DPG at temperatures above 10°C was observed. This result confirms that ACD blood should be cooled immediately after collection. As outlined before, Prins and Loos, Proc.
Int. Symp. of Modern Problems of Blood Preservation, Frankfurt,
1969 (in press), it may sometimes be difficult to achieve rapid
cooling, e.g. after blood collection by mobile teams. Even at low
temperature there is a considerable loss of DPG during one week of
storage. (see Table IV).

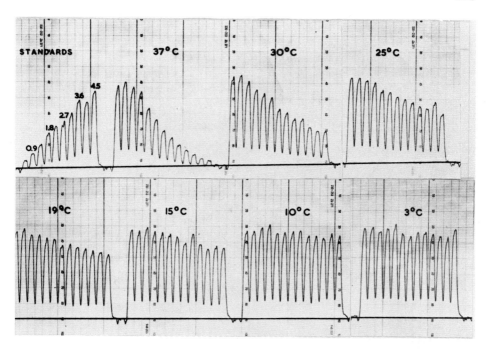

Fig. 2 - Recorder track of DPG determinations in blood samples
during incubation of ACD blood at different temperatures.

ACD blood was divided into 7 portions immediately after collection
and each portion was stored at constant temperature (37, 30, 25, 19,
15, 10, and 3°C, resp.) during 12 hours. Each hour samples were taken
and diluted with 1 mM ammonia. DPG determinations were performed in
the diluted samples in one run.

Table III - Temperature dependence of DPG loss.

Temperature (°C)		37	30	25	19	15	10	3
DPG loss	ACD blood 1	0.54	0.32	0.21	0.12	0.07	0.04	0.04
(mmole/l cells/h)	ACD blood 2	0.55	0.29	0.24	0.12	0.02	0.03	0.02
	CPD blood 1	0.52	0.32	0.18	0.08	0.01	-0.02	-0.03
	CPD blood 2	0.74	0.31	0.17	0.06	-0.03	-0.02	-0.01
Defibrinated blood 1		0.04	-	-	-	-	-	-
Defibrinated blood 2		0.04	-	-	-	-	-	-

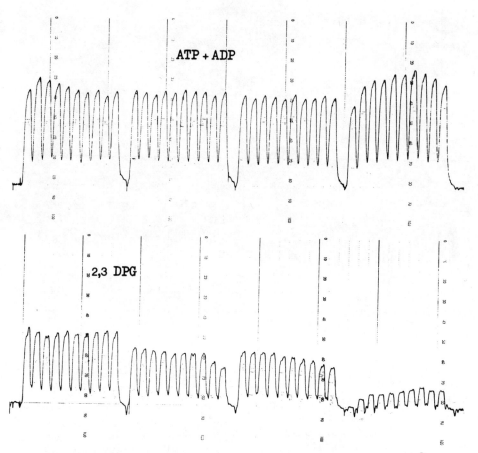

Fig. 3 - Effect of different additives on blood at 37°C.

Blood was taken from one donor; one part was defibrinated, the other
part was collected in ACD. Of the ACD blood one half was incubated
without addition, the other half was incubated with 8.9 mM $MgCl_2$.
Along with the three portions, DPG-poor ACD blood from another donor
was incubated with 8.9 mM $MgCl_2$ + 6.2 mM adenosine.
Samples were taken after 0, 15, 30, 60, 90, 120, 150, 180, 210 and
240 minutes.
From left to right: defibrinated blood, ACD blood, ACD-blood + Mg$^{\cdot\cdot}$,
DPG-poor blood + Mg$^{\cdot\cdot}$ + adenosine.

When we incubated DPG-poor ACD blood at 37°C with adenine +
inosine + glucose, according to Åkerblom et al, Scand. J. Clin. Lab.
Invest. 21:245, 1968, with adenosine, and combinations of adenosine,
pyruvate, ascorbate, aneurine and glucose, DPG resynthesis never
exceeded 1 mmole/L cells. Resynthesis was somewhat better (1.4
mmole/L) in the presence of adenosine and $MgCl_2$ (Fig. 3).

Table IV - 2,3-Diphosphoglycerate and Energy-Rich Phosphate in
Packed Cells after Different Periods of Storage.

		2,3-DPG (mmole/l cells)			ATP + ADP (mmole/l cells)		
		n	mean	σ	n	mean	σ
ACD	1 day after collection	10	4.8	0.46	10	1.75	0.17
	8 days after collection	9	1.3	0.44	9	1.61	0.10
	15 days after collection	10	0.2	0.16	10	1.45	0.07
	22 days after collection	8	0.0	0.1	8	1.09	0.10
CPD	1 day after collection	10	4.4	0.8	10	1.59	0.17
	8 days after collection	10	4.2	0.6	10	1.23	0.07
	15 days after collection	10	2.3	0.9	10	1.19	0.17
	23 days after collection	9	0.3	0.17	9	1.20	0.2

Similar experiments were performed with blood that had been collected in CPD solution. Although at 37°C no significant differences
with ACD blood were observed (Table III), at room temperature DPG
loss in CPD blood is slower. On storage at 0-4°C (Table IV) the DPG
level remained almost constant during the first week; during the
second week the loss was 50 percent. The effect of CPD may partially
be due to the higher pH of CPD blood immediately after collection
(7.8 at 0°C instead of 7.4 in ACD blood): lactate production was
considerably higher during the period of storage.

In another experiment blood was defibrinated with glass beads,
according to Wilson and Grimes, Nature 218:178, 1968, and then
divided into two portions. To one portion 125 mmole glucose/L cells
was added. The two portions were incubated at 37°C for 24 hours.
DPG, ATP+ADP and GDP were constant until the samples ran out of
glucose. It was noteworthy, furthermore, to see that in defibrinated
blood lactate production was twice as high as in ACD blood from the
same donor.

Restoration of 2,3-DPG and ATP + ADP

Another well-known approach is to counteract loss of 2,3-DPG
and ATP by addition of suitable substrates (Chanutin, Transfusion
7:120, 1967, and Åkerblom et al., Scand. J. Clin. & Lab. Invest.
21:245, 1968). We performed some experiments, trying to prevent loss
of DPG in freshly collected ACD blood on incubation at 37°C after
addition of Mg⁺⁺ in order to reactivate Mg⁺⁺-dependent kinases,
which had been blocked by citrate (although this Mg⁺⁺ concentration
did not induce clotting, it completely restored leucophagocytic activity in ACD blood). However the rate of DPG loss was not influenced
by this addition (Fig. 3).

Table V - Changes of DPG and energy-rich phosphate in washed red cells after suspension in Ringer-NaF solution, containing 3.9 mM adenosine + 1.5 mM pyruvate, during incubation at 37°C.

Time (minutes)	0	10	20	30	40	60	80	120
ATP+ADP (mmole/L cells)	1.33	1.38	1.33	1.14	0.96	0.48	0.21	0.14
2,3-diPG(mmole/L cells)	1.6	2.3	2.9	2.8	3.1	3.3	3.1	3.1

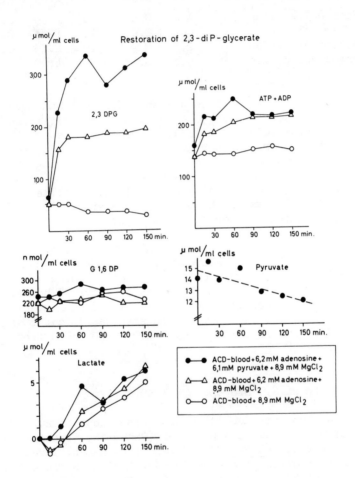

Fig. 4 - Changes in DPG, ATP+ADP, GDP, lactate and pyruvate during incubation of DPG-poor ACD blood with MgCl$_2$, MgCl$_2$+adenosine, and MgCl$_2$+adenosine+pyruvate.

Table VI - Loss and restoration of organic phosphates in defibrinated
          blood.

Defibrinated blood was incubated without (I) and with (II) extra
glucose (125 mmole/l cells). After 24 hours of incubation at 37°C
$MgCl_2$, adenosine, and pyruvate were added (final concentrations
8.9, 6.2, and 6.1 mM, resp.) and incubation was continued.

Time of incubation	ATP + ADP (mmole/lcells)		2,3-DPG (mmole/l cells)		GDP (mmole/l cells)	
	I	II	I	II	I	II
0 h	1.78	1.70	3.9	3.8	0.25	0.23
5 h	1.80	1.47	3.7	3.6	0.24	0.18
10 h	1.00	1.30	0.6	3.1	0.17	0.20
22 h	0.31	1.28	0.0	0.2	0.14	0.21
24 h	0.26	1.40	0.2	0.2	0.13	0.24
24 h + 5 min	0.35	1.58	0.2	0.6	0.22	0.22
24 h + 10 min	0.42	1.58	0.4	1.0	0.12	0.19
24 h + 20 min	0.46	1.63	1.1	1.7	0.11	0.21
24 h + 40 min	0.54	1.69	1.6	2.1	0.11	0.21
24 h + 60 min	0.61	1.84	1.8	2.3	0.11	0.22
24 h + 80 min	0.72	2.02	1.7	2.9	0.10	0.31

The only way of nearly complete DPG restoration we knew so far,
was the incubation of washed red cells with fluoride, adenosine and
pyruvate (Loos et al. , Hereditary Disorders of Erythrocyte Metabolism,
E.Beutler, Ed., Grune and Stratton, New York, p.280, 1968). Pyruvate is
added in order to avoid exhaustion of NAD during DPG production in red
cells in which the enolase reaction is blocked. In Table V the result
of such an incubation with DPG-poor ACD cells is represented. Although
these conditions cannot be applied in the blood bank, the result led
us to try a combination of $Mg^{\cdot\cdot}$, adenosine and pyruvate. In the
experiment which is represented in Fig. 4, DPG-poor ACD blood was
incubated with $MgCl_2$, $MgCl_2$ + adenosine, and $MgCl_2$ + adenosine +
pyruvate, resp. The best results were obtained with the third combination; the results may help us in finding a practical method for
restoration of DPG and ATP in red cells, derived from old ACD blood.
In a similar experiment 5 different blood samples were incubated with
$MgCl_2$ + adenosine + pyruvate; 5 other blood samples were incubated
with inosine + $MgCl_2$ + pyruvate. 80 minutes of incubation with the
first combination resulted in the synthesis of 2.68 $\pm$ 0.44 mmole DPG/L
cells and 0.78 $\pm$ 0.09 mmole ATP+ADP/L cells; in the inosine-containing
mixtures these increases were 2.50 $\pm$ 0.39 and 0.14 $\pm$ 0.04, respectively.

In an experiment with defibrinated blood, considerable restoration
of DPG and ATP + ADP was observed on incubation with $MgCl_2$ + pyruvate
+ adenosine (Table VI).

No special reference has been made so far to the application of
the glycerol determination. It will be clear, however, that the estimation was adopted to be used in studies on deglycerolisation. The
presentation of some results of our studies about loss and restoration
of energy-rich phosphates and DPG in red cells was not based primarily
on the eventual scientific significance of those results; the intention was rather to demonstrate that with our mechanized system the
number of determinations to be performed is no longer a bottle-neck,
and that therefore in an incubation study the concentrations of the
various compounds can be followed as a function of time, even in a
series of incubation mixtures. We also want to emphasize that quality
control in the blood bank is not necessarily restricted to a small
number of determinations in randomly taken samples.

SUMMARY

1. A mechanised system was developed for the enzymatic determination
of ATP + ADP, 2,3-diP-glycerate, glucose-1,6-diP, lactate, pyruvate
and glycerol + glycerol-1-P with a frequency of 1 sample per minute.
2. Determinations are performed in samples, obtained by 900-27,000
fold dilution of 0.1 ml quantities of blood in 1 mM ammonia with a
semi-automatic diluting device.
3. With this system we studied biochemical changes in red cells after
collection and transport of blood and during storage of red cell
concentrates at different conditions.
4. It was found that in ACD and CPD blood loss of 2,3-DPG increases
rapidly with increasing temperature. In defibrinated blood no appreciable loss of 2,3-DPG was observed for many hours, even at $37^{\circ}C$, as
long as glucose was present.
5. Complete restoration of energy-rich phosphate and 2,3-DPG was
observed in ACD blood and defibrinated blood on incubation at $37^{\circ}C$
with adenosine + pyruvate + $MgCl_2$.
6. We expect that the described mechanised system can be useful in
the pretransfusion quality control on stored and processed blood.

ACKNOWLEDGEMENT

This study was partly supported by financial aid of the
Netherlands Organisation for the Advancement of Pure Research
(Z.W.O.), The Hague, The Netherlands, grant nr 534-12.

RED CELL 2,3 DPG, ATP, AND CREATINE LEVELS IN PRESERVED RED CELLS

AND IN PATIENTS WITH RED CELL MASS DEFICITS OR WITH CARDIOPULMONARY

INSUFFICIENCY

C. Robert Valeri and Normand L. Fortier

Naval Blood Research Laboratory, Chelsea, Mass.   02150

INTRODUCTION

The therapeutic effectiveness of red cell preservation (either by liquid or freezing procedures) has been evaluated primarily by the measurements of 24-hour posttransfusion survival (Jones et al., 1957; Szymanski and Valeri, 1968). Since the main reason for transfusing preserved red cells is to increase the oxygen carrying capacity of the recipient's blood, the circulating preserved red cells should at the time of transfusion have normal oxygen uptake and oxyhemoglobin dissociation characteristics. Valtis and Kennedy, (1954) observed that human red cells stored in acid-citrate-dextrose (ACD, National Institutes of Health, Formula A) longer than one week had progressive shifts in oxyhemoglobin toward higher oxygen affinities. Following transfusion, the red cells that exhibited this higher in vitro affinity for oxygen were incapable, usually for several hours, of releasing in vivo as large a quantity of oxygen to tissue as did normal red cells. The time required for in vivo restoration of the red cells' oxygen affinity to normal was related to both the volume and the duration of storage of the transfused blood.

Two phosphate compounds, adenosine triphosphate (ATP) and 2,3

This work was supported by the U. S. Navy.

The opinions or assertions contained herein are those of the authors, and are not to be construed as official or reflecting the views of the Navy Department or the Naval Service at large.

diphosphoglycerate (2,3 DPG) have been shown to facilitate the
release of oxygen from hemoglobin (Benesch et al., 1968; Chanutin
and Curnish, 1967). Benesch et al (1968) were the first to demonstrate that 2,3 DPG forms a complex with purified deoxyhemoglobin
and thereby reduces the affinity of hemoglobin for oxygen. Chanutin
and Curnish (1967) also reported that the affinity of a hemoglobin
solution for oxygen may be decreased by its interaction with organic
phosphates, particularly 2,3 DPG.

Storage of blood in acid-citrate-dextrose (ACD) solution at 4 C
leads to progressive decreases in the levels of organic phosphates
(Rapoport, 1947), whereas the 2,3 DPG level decreases rapidly during
the first two weeks of storage, the ATP concentration decreases
slowly (Bartlett and Barnet, 1960).

Akerblom et al (1968) and Bunn et al (1969) have emphasized the
relationship in preserved red cells between oxygen affinity and the
sum of the levels of the organic phosphate compounds 2,3 DPG and
ATP.

In Vivo and In Vitro Restoration of Organic Phosphates in Liquid
Red Blood Cells.

Our laboratory has reported on the restoration to normal in
vivo of erythrocyte adenosine triphosphate, 2,3 diphosphoglycerate,
potassium ion, and sodium ion concentrations following the transfusion of acid-citrate-dextrose-collected human red blood cells that
had been stored for 15 days at 4 C (Valeri and Hirsch, 1969;
Valeri et al., (in press)). A manual differential agglutination
procedure was used to identify red cells transfused to group A_1
recipients. A significant increase in cellular 2,3 DPG in the donor
population was found immediately at the completion of the 2-3/4 hour
transfusions. Within three hours following the end of transfusion
the level of 2,3 DPG rose to at least 25% of the final level (3.48
u moles/g Hb or 0.233 moles/mole Hb). The level of 2,3 DPG was
greater than 50% of the final level within 24 hours after the end
of transfusion, after which it gradually continued to increase up
to 11 days (Figure 1). During this period significant increases
in the donor cell ATP concentration also occurred. These results
support earlier observations that preserved red cells that have
circulated for 24 hours following transfusion usually have normal
oxygen uptake and oxyhemoglobin dissociation (Valtis and Kennedy,
1954; O'Brien and Watkins, Jr., 1960).

Other information suggests that the condition of the recipient,
in addition to the quality and quantity of the blood itself, is an
important determinant of the time required for preserved red cells
to recover normal oxygen affinity after transfusion. The data of
O'Brien and Watkins (1960) indicate that restoration of the organic
phosphates, 2,3 DPG and ATP, depends not only on the metabolic state

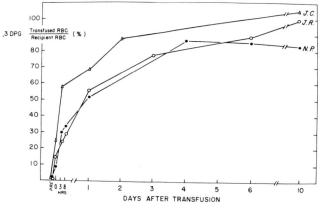

FIGURE 1

The *in vivo* restoration of 2,3 DPG-depleted transfused human
red cells is shown as a percentage of recipient's level of 2,3 DPG
in each of the three patients.

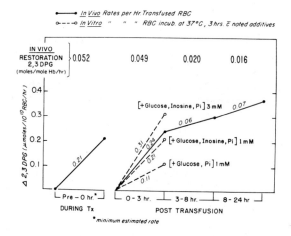

FIGURE 2

The *in vivo* rates of restoration of transfused red cell 2,3
DPG during the transfusion period; and the 0-3 hour, 3-8 hour, and
8-24 hour periods following transfusion. The rates calculated during
the transfusion are minimal estimates. The *in vitro* rates of 2,3
DPG restoration for preserved red cells incubated at 37 C with three
different media are also shown.

of the cells transfused, but also on the ability of the recipient
to replenish these depleted cellular intermediates.

Factors other than the organic phosphate intermediates (ATP and
2,3 DPG) may participate in the unloading of oxygen from hemoglobin
under physiological conditions. Reduced glutathione has also been
considered important in the transport of oxygen by hemoglobin.
Horejsi (1967) reported that reduced glutathione (GSH) affected both
the shape and location of the dissociation curve of oxyhemoglobin,
a higher concentration of reduced glutathione in blood causing a
shift of the dissociation curve to the right (indicating that a
given amount of blood liberates more oxygen at decreased partial
pressures of oxygen). However, in a study of hemoglobin function
in stored blood, Bunn et al (1969) failed to confirm this. Inorganic
phosphate also reduces the oxygen affinity of hemoglobin, but the
effect is much weaker than that of 2,3 DPG and ATP (Chanutin and
Curnish, 1967; Benesch and Benesch, 1967).

The liberation of oxygen from oxyhemoglobin is facilitated by
increases in pCO_2 and decreases in blood pH (Bohr effect). Moreover,
Valtis and Kennedy (1953) reported the beneficial effect of adding
sodium chloride to stored blood prior to its administration to
correct the abnormality of the oxygen dissociation curve.

In our study the rate of restoration of 2,3 DPG in vitro at 37 C
in a medium that contained lmM each of glucose, inorganic phosphate,
and inosine was similar to that observed in vivo (Figure 2) (Valeri
et al., (in press)). These observations suggest that the recipient's
intravascular environment provide substrates in addition to glucose
for the rapid restoration in vivo of the transfused red cell 2,3 DPG
level. In addition, circulation of the transfused red cells through
hypoxic tissue may stimulate the restoration of the cellular intermediates as a consequence of tissue oxygen requirements.

The therapeutic significance of the increased oxygen affinity
of stored blood is uncertain. Nevertheless one may speculate that
in clinical situations when large volumes of red cells are urgently
needed, there may not be sufficient time for in vivo restoration of
donor cells depleted of 2,3 DPG and ATP and normalization of oxyhemoglobin dissociation.

Maintenance of Preserved Red Cell 2,3 DPG and ATP Levels at the time
of Transfusion.

Many authors have reported that red cell ATP and 2,3 DPG levels
can be maintained by supplementation of either of the two chief blood
preservative solutions (acid-citrate-dextrose and citrate-phosphate-
dextrose) with purine nucleosides (principally adenine and inosine)
at various periods during storage at 4 C (Akerblom et al., 1968;
Bunn et al., 1968; Rubinstein et al., 1959; Chanutin, 1967;

Bartlett and Shafer, 1961; Seidl, (t0 be published); Shafer and
Bartlett, 1961; Akerblom et al, 1969). However, the amount of inosine
required commonly produces hyperuricemia for approximately 24 hours,
in patients given three or four units of such blood (Seidl, (to be
published). In addition, the possible renal toxicity of 2,8
dioxyadenine, a metabolite of adenine, is a cause of some concern.

The present methods for freeze-preservation of human red cells
either by high-concentration of glycerol and the slow freeze-thaw
technic or by low-concentration glycerol and rapid freeze-thaw
technic can maintain normal levels of these organic phosphates.
O'Brien and Watkins (1960) demonstrated that heparinated red cells
and ACD-collected red cells frozen within five hours after
collection (with a high-concentration of glycerol and the slow
freeze-thaw technic) had normal oxyhemoglobin dissociation characteristics after thawing, deglycerolization, and resuspension. Zemp
and O'Brien (1960) reported maintenance of normal levels of the
organic phosphate compounds in these previously frozen red cells
immediately following deglycerolization and resuspension.

The following variables may reasonably be expected to affect
the levels of organic phosphates in washed, previously frozen red
cells at the time of transfusion: the anticoagulant used for
collection, the length of storage and the temperature of storage of
the blood prior to freezing, the pH of the glycerolizing solution,
the pH of the wash solutions required to remove the glycerol, the
composition and pH of the resuspension medium, and the length of
storage of the washed red cells at 4 C prior to transfusion. Higher
red cell 2,3 DPG levels are observed when the pH levels of the
preservative and wash solutions are increased from 5.5 to 7.5 whereas
these higher pH levels adversely affect the ATP levels (Beutler et
al., 1969).

Since current methods for freeze-preservation of human red cells
use the intracellular cryoprotective substance, glycerol, post-thaw
washing is essential (Valeri et al., 1969). It is now possible to
combine both liquid and freeze-preservation methods in order to
provide functioning red cells and help resolve problems of unbalanced
supply and demand for human red cells (Hogman (to be published)).
If a period of liquid storage at 4 C is sufficient to meet current
needs of the blood bank, one can collect and store blood in CPD-
adenine for at least two weeks. If the blood is not used during this
initial period, inosine can then be added to restore the 2,3 DPG
pool, after which the red cells can be frozen using one of the
glycerol procedures. The post-thaw washing will reduce the amount
of adenine and inosine that might otherwise produce untoward side
effects following multiple unit transfusions.

However, the freezing of human red cells immediately following
collection would avoid the need for any supplementation with the

purine nucleosides. Moreover, freezing of human red cells immediately after collection would permit the separation of whole blood into its components (red cells, platelets, antihemophilic factor or cryoprecipitate, albumin, and gamma globulin). Each blood component would be then stored separately using the specific technic appropriate for optimal preservation of the individual component.

Clinical Observations on the Levels of Red Cell 2,3 DPG, ATP, Reduced Glutathione, and Creatine in Patients With Red Cell Mass Deficits or With Cardiopulmonary Insufficiency.

Substantial reductions in red cell mass have been observed in patients returned from Vietnam with traumatic injuries. The patients were usually one to two months post-severe disabling wounds of the extremities and had experienced at least a 10-pound weight loss. In some of these patients cardiac arrest or hypotension occurred during surgical procedures requiring general anesthesia. These cardiovascular complications of surgery were apparently related to undiagnosed pre-operative hypovolemia, although venous hematocrit values were usually within the normal range or only slightly reduced.

Because of these observations, we have undertaken routine measurements of pre-operative red cell volumes using ^{51}Cr labelling of autologous red cells. The red cell volume deficit was taken to be the difference between the theoretical red cell volume (estimated from the patient's actual weight and height) and the measured ^{51}Cr volume. The deficit was corrected pre-operatively with the transfusion of at least two units of washed red cells. After this type of hemotherapy approximately 100 patients have tolerated surgical procedures without incident. Moreover, in most patients clinical improvement (e.g., in appetite and mental status) was usually observed within 24 hours following transfusion, together with a subsequent decrease in requirement for analgesia, an increase in strength, and an apparent improvement in wound healing. Creatinuria present in some of these patients disappeared following therapeutic transfusion to correct red cell mass deficits.

Clinical improvement following transfusion of washed red cells in these cases might be termed a non-specific or "tonic" effect of transfusion, as objectionable as this idea may currently appear. In an attempt to collect objective data supporting these clinical observations, we studied red cell ATP, 2,3 DPG, reduced glutathione and creatine levels, and whole blood lactate, in these patients prior to and after transfusion.

A change in heparinized venous hematocrit levels from approximately 45 to 40% v/v represented a red cell mass deficit of approximately 140 g (approximately two to three units of red cells); this deficit was associated with a mean increase in the red cell 2,3 DPG level from 0.79 ± 0.01 to 1.06 ± 0.20 moles/mole Hb

Means of 4 Groups, ~10 Patients in Each Group

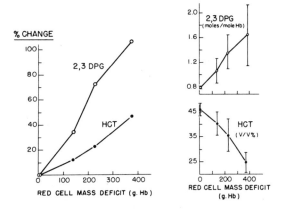

FIGURE 3

Figure 3 shows the relationships between the red cell mass deficit and both the venous hematocrit (v/v%) and the red cell 2,3 DPG level (moles/mole Hb) in 62 patients. In addition, the red cell mass deficit is related to both the percentage change in hematocrit and red cell 2,3 DPG level. (Two patients of the original 64 were excluded; each had cardiopulmonary insufficiency with normal red cell mass and an elevated level of red cell 2,3 DPG).

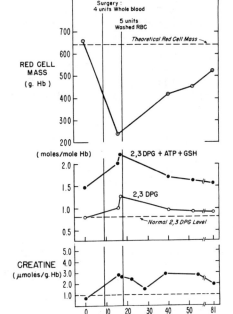

FIGURE 4

Figure 4 depicts the measurements of red cell mass (g Hb) in the patient S.S. related to his red cell level of 2,3 DPG, creatine, and the summated levels of ATP, 2,3 DPG, and GSH.

(Figure 3). The change in red cell 2,3 DPG level is approximately 2-1/2 to 3 times more sensitive to red cell volume depletion than the peripheral venous hematocrit values (Figure 3). Our data again demonstrate the limited reliance which may be placed on a venous hematocrit reading in the so-called "normal range" (of 40 and 45% v/v for males) for the diagnosis of the magnitude of a possible red cell mass deficit (Figure 3). Moreover, the need to measure red cell mass may not be obvious in patients who require surgical procedures and whose hematocrit is normal or only slightly reduced.

Figure 4 shows the results observed in the patient, S.S., who had traumatic injuries of both lower limbs. The pre-operative red cell mass was normal with normal levels of 2,3 DPG, creatine, and summated ATP, 2,3 DPG, and GSH. The surgical procedure involved inserting a prosthesis in the right hip, during which four units of whole blood were administered to replace the estimated "non excessive" blood loss. Post-operatively the patient was pale, weak, sleepy, and had persistent tachycardia without hypotension. Measurements made at this time demonstrated a marked reduction in red cell mass and elevated erythrocyte levels of 2,3 DPG, creatine, and summated ATP, 2,3 DPG, and GSH over the four day post-operative period (red cell 2,3 DPG level rose from 0.8 to 1.25 moles/mole Hb and red cell creatine rose from 0.8 u moles/g Hb to 2.9 u moles/g Hb). The patient received five units of washed red cells (stored as whole blood at 4 C for approximately ten days) with excellent clinical improvement. About two weeks following the transfusion the patient developed low grade fever associated with wound infection. Following the transfusion a gradual increase in red cell mass was observed together with the gradual restoration towards normal of red cell 2,3 DPG and creatine levels.

Figure 5 shows the findings in another patient, P.T., with traumatic injuries. Transfusion of three units of washed red cells depleted of 2,3 DPG and with normal creatine levels (representing 37% of the circulating red cells following transfusion) produced a decrease in the red cell 2,3 DPG and creatine levels 24 hours after transfusion. The increase in red cell 2,3 DPG level five days after transfusion was consistent with in vivo restoration of the 2,3 DPG level in the depleted donor erythrocytes. When the red cell mass of this patient eventually returned to normal, the red cell levels of 2,3 DPG, creatine and summated 2,3 DPG, ATP, and GSH likewise were within normal limits.

Elevated erythrocyte levels of ATP, 2,3 DPG, creatine, and reduced glutathione - principally 2,3 DPG and creatine - proved to be sensitive indicators of red cell mass deficiency in patients without cardiopulmonary disease. Therefore, in patients free of cardiopulmonary disease, knowledge of the level of red cell 2,3 DPG and creatine would be helpful in interpreting the red cell mass measurements, when evaluating the necessity for therapeutic transfusions.

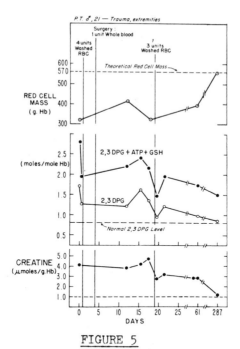

FIGURE 5

Figure 5 depicts the changes in red cell mass in patient P.T. together with red cell levels of ATP, 2,3 DPG, creatine, and GSH. Transfusion of red cells depleted of 2,3 DPG causes an immediate decrease (24 hours following transfusion) in circulating red cell 2,3 DPG level and then an increase for up to five days following transfusion.

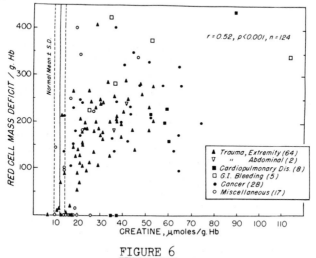

FIGURE 6

Figure 6 shows the relationship between the red cell mass deficit and red cell creatine level.

The adequacy of red cell transfusion in restoring red cell mass may
be estimated by the posttransfusion red cell 2,3 DPG and creatine
levels. However, as noted in patient, P.T., (Figure 5) the transfusion of red cells depleted of 2,3 DPG will produce an immediate
posttransfusion lowering of the 2,3 DPG level, although in vivo
restoration of these cells occurs as described previously (Valeri
and Hirsch, 1969; Valeri et al., (in press)).

On the other hand, elevation of red cell 2,3 DPG and creatine
may be observed in patients who have cardiopulmonary insufficiency
without red cell volume deficiency. These data suggest that
increases in red cell 2,3 DPG reflect an attempt by circulating red
cells to compensate for any impairment in oxygen supply to tissue,
while the elevation of red cell creatine remains obscure.

The adaptive mechanisms provided by the body in attempting to
supply adequate oxygen to satisfy tissue demands in patients with
either decreased red cell mass, cardiac disease, or pulmonary
insufficiency include augmentation of cardiac output (Backman,
1961; Blumgart and Altschule, 1948; Sproule et al., 1960; Whitaker,
1956), greater flow to more important organs (Backman, 1961;
Whitaker, 1956; Kety, 1950), and increased release of oxygen from
hemoglobin (Rodman et al., 1960; Edwards et al., 1968). Many recent
reports (Benesch et al, 1968; Benesch and Benesch, 1967; Benesch and
Benesch, 1969; Chanutin and Hermann, 1969; Lenfant et al, 1968;
deVerdier and Garby, 1969; Rorth, 1968; Weatherall, 1969; Bellingham
and Huehns, 1968) and editorials (Astrup et al, 1968; Beutler, 1969;
Benesch, 1969; deVerdier et al, 1969) have discussed the physiological
importance of the oxyhemoglobin dissociation curve in regulating
oxygen transport to tissue.

No disscussion of these adjustments is now complete without
consideration of the reports that have emphasized the significant
inverse relation in the human erythrocyte between hemoglobin
concentration and the intracellular concentration of 2,3 DPG
(Hjelm, (in press); Eaton and Brewer, 1968; Valeri and Fortier,
(in press,a)) the elevated level of red cell 2,3 DPG in proportion
to the degree of red cell mass deficiency in patients who were not
suffering from cardiopulmonary insufficiency (Valeri and Fortier,
(in press,a)), and the increased red cell 2,3 DPG in patients with
cardiopulmonary diseases who had no red cell deficits (Valeri and
Fortier, (in press,a)). Recent studies by Oski et al (1969) have
confirmed the observation that red cell 2,3 DPG levels are elevated
in patients with chronic hypoxemia.

Our present report enlarges on our earlier suggestion that
measurement of red cell 2,3 DPG level may serve as a functional
biopsy for the determination of the adequacy of tissue oxygenation.
We have also included measurements of red cell creatine concentration
(Valeri and Fortier, (in press,b)).

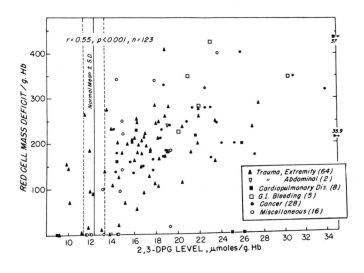

FIGURE 7

Figure 7 shows the relationship between the red cell mass deficit and red cell 2,3 diphosphoglycerate (2,3 DPG) level.

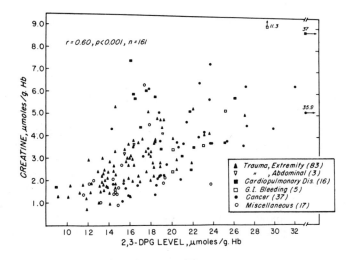

FIGURE 8

Figure 8 shows the relationship between creatine and 2,3 diphosphoglycerate concentrations in human erythrocytes.

The individual case data discussed earlier are now supported
by observations on 161 male patients whose ages ranged from 18 to
65, with a mean of 28 years. These patients suffered from a variety
of diseases including traumatic injuries (86); cardiopulmonary
diseases (16); gastrointestinal bleeding (5); carcinoma (37); and a
miscellaneous group encompassing uremia, hepatitis, cirrhosis,
epilepsy, cerebrovascular diseases, toxic myositis, and lympho-
proliferative disorders (17). Ten healthy male donors were also
studied.

In our group comprising ten healthy donors with normal red cell
masses, and ten patients with traumatic injuries and cellular hemoglobin deficits of 100 $\pm$ 50 g, creatine was found to be located
predominantly in the red cells. The reticulocyte counts were only
slightly elevated in some of the 109 patients studied.

Red cell creatine levels (u moles/g Hb) were significantly
related to the red cell mass deficits (r = 0.52, p<0.001) (Hays,
1963) in 124 patients with various diagnoses (Figure 6). Two
patients with cardiopulmonary disorders but without red cell
deficits showed increased red blood cell creatine concentrations.
The relation between the red cell 2,3 DPG level and the red cell mass
deficit was also significant (r = 0.55, p<0.001, n = 123) (Figure 7).
Likewise, there was a significant correlation between red cell
creatine and 2,3 DPG concentration in 161 patients (r = 0.60,
p<0.001) (Figure 8).

Whole blood lactic acid concentrations varied from 0.5 u moles
to 3.0 u moles per ml in 123 patients with varying degrees of red
cell mass deficit. However, the correlation was not significant
(r = 0.12, p>0.05, n = 123), a finding similar to that reported by
Seibert et al (1967). The highest lactic acid concentrations were
observed in the 28 patients with carcinoma.

Griffiths and Fitzpatrick (1967) observed elevated creatine
levels in the blood of patients suffering from anemia, and reported
the creatine to be present predominantly in the red cells, a finding
that we corroborate. However, they related the elevated red cells
creatine to the reticulocytosis observed in their patients, whereas
the creatine elevations in our patients cannot be so explained. The
mechanism of the creatine accumulation (from 1.0 to 11 u moles/g Hb)
in our patients is not known. Altschule has discussed the earlier
observations that patients with cardiac decompensation usually had
creatinuria, and that the creatinuria regressed with clinical improvement. The mechanism of the creatinuria was not established, but it
was thought to be a manifestation of skeletal muscle hypoxia
(Altschule, 1954). The majority of our patients were suffering from
weight loss, and the elevated creatine in the red cells might
represent creatine transferred from muscle into circulating mature

red cells. Since Griffiths (1968) has shown that the red cell membrane is impermeable to plasma creatine in vitro, the existence of an as yet undefined circulating substance affecting red cell permeability to creatine in vivo is one explanation of the results of our studies. Another possible explanation is that circulating mature red cells synthesize creatine de novo; to support this speculation, however, no data are available.

We interpret our data as supporting the view that the increased 2,3 DPG concentration in erythrocytes is a compensatory mechanism for delivering more oxygen to the tissues. Although the mechanisms of the observed increases in red cell creatine and 2,3 DPG concentrations are not known, the clinical importance of these red cell compounds deserves evaluation because of their possible application both as diagnostic aids and for measuring the effectiveness of therapy.

Prins and Loos (submitted for publication) have recently automated the measurements of red cell ATP, 2,3 DPG, and lactate. However, Astrup (in press) has cautioned that the measurement of red cell 2,3 DPG is affected by changes of acid-base balance because acidosis decreases the red cell 2,3 DPG level while alkalosis increases it (Guest and Rapoport, 1939; Guest, 1942; George et al., 1964). Since the measurement of 2,3 DPG is technically difficult and because there is an excellent correlation between red cell levels of 2,3 DPG and creatine, the red cell creatine measurement may represent a simpler clinical assay for evaluating tissue hypoxia--as a manifestation of both cardiopulmonary insufficiency and decreased circulating red cell mass.

ACKNOWLEDGEMENT

The authors gratefully acknowledge the excellent technical assistance of Linda Pivacek, Kenneth Patti, and Robert Norton.

REFERENCES

Akerblom, O., deVerdier, C. H., Garby, L. and Hogman, C. (1968). Scand. J. Clin. & Lab. Invest. 21:245.
Akerblom, O., deVerdier, C. H., Eriksson, A., Garby, L. and Hogman, C. (1969). Folia. Hematologica 9:142.
Altschule, M. D. (1954). Physiology in Diseases of the Heart and Lung. Cambridge-Harvard University Press, Cambridge, Mass.
Astrup, P., Garby, L. and deVerdier, C. H. (1968). Scand. J. Clin. & Lab. Invest. 22:171.
Astrup, P. Forsvarsmedicin. (In press).
Backman, H. (1961). Scand. J. Clin. & Lab. Invest. 13:1.
Bartlett, G. R. and Barnet, H. N. (1960). J. Clin. Invest. 39:56.

Bartlett, G. R. and Shafer, A. W. (1961). J. Clin. Invest. 40: 1185.

Bellingham, A. J. and Huehns, E. R. (1968). Nature (London). 218:924.

Benesch, R. (1969). New Eng. J. Med. 280:1179.

Benesch, R. and Benesch, R. E. (1967). Biochem. Biophys. Res. Commun. 26:162.

Benesch, R., Benesch, R. E. and Yu, C. I. (1968). Proc. Nat. Acad. Sc. 59:526.

Benesch, R. and Benesch, R. E. (1969). Nature 221:618.

Beutler, E. (1969). Blood 33:496.

Beutler, E., Meul, A. and Wood, L. A (1969). Transfusion 9:109.

Blumgart, H. L. and Altschule, M. D. (1948). Blood 3:329.

Bunn, H. F., May, M. H., Kocholaty, W. F. and Shields, C. E. (1969). J. Clin. Invest. 48:311.

Chanutin, A. (1967). Transfusion 7:120.

Chanutin, A. and Curnish, R. R. (1967). Arch. Biochem. Biophys. 131:96.

Chanutin, A. and Hermann, E. (1969). Arch. Biochem. Biophys. 131:180.

deVerdier, C. H. and Garby, L. (1969). Scand. J. Clin. & Lab. Invest. 23:149.

deVerdier, C. H., Garby, L. and Hjelm, M. (1969). New Eng. J. Med. 280:1360.

Eaton, J. W. and Brewer, G. J. (1968). Proc. Nat. Acad. Sc. 61:756.

Edwards, M. J., Novy, M. J., Walters, C. L. and Metcalfe, J. (1968). J. Clin. Invest. 47:1851.

George, W. T., George, W. D., Smith, J. P., Gordon, F. T., Baird, E. E. and Mills, G. C. (1964). New Eng. J. Med. 270:726.

Griffiths, W. J. and Fitzpatrick, M. (1967). Brit. J. Haemat. 13:175.

Griffiths, W. J. (1968). Brit. J. Haemat. 15:389.

Guest, G. M. and Rapoport, S. (1939). Am. J. Dis. Child. 58:1072.

Guest, G. M. (1942). Am. J. Dis. Child. 64:401.

Hays, W. L. (1963). Statistics for Psychologists. Holt, Rinehart and Winston, New York.

Hjelm, M. Forsvarsmedicin. (In press).

Högman, C. and Åkerblom, O. (1969). Reported at the International Symposium of Modern Problems of Blood Preservation, Frankfurt, Germany. G. Fischer, Verlag, Stutgart. (To be published).

Horejsi, J. (1967). Hematologia 1:35.

Jones, N. C. H., Mollison, P. L. and Robinson, M. A. (1957). Proc. Roy. Soc. London Series B. 147:476.

Kety, S. S. (1950). Am. J. Med. 8:205.

Lenfant, C., Torrance, J., English, E., Finch, C. A., Reynafarje, C., Ramos, J. and Faura, J. (1968). J. Clin. Invest. 47:2652.

O'Brien, T. G. and Watkins, Jr., E. (1960). J. Thoracic &
    Cardiovas. Surg. 40:611.
Oski, F. A., Gottlieb, A. J., Delivoria-Papadopoulos, M. and
    Miller, W. W. (1960). New Eng. J. Med. 280:1165.
Prins, H. K. and Loos, G. A. (Submitted for publication).
Rapoport, S. (1947). J. Clin. Invest. 26:591.
Rodman, T., Close, H. P. and Purcell, M. K. (1960). Ann. Int.
    Med. 52:295.
Rorth, M. (1968). Scand. J. Clin. & Lab. Invest. 22:208.
Rubinstein, D., Kashket, S., Blostein, R. and Dendstedt, O. F.
    (1959). Canad. J. Biochem. Physiol. 37:69.
Seibert, D. J. and Ebaugh, Jr., F. J. (1967). J. Lab. Clin. Med.
    69:177.
Seidl, S. (To be published).
Shafer, A. W. and Bartlett, G. R. (1961). J. Clin. Invest.
    40:1178.
Sproule, B. J., Mitchell, J. H. and Miller, W. F. (1960). J.
    Clin. Invest. 39:378.
Szymanski, I. O. and Valeri, C. R. (1968). Transfusion 8:74.
Valeri, C. R. and Hirsch, N. M. (1969). J. Lab. Clin. Med.
    73:722.
Valeri, C. R., Runck, A. H. and Brodine, C. E. (1969). J. Am.
    Med. Assoc. 208:489.
Valeri, C. R., Hirsch, N. M. and Fortier, N. L. Forsvarsmedicin.
    (In press).
Valeri, C. R. and Fortier, N. L. (1969, a). Forsvarsmedicin.
    (In press).
Valeri, C. R. and Fortier, N. L. (1969, b). New Eng. J. Med.
    (In press).
Valtis, D. J. and Kennedy, A. C. (1953). Glasgow M. J. 34:521.
Valtis, D. J. and Kennedy, A. C. (1954). Lancet. 266:119.
Weatherall, D. J. (1969). New Eng. J. Med. 280:604.
Whitaker, W. (1956). Quart. J. Med. 25:175.
Zemp, J. W. and O'Brien, T. G. (1960). Proc. VIIIth Int. Congr.
    Haematol. 2:1189.

THE HEMOGLOBIN FUNCTION OF BLOOD STORED AT 4° C

R. Ben Dawson, Jr., MAJ, MC

Blood Transfusion Division, USAMRL

Fort Knox, Kentucky

INTRODUCTION

It is appropriate that this First International Conference on Red Cell Metabolism and Function is dedicated to A. C. This investigator noted that a slow moving electrophoretic component (B) decreased at the same rate as red cell organic phosphate concentrations during the storage of blood (Berry and Chanutin, 1958). This was assumed to be a hemoglobin-organic phosphate complex. After Bartlett and Barnett (1960) found that 2,3-DPG became rapidly depleted in ACD-stored blood, component B was found to be composed chiefly of DPG and ATP (Sugita and Chanutin, 1963; Chanutin and Curnish, 1964, 1965a). Further work showed that this complex was capable of decreasing the affinity of oxygen to hemoglobin (Chanutin, 1966). Since DPG is present in large amounts in the red cell, it was clear that the Hb-DPG complex is important for decreasing the affinity of O_2 to hemoglobin. This effect was confirmed (Chanutin and Curnish, 1967; Benesch and Benesch, 1967), and recent studies have shown binding of 2,3-DPG to both oxyhemoglobin and deoxyhemoglobin, using equilibrium dialysis (Chanutin and Hermann, 1969) and ultracentrifugation (de Verdier and Garby, 1969).

It has been known for some time (Valtis and Kennedy, 1953, 1954; Gullbring and Strom, 1956), that the oxygen affinity of blood increases during storage in ACD, as shown by a significant shift to the left of the hemoglobin oxygen dissociation curve.

This defect or impairment of hemoglobin function develops during the first few days of storage and persists throughout the storage period. When this blood is transfused it does not release oxygen normally to the tissues until the metabolism of the recipient has corrected the defect. Valtis and Kennedy calculated that a transfusion of 3 units of 7-day-old ACD blood, sufficient to raise the hematocrit from 35% to 55%, actually decreased the oxygen delivered to the tissues for several hours after transfusion; and at 24 hours, the patient's oxygen dissociation curve was still slightly shifted to the left. Valeri and Hirsch (1969) have shown that regeneration of 2,3-DPG after transfusion is more than 50% complete at 24 hours, but normal concentrations are not reached for several days. This defect might be critical for a patient who depends on normal oxygen transport to the tissues.

Improvements in the preservative solution for storing blood at 4° C have been directed toward maintaining adequate ATP levels, necessary for red cell viability. Adenine was found to be very effective in small concentrations for maintaining red cell ATP content and viability (Nakao, 1962; Simon, et al., 1962; de Verdier, 1964). A lack of toxicity of adenine containing solutions was confirmed in humans (Shields, 1967). Further studies with blood collected into ACD and CPD (Citrate-Phosphate-Dextrose) containing adenine gave acceptable post-transfusion survivals of 70% of the red cells 24 hours after transfusion, when the blood had been stored for 5 weeks (Simon, 1962; de Verdier, 1964; Shields, 1968).

However, it was known that adenine seemed to maintain ATP at the expense of 2,3-DPG during storage at 4° C. This was confirmed by comparative studies under blood banking conditions using blood collected into ACD and ACD-adenine, and the lower levels of 2,3-DPG in the adenine blood correlated closely with a greater oxygen affinity or lower p_{50} (Bunn, 1969). Now that 2,3-DPG is known to be important for hemoglobin to function normally, it has become important to maintain 2,3-DPG levels during storage as well as ATP.

The maintenance of acceptable DPG levels during storage may be attained in the presence of inosine and by elevating the blood pH. Inosine, which will maintain 2,3-DPG through the pentose phosphate pathway, can be included in the adenine containing preservative. Also, inosine can be added during the storage period to resynthesize 2, 3-DPG prior to transfusion (Akerblom, et al., 1968). Inosine is essentially non-toxic, and has been used in transfusion practices in Europe for several years to supplement stored blood. The pH of blood in CPD, 0.5 pH units higher than blood in ACD, is maintained throughout storage and is associated with higher levels of 2, 3-DPG during most of the storage period (Chanutin and Curnish, 1965b). It is possible therefore, to utilize media containing adenine, inosine and CPD which will provide conditions for maintaining the red cell ATP and DPG concentrations at functional levels.

The studies reported here have two purposes. First, the relationship between 2, 3-DPG and the oxygen affinity of hemoglobin is extended by experiments in CPD blood. Further, the oxygen dissociation curves and concentrations of 2, 3-DPG and ATP have been studied at intervals during the storage period in CPD blood which has been supplemented with adenine and inosine. In the second group of studies, experiments with added neutral salts, some of which are known to influence the oxygen affinity of hemoglobin, were performed using whole blood. It is hoped that these studies will help to define the conditions, especially 2, 3-DPG and ionic environment, which determine the normal function of hemoglobin in the red cell.

METHODS

Blood was drawn as units (450 ml) from young male, non-smoking volunteers into two or more Fenwal plastic bags[*], containing the preservatives to be compared. These half or quarter units were stored at $4 \pm 1°$ C in a blood bank refrigerator. At regular intervals during storage, usually weekly, aliquots were removed for study. Anaerobic and aseptic techniques were used during collection, storage and sampling.

Oxygen dissociation curves were done on whole blood by the Van Slyke manometric method in most experiments, or by

---

[*]Fenwal, Inc. , Morton Grove, Ill.

spectrophotometry[*]. The manometric technique and tonometer developed in this laboratory have been described by Bunn et al. (1968, 1969). An improved tonometer[*] using similar volumes and the same water bath temperature, 37°C, allowed equilibration of several samples simultaneously and gave similar results. The gas mixtures contained 40 mm Hg of CO_2 and varying proportions of oxygen and nitrogen. In the original vacuum filled tonometer, the blood sample was equilibrated with each gas mixture for 20 minutes. In the improved flow-through tonometer, a 10-minute equilibration period was adequate. Upon completion of tonometry the oxygen content or percent oxyhemoglobin was determined by manometry, except where the spectrophotometric method is specified in the results. The pH of each equilibrated sample was measured anaerobically at 37°[*]. Hemoglobin concentrations were determined from the absorbance at 540 mu in Drabkin's solution, or at 548, 568 and 578 mu after dilution in a solution of Triton X100[*]. The partial pressure of oxygen, pO_2, of the mixtures was measured by amperometric blood gas analysis[*], and was corrected to the whole blood pH value of 7.40 by the Severinghaus nomogram. Oxygen dissociation curves were drawn as linear plots using logarithmic values from the Hill equation. Four to 7 points were adequate for plots from which reliable values for P_{50} (HbO_2 = Hb) could be derived.

Concentrations of 2,3-DPG, ATP, and G6P (glucose-6-phosphate) were determined in duplicate samples by fluorometric assays of enzymatically coupled reactions (Keitt, 1966). The techniques, originally described by Lowry (1964) were first used in this laboratory by Bunn, et al. (1968).

RESULTS

2,3-DPG Studies

Storage of blood in either ACD or CPD results in a progressive increase in oxygen affinity, shown in Figure 1 as a decrease in p_{50}, the partial pressure of oxygen at which hemoglobin is 50 percent saturated. Blood from two donors is represented; each unit was split into half units for comparison of the two

---

[*]Instrumentation Laboratories, Lexington, Mass.

preservatives, and each half unit was sampled at three times
during the storage period. In CPD, the p_{50} values are consistently greater during the 3 week storage period, than those
observed in ACD blood. The changes in 2, 3-DPG concentrations
in the red cell approximately parallel the changes in p_{50}. The
relationship between p_{50} and 2, 3-DPG concentrations for these
experiments is shown in Figure 2.

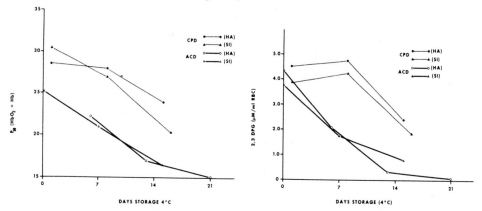

Fig. 1. Values for p_{50} and concentrations of 2, 3-diphosophy-
glycerate (2, 3-DPG) during storage of blood preserved in ACD
and CPD. The letters, HA and SI indicate the donors.

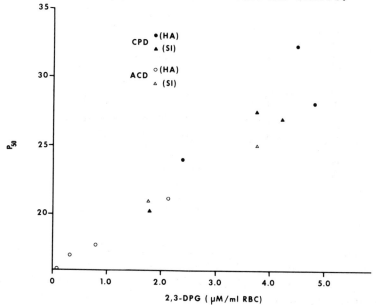

Fig. 2. The relationship between p_{50} and 2, 3-DPG concentration
of blood preserved in ACD and CPD.

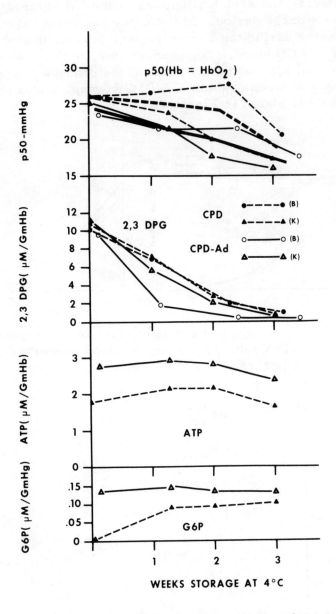

Fig. 3. Oxygen affinity (p_{50}), 2,3-DPG, ATP, G6P (glucose-6-phosphate) of blood at 1, 2 and 3 weeks of storage in CPD and CPD-adenine. The dotted lines represent values in CPD stored blood and the solid lines changes in CPD adenine blood. Heavy lines represent average values of p_{50} for the two donors.

The oxygen affinity and 2, 3-DPG data for CPD and CPD-adenine blood are shown in Figure 3. The differences in p_{50} values between these preservatives are small compared to the difference between CPD and ACD stored blood. The values are slightly higher in blood preserved in CPD than in CPD adenine. The 2, 3-DPG concentrations are somewhat higher throughout the storage period in CPD. The ATP concentrations for one of these units are also shown in Figure 3. ATP is better maintained in the adenine containing blood. The higher concentration of glucose-6-phosphate (G6P) in the adenine containing blood is also expected when sufficient adenine is present (0.47 millimolar) to maintain higher ATP concentrations.

The p_{50} values and concentrations of 2, 3-DPG, ATP, G6P for blood stored in CPD-adenine-inosine are shown in Figure 4. The presence of inosine (3.6 millimolar) allows the p_{50} to remain near normal for almost two and one-half weeks. Further, when this concentration of inosine was added to CPD adenine half units from the same donors, the p_{50} increased substantially. Here, the inosine was added after 25 days of storage in 10 ml of .15 M sodium chloride and the blood was not incubated, but kept at 4°.

Salt Studies

The effect on the oxygen dissociation curve of adding one volume of 1 M sodium chloride to 10 volumes of outdated bank blood is shown in Figure 5. The curve is shifted to the right and the p_{50} which had been 16.5 was increased to 18.8. Further, when these points, obtained from CPD adenine blood which was 21 days old, are graphed logarithmically according to the Hill equation, the (n) value, denoting heme-heme interaction, is seen to have increased from 2.50 to 3.00 after addition of the salt. The concentration of 2, 3-DPG was very low, less than 0.1 uM/Gm of Hb, and did not change after addition of the salt.

The oxygen affinity data shown in Figure 6 were obtained by the spectrophotometric determination of percent oxyhemoglobin. The salt solutions were added to 21-25 day old ACD blood. The p_{50} values, without addition of salt, for these units were in the range of 12 to 17. These have been adjusted to a control value of 15 for a clear graphical presentation, and the experimental data were adjusted by the same magnitude. The volume of salt

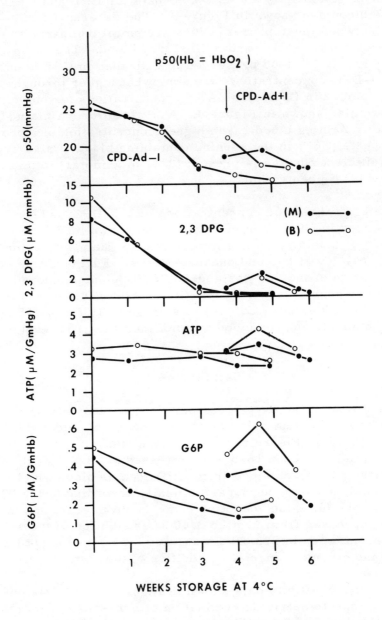

Fig. 4. Values for p_{50}, 2,3-DPG, ATP, and G6P during storage in CPD-adenine-inosine over 5 to 6 weeks. The arrow at 25 days indicates addition of inosine to CPD-adenine blood from the same donors.

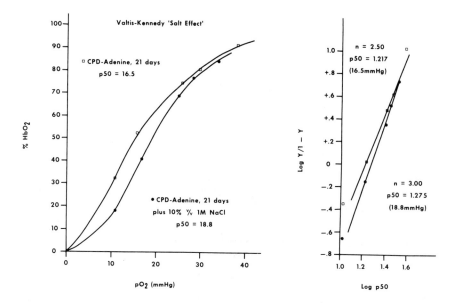

Fig. 5. Oxygen dissociation curves of 21 day old CPD adenine stored blood before and after addition (same day) of 1/10 volume 1 M sodium chloride. Details are given in the text.

was 10% of the blood in each experiment and the oxygen dissociation curves were performed on the same day, unless otherwise noted. The increases in p_{50} obtained with 0.5 and 1 M concentrations of NaCl, KCL, and NH_4Cl were similar. Magnesium chloride had less effect and calcium chloride had no effect except in a 2 M concentration. Five molar sodium chloride increased the p_{50} to a normal value of 26. The same value was obtained by adding 5 M sodium chloride to fresh ACD blood. Sodium and potassium acetate had effects similar to their chloride salts. The p_{50} values with the acetate salts had diminished when they were measured 24 hours later.

DISCUSSION

The deterioration of hemoglobin function during blood storage noted by Valtis and Kennedy (1953) and Gullbring and Strom (1956) has only recently been related to the progressive decline in red cell concentrations of 2,3-DPG. The present studies confirm and

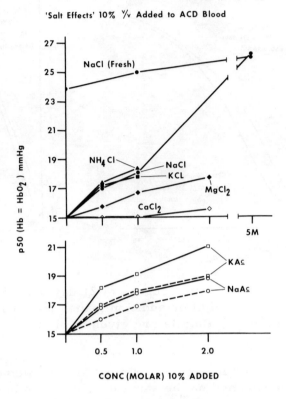

Fig. 6.   Increases in p_{50} of outdated ACD blood produced by
adding 1/10 volume of various salts in the concentrations indicated.
The dotted lines are used to join p_{50} values which were obtained
24 hours after salt addition.   The other values were obtained
within 2-3 hours of salt addition.

extend the dependence of normal hemoglobin function on 2, 3-DPG
(Chanutin, 1966; Benesch and Benesch, 1967; Chanutin and
Curnish, 1967).   Hemoglobin function expressed as p_{50}, is better
maintained during storage in CPD than in ACD.   This conclusion
is supported by higher 2, 3-DPG concentrations in CPD blood.
Further, the slightly higher ATP levels in CPD blood are in
agreement with this finding by previous workers.   Evidence has
been presented by Chanutin (1965) that the pH of CPD blood, 0.5 pH
units higher than ACD blood, is responsible for the higher 2, 3-DPG
concentrations.

The slightly lower concentrations of 2, 3-DPG in adenine containing CPD blood was expected since adenine had this effect on blood stored in ACD (Bunn, 1969). Further, when inosine was included in the CPD adenine preservative or added late to the CPD adenine blood, 2, 3-DPG was better maintained or regenerated so that hemoglobin function was controlled for a longer period than in preservatives which lack inosine.

Apart from 2, 3-DPG, other important variables which affect hemoglobin function during blood storage are pH, temperature, and the salt environment. In the preservative studies, comparing CPD with ACD and with CPD-adenine and CPD-adenine-inosine, adjustments in temperature and pH to normal whole blood values have been made by accepted methods (Bunn, et al., 1969). Thus, for these variables the hemoglobin function data can be considered relevant for physiologic or transfusion considerations. Also, the changes in red cell salt concentrations which are known to occur in stored blood do not appear to be significant in the present 2, 3-DPG studies nor in previous studies which have shown a direct correlation between decreasing hemoglobin function or p_{50} and decreasing concentrations of 2, 3-DPG during storage (Akerblom, et al., 1968; Bunn, et al., 1969).

The effects of salts on the oxygen affinity of hemoglobin and the shape of the dissociation curve have been known for a long time. Important early studies using hemoglobin solutions (Taylor and Hastings, 1942; Rossi Fanelli, et al., 1961) showed an increase in p_{50} with various salts, several of which contain chloride. These effects were confirmed in whole blood which had been stored 21 days in ACD (Valtis and Kennedy, 1963). They also showed that the increase in p_{50} resulting from the addition of a 10% solution of 1 M sodium chloride was maintained in the recipient of this blood which we now know to have been depleted of 2, 3-DPG. This finding may be important because several hours are required for regeneration of 2, 3-DPG by the recipient after transfusion and normal hemoglobin function might be provided during this interval by the addition of an appropriate salt just prior to transfusion.

In the present report, the salt effect is much more pronounced in blood that is depleted of 2, 3-DPG. This supports a similar finding using hemoglobin solutions, and the converse as well; a sufficient concentration of 2, 3-DPG makes the oxygen affinity

essentially independent of the salt concentration (Benesch, et al.,
1969). It appears, therefore, that the salt effects reported here
do not result primarily from changes in red cell size, and thus in
hemoglobin concentration (Dawson, in preparation). However,
further work is needed in order to understand the mechanism of
the salt effects on intact red cells. The evidence presented
supports a view that the ionic environment of hemoglobin, as well
as the concentration of 2, 3-DPG, in the red cell might be favorably
altered in stored blood to provide the recipient with normally
functioning hemoglobin.

SUMMARY

Blood was collected in citrate-phosphate-dextrose (CPD) and
acid-citrate-dextrose (ACD) media supplemented with adenine,
inosine and inorganic salts in order to affect the levels of ATP,
DPG and the ionic environment of the red cell during storage in
the cold. The oxyhemoglobin dissociation curves of whole blood
were determined and related to the 2, 3-DPG concentrations. The
P_{50} (the pO_2 at which Hb is 50% oxygenated) and the 2, 3-DPG
concentrations were higher in blood stored in CPD than in ACD
bloods. These values declined rapidly in the presence of adenine.
Blood collected in CPD supplemented with adenine and inosine
maintained the P_{50} and 2, 3-DPG at near normal levels during a
three week storage period. The addition of salts increased the
P_{50} levels of three week old ACD blood and thus confirmed the
findings of Valtis and Kennedy.

REFERENCES

Akerblom, O., de Verdier, C.H. Garby, L. and Hogman, C.
    (1968). Scand. J. Clin. and Lab. Invest. 21:245.
Bartlett, G.R. and Barnet, H.N. (1960). J. Clin. Invest. 39:56.
Benesch, R. and Benesch, R.E. (1967). Biochem. Biophys. Res.
    Commun. 26:162.
Benesch, R.E., Benesch, R. and Yu, C.I. (1969). Biochemistry
    8:2567.
Berry, E.R. and Chanutin, A. (1958). J. Clin. Invest. 37:974.
Bunn, H.F., May, M.H., Kocholaty, W.F. and Shields, C.E.
    (1969). J. Clin. Invest. 48:311.

Bunn, H. F., May, M. H., Lenzi, D. and Taylor, J. F. (1968).
    USAMRL, Ft. Knox, Ky., Report # 785.
Chanutin, A. and Curnish, R. R. (1964). Arch. Biochem. Biophys.
    106:433.
Chanutin, A. and Curnish, R. R. (1965a). Proc. Soc. Exp. Biol.
    (N. Y.) 120:291.
Chanutin, A. and Curnish, R. R. (1965b). Transfusion 5:254.
Chanutin, A. (1966). U. S. Army Report, R & D Command
    (Washington, D. C.) 30 June 1966.
Chanutin, A. and Curnish, R. R. (1967). Arch. Biochem.
    Biophys. 121:96.
Chanutin, A. and Hermann, E. (1969). Arch. Biochem. Biophys.
    121:180.
de Verdier, C. H., Hogman, C., Garby, L. and Killander, J.
    (1964). Acta Physiol. Scand. 60:141.
de Verdier, C. H. and Garby, L. (1969). Scand. J. Clin. Lab.
    Invest. 23:149.
Gullbring, B., and Strom, G. (1956). Acta. Med. Scand. 155:413.
Keitt, A. S. (1966). Am. J. of Med. 41:762.
Lowry, O., et al. (1964). J. Biol. Chem. 239:18.
Nakao, K., Wada, T. and Kamiyama, T. (1962). Nature 194:877.
Rossi-Fanelli, et al. (1961). J. Biol. Chem. 236:397.
Shields, C. E., Dennis, L. H., Eichelberger, J. W., and Conrad,
    M. E. (1967). Transfusion 7:133.
Shields, C. E., and Camp, F. R. (1968). Transfusion 8:1.
Simon, E. R., Chapman, R. G., and Finch, C. A. (1962). J. Clin.
    Invest. 41:351.
Sugita, Y. and Chanutin, A. (1963). Proc. Soc. Exp. Biol. (N. Y.)
    112:72.
Taylor, J. F. and Hastings, A. B. (1942). J. Biol. Chem. 144:1.
Valeri, C. R. and Hirsch, N. M. (1969). J. Lab. Clin. Med.
    73:722.
Valtis, D. J., and Kennedy, A. C. (1953). Glasgow Med. J. 34:521.
Valtis, D. J. and Kennedy, A. C. (1954). Lancet 1:119.

APPENDIX - DISCUSSION OF PAPERS

EDITORS NOTE: The recording, typing and editing of symposium
discussions is, I find, a very imperfect science. The material
included in this Appendix has been partly but not completely
reviewed by the discussants. It is offered for the information
and interest of the reader, but it should not be quoted in the
literature without permission of the discussants since many
inaccuracies may be present through no fault of theirs. I
apologize for such errors, but I have chosen to minimize correspondence with discussants in order to have the volume published
promptly.

DISCUSSION OF PAPER BY GARBY AND DEVERDIER

Dr. Bunn: You made a very interesting point, Dr. Garby, about abnormal hemoglobins interacting with 2,3-DPG. One would think that if one prepared Hiroshima on a column and looked at its oxygen equilibrium you could tell whether or not the isolated hemoglobin is intrinsically of high affinity or whether it depends on an interaction with organic phosphates for its high affinity. Unfortunately, the experiments that have been done in Japan used 0.1 M phosphate, and as Dr. Chanutin has nicely shown, 0.1 M phosphate will itself cause a tremendous decrease in affinity. So one can't tell from the published data, as yet, whether Hiroxhima has an intrinsically high affinity or whether it just doesn't interact with phosphate. This past year at the Albert Einstein College of Medicine we have looked at hemoglobin Chesapeake with Dr. Charache, and have found that Chesapeake, stripped of phosphate, by G-25 Sephadex, has itself a high affinity. The addition of 2,3-DPG to Chesapeake causes a normal decrease in oxygen affinity, so the reactivity with Chesapeake with DPG in terms of oxygen equilibrium appears to be normal.

Dr. Chanutin: Dr. Garby, you have pointed out that histidine in position number 21 in the beta chain is the probable site of binding for these phosphate compounds. Is that correct?

Dr. Garby: It is a possible one.

Dr. Chanutin: From work done in our laboratories at Charlottesville and Uppsala, there appears to be evidence that at least 3 sites are available for binding phosphate compounds. Would you agree that amino acid residues other than histidine are capable of binding phosphorylated compounds?

Dr. Garby: Yes. That must be so. However, one must remember that in speaking about DPG binding in relation to oxygen binding, it may well be that some of the binding sites have nothing to do with oxygen affinity. So this is difficult to discuss.

Dr. Chanutin: We found that certain phosphate compounds that had no effect on the oxygen dissociation curve could be bound in appreciable amounts to both reduced and oxyhemoglobin. Perhaps one site may be involved in the actual release of oxygen from hemoglobin and other sites may be inactive in this respect.

Dr. Garby: Yes.

Questioner: Dr. Garby, could you give us some idea of the difference between the affinity of 2,3-DPG of fetal hemoglobin as opposed to adult human hemoglobin?

<u>Dr. Garby</u>: We haven't calculated affinity constants for DPG to
these 2 hemoglobins, partly because the experiments were done at
zero degrees, and I'm not sure that affinity constants calculated
at that temperature would make much sense in the intact living
cells. The experimental data are given in a paper published in
Scan. J. Lab. Clin. Med. <u>23</u>, 149, 1969.

<u>Dr. Brewer</u>: Do you have evidence that ATP and DPG are competing
for the same binding site?

<u>Dr. Garby</u>: We have studied the effect of DPG on ATP binding, and
addition of DPG lowers the binding of ATP to deoxygenated hemoglobin, but increases the binding of ATP of ATP to oxygenated
hemoglobin. However, the effects are small, so that from the
point of view of metabolic regulation we are not in a position to
help you very much.

<u>Dr. Brewer</u>: And I assume you're not in a much better position
with regard to glutathione. Dr. Chanutin has shown that glutathione
increased his electrophoretic component B, as did DPG and ATP.
Also, Dr. Horejsi's data suggests that glutathione shifts the
dissociation curve to the right. Do we have any information on
whether glutathione is binding at a completely different site?

<u>Dr. Garby</u>: We have no information on that.

DISCUSSION OF PAPER BY HOREJSI

Unidentified Questioner: I would like to ask you first, were the dissociation curves you showed on the slides done at constant pH and constant pO_2?

Dr. Horejsi: Certainly, under very strict experimental conditions.

Questioner: Could the change in the position of the dissociation curve when you add carbonic anhydrase and carbonic anhydrase plus Diamox[R] be due to changes in the carbaminohemoglobin or bound CO_2?

Dr. Horejsi: This we have not tested. I can't answer that.

Questioner: Was there any change in the hydrogen ion concentration between the plasma and the cell after addition of the glutathione? That is, a change in the hydrogen ion gradient - the pH gradient - between plasma and the cell?

Dr. Horejsi: We have not tested that.

Dr. Astrup: Thank you very much, Dr. Horejsi, for your very interesting lecture. Your results concerning the influence of glutathione on the survival of dogs is very important and should be tested in other laboratories.
I disagree with you a little concerning your explanation of the effects of glutathione. We were interested some years ago in the effect of glutathione on the oxyhemoglobin dissociation curve and we added reduced glutathione to whole blood, but we didn't get any effect at all on the oxyhemoglobin dissociation curve. This we explained in the way that glutathione does not penetrate the red cell membrane. We had some effect with ascorbic acid, but in very high and unphysiological concentrations. We had a small effect with cysteine. I would like to ask· How did you determine your oxyhemoglobin dissociation curves? Did you equili-brate the blood with an oxygen mixture in a tonometer and did you equilibrate it before or after lysis of the red cells?

Dr. Horejsi: Yes, both examinations have been made and always the dissociation curve has been determined by the classical method equilibrating the blood with a well-defined mixture of gases. At least 3 points of the curve were always determined and from that the Hill's constant has been calculated.

Dr. Astrup: Yes, but did you equilibrate hemolysate or whole blood?

Dr. Horejsi: Both whole bloods and hemolysates also.

Dr. Astrup: Yes, I understand that you can obtain the results if you equilibrate erythrolysates, but I cannot understand that you can obtain the results when you equilibrate whole bloods.

Dr. Horejsi: Yes, with the whole bloods also.

Dr. Astrup: Well, we couldn't find it.

Dr. Horejsi: And also in the experiments in dogs I have mentioned. We have taken the blood after the infusion of preparation with glutathione and equilibrated the whole blood directly.

Dr. Loos: Is it possible to explain the effect of vitamin C on the basis of a higher oxygen pressure inside the red cells? It is known that vitamin C gives rise to the production of hydrogen peroxide and since in your experiments catalase was not inhibited it may be expected that oxygen is generated inside the red cells.

Dr. Horejsi: That's a possible hypothesis, but we have not tested it. I can't answer that on the basis of experiment.

Dr. Loos: You explained the favorable effect of glutathione outside the red cell on the basis of a change in the electric charge of the membrane. Could it also be explained by localization of the enzyme glutathione reductase in the membrane allowing transport of reducing equivalents across the membrane?

Dr. Horejsi: Well, I think this could be some contribution to the explanation. Some time ago there was a paper published, that the change of reduced and oxidized hemoglobin can be caused without oxygen intermediate but by changes of electron charges.

Dr. Loos: Have you tried the effect of N-ethylmaleimide on the oxygen dissociation curve?

Dr. Horejsi: No, not yet.

DISCUSSION OF PAPER BY EATON ET AL.

Dr. Engel: I first would like to congratulate you very much on
this elegant method for measurements of oxygen release. I think
it's the first time we really have seen experiments carried out on
the effects of variation of red cell levels of 2,3-DPG. I would
like to suggest an alternative explanation of the increase of 2,3-DPG
in exercise. We know that the spleen releases reduced hemoglobin
during exercise, and if 2,3-DPG is more tightly bound to reduced
hemoglobin, then the average 2,3-DPG concentration in the circulating blood could increase because of release of new red cells from
the spleen.

Dr. Eaton: I think it's possible that a release of the splenic
reserve might be a very small factor in the increase of DPG.
However, the mass of red cells released by the spleen probably is
not large enough to account for the differences we've seen.

Dr. Necheles: I was curious as to whether you had any children
with high hemoglobin concentrations with congenital cyanotic
heart disease, and what you found in these children.

Dr. Eaton: I'm sorry, we have not done any children. I would
expect that there are elevations in DPG in children with cyanotic
heart disease. Do you have data to the contrary?

Dr. Necheles: Actually, we have data on children with cyanotic
heart disease aged about 3 to 8 years. Surprisingly enough,
the 2,3-DPG levels are very low, and we're not certain whether this
is related to the acidosis which many of these children have, or
what actually is going on.

Dr. Oski: Our data is perfectly at variance with Dr. Necheles.
We have found, in a study of 50 children and infants with cyanotic
heart disease ranging in age from about 1 day to about 16 years,
that after about one month of age a very significant elevation occurs
in the 2,3-DPG level. This seems directly related to the decrease
in arterial pO_2. Under a month of age, there is not the expected
response to hypoxia as reflected in elevation of 2,3-DPG level.

Dr. Eaton: Well, part of that early lack of response may be due
to the presence of high levels of fetal hemoglobin.

Dr. Necheles: We feel very strongly that it is the lack of
significant binding of DPG by fetal hemoglobin in these infants
under a month of age which accounts for the lack of response.

Dr. Eaton: Unfortunately, we have no data on cyanotic children,
so I think that you'll have to fight it out between the two of you.

<u>Dr. Harkness</u>: I, too, think that your machine is very elegant, though I would like to caution the interpretation that you're measuring everything that takes place in an extremity. In an anemic person, the rate of circulation is going to be quite increased, and you're doing all of your experiments at one flow rate. It may be that this compensation by the increased rate in delivery of oxygen with increased levels of 2,3-DPG may not compensate as much as you'd like. You'd have to do measurements on both the arterial and venous side to evaluate what really happens.

<u>Dr. Eaton</u>: Right. I wasn't trying to say we had built an animal. We've just built a device that is, though admittedly not perfect at representing the organism, better than what we had before.

<u>Dr. Astrup</u>: Thank you for your nice paper. I was very much interested in your results concerning lactic acidosis (which I'll come back to in my paper. I think we have to distinguish between lactic acidosis and other kinds of acid base disturbances. I would like to ask some of the biochemists here: How can an increase of lactic acid in the blood increase the 2,3-DPG level?

<u>Dr. Eaton</u>: Well, I wasn't suggesting, if I may interject, that the two were causally connected. Lactic acid increase has been used by physiologists for quite a while as a measure of physiologic stress during exercise, and that's what we were using it as in this situation. I think that what that relationship tells us is that the greater the stress produced by the exercise the more likely a significant increase in DPG.

<u>Dr. Astrup</u>: Yes, but can the relationship between DPG and lactate change be explained biochemically?

<u>Unidentified Speaker</u>: That's just the hypoxia effect that's causing the increase in DPG. We haven't had long enough for the pH to have any effect. Lactic acidosis is merely a measure of the degree of hypoxia that the person has had.

<u>Dr. Garby</u>: I may have a suggestion for you. What happens to the pyruvate lactate ratio in this experiment? If the pyruvate/ lactate ratio increases, then you would have a biochemical mechanism.

<u>Dr. Eaton</u>: Unfortunately, there's no consistent change in the ratio even in the most stressed individuals. If you're thinking of pyruvate elevation proportionately changing DPG through a shift in the DPN-DPNH ratio, it apparently doesn't work in this situation.

<u>Dr. Chanutin</u>: You said rats exposed to hyperoxia had a decrease in DPG. Was this an appreciable drop?

<u>Dr. Eaton</u>: Well it depended on how the hyperoxia was administered and whether or not we got around the atelectasis frequently caused by high oxygen pressures. We found maximal decreases in ATP, as I remember, down to 50% of normal levels and the DPG dropped about the same amount.

<u>Dr. Chanutin</u>: Would you be willing to postulate or perhaps you know the answer. What happens to an astronaut exposed to pure oxygen not at high pressure?

<u>Dr. Eaton</u>: I think that an increase of up to 50% above atmospheric in the pO_2 may not be great enough to produce significant change. In other words putting more oxygen in solution in the plasma increases the average saturation of the circulating hemoglobin, through making the plasma act as a substitute oxygen carrier. Unless the oxygen or air is under high tension, the solubility of oxygen in the plasma will not be increased much. Therefore, you don't get the increased oxygen carrying capacity of the plasma and the correspondingly increased average saturation of the circulating blood.

<u>Dr. Garby</u>: Did you use constant value of hematocrit in your machine in all your experiments, or did the hematocrit values vary?

<u>Dr. Eaton</u>: In the data we reported here, we left the hematocrits fall where they may, just as the blood came out of each individual, because we were interested in working with physiologic blood. However, after this we did some adjusting of hematocrits, and the results were what one would predict from the correction factor.

DISCUSSION OF PAPER BY GRISOLIA ET AL.

<u>Dr. Diederich</u>: I wish to present data from studies recently completed which extend the findings already presented. Table 1 summarizes the binding of DPG by several additional abnormal hemoglobins as well as fetal hemoglobin.

Quite striking is the increased DPG binding by hemoglobins Zurich and Chesapeake and the extremely low DPG affinity of fetal hemoglobin when compared to that of Hb A. The data in Table 1 also demonstrate that passing hemolysates through DE Sephadex, utilizing the conditions described by T. Huisman and A. Dozy (J. of Chromatography, 19,160 (1965), separates phosphoglyceromutase from the hemoglobin and also removes in essence all of the DPG from the hemoglobin. This latter observation has been confirmed by additional studies on normal adult hemoglobin. The residual DPG bound to hemoglobin after passage through Sephadex G-25 column can also be removed by passage through DE Sephadex.

Table 2 demonstrates the lack of correlation between DPG affinity of several abnormal hemoglobins and the reported blood oxygen affinity for the respective hemoglobin disorder. Sickle cell hemoglobin, with decreased whole blood oxygen binding affinity binds significantly less DPG than does Hb A, whereas, hemoglobins Zurich and Chesapeake, possessing increased oxygen affinity, demonstrate also increased affinity for DPG.

<u>Dr. Keitt</u>: For those who prefer to use an endpoint assay rather than a rate assay for measuring a substrate, the fluorometric method of Lowry can be adapted to the spectrophotometer. The assay utilizes the 2,3-DPG phosphatase activity which is present in commercial preparations of muscle monophosphoglycerate mutase. This phosphatase activity has been shown by Dr. Harkness to be selectively stimulated by pyrophosphate. If 10 mM pyrophosphate is included in the assay the assay goes to completion in about 20 to 25 minutes, depending on the 2,3-DPG concentration. The procedure is performed on neutralized PCA extracts.

<u>Dr. Loos</u>: I completely agree with Dr. Keitt when he says that it is difficult to apply systems of estimation in which a rate is used as a function of concentration. However, this only holds true when these estimations are performed by hand; using an autoanalyzer, reproducibility becomes as good as with endpoint determinations. Systems of estimation in which a rate is used as a function of concentrations are much more sensitive than endpoint determinations and the high sensitivity of these estimations allowed us to determine e.g. 2,3-diP-glycerate in one million human lymphocytes.

<u>Dr. Grisolia</u>: May I comment again, that life is too short to modify a method <u>ad</u> <u>infinitum</u>. The question is, what is the simplest method, and how fast it can get reliable data for

TABLE 1. RESUME OF MUTASE, DPG PHOSPHATASE, RESIDUAL DPG AND DPG BINDING
BY SEVERAL HEMOGLOBINS

Type HB	Mutase Units/mg Hb	Phosphatase μmoles/mg Hb/hr	Residual DPG Molar Ratio	DPG Binding in 0.02 M NaCl Molar Ratio
A	0.086	0.0011	0.063	1.03
A*	0.0	0.0010	0.003	1.03
J Baltimore*	0.0	0.0006	0.001	1.09
Kansas	0.091	0.0018	0.106	1.21
Chesapeake*	0.0	0.0014	0.005	2.56
Zurich*	0.0	0.0	0.001	1.73
Fetal	0.068	0.0016	0.097	0.10
SS	0.100	0.0	0.018	0.41

*Passed through DE Sephadex column

TABLE 2 .   RESUME OF RESIDUAL 2,3 DPG, 2,3 DPG BINDING
AND OXYGEN AFFINITY OF SEVERAL HEMOGLOBINS

Type Hb	Residual 2,3 DPG	2,3 DPG Binding in 0.02 M NaCl	Blood O_2 Affinity
A	0.003* 0.063	1.03	Normal
F	0.0974	0.10	Increased
K	0.106	1.21	Decreased
Zurich	0.0014*	1.73	Increased
Chesapeake	0.0047*	2.56	Increased
J Baltimore	0.0015*	1.09	Normal
SS	0.018	0.41	Decreased

* Passed through DE Sephadex column

whatever you want.

<u>Dr. Charache</u>:   I don't speak biochemistry; I think maybe I'm here for comic relief.

Our interest has been in sickle cell anemia; the oxygen affinity of the blood of patients with sickle cell anemia is decreased, as many of you know, although the hemoglobin has the same oxygen affinity as hemoglobin A. When we first heard about diphosphoglycerate, it sounded like this was going to be the answer. So we collected blood from a number of patients in Baltimore, froze it at -70° and sent it to Kansas City packed in dry ice where the DPG levels were measured.

Studies in animals, and in some patients with anemia, have shown a correlation between severity of anemia and increase in DPG concentration. Bromberg and Jensen related oxygen affinity to hemoglobin concentration in sickle cell anemia, and we expected to find the highest DPG levels in our most anemic patients. We did not find such a relationship (Fig. 1A). The binding of DPG to hemoglobin and the activities of the enzymes of DPG metabolism are affected by DPG concentration, pH, and particularly by ionic strength of the system. Our patients with sickle cell anemia, although ambulatory, were not in good health, and it seems likely that unmeasured biochemical abnormalities of many types were the cause of the apparently random scatter of their DPG concentrations.

A similar explanation may underlie our inability to correlate DPG levels with reticulocyte counts (Fig. 1B). DPG concentrations are said to be increased in reticulocyte-rich blood, but that is not true of the reticulocytes of patients with hereditary spherocytosis. In that case, increased splitting of DPG was observed, and related to decreased pH within red cells.

Studies in which DPG was added to lysed normal red cells, and our comparisons of lysed normal and SS red cells, suggest that levels of DPG found in SS cells may be one cause of decreased oxygen affinity in sickle cell anemia.   The differences between the observed pO_2, and that of normal whole blood at the same intracellular pH and % oxygen saturation, are expressed as ΔA. Although the oxygen affinity of hemolysates was equivalent to that of normal blood at DPG concentrations found in normal red cells, an oxygen affinity as low as that found in SS patients ($\Delta A = 4\text{-}6$) was found only at DPG concentrations in excess of 8 µmole/ml. Only one SS patient had a DPG level that high. Oxygen affinity of blood from our patient with pyruvate kinase deficiency, and that of other patients with the same disease, is also difficult to explain on DPG concentration alone, for oxygen affinities as low as those found in these patients (ΔA 12-14) were not found at the DPG levels found in their red cells (6.6-14.9 µmole/ml).

Abnormal aggregation of molecules of hemoglobin S, independent of DPG concentration, has been suggested as a cause of abnormal oxygen affinity of SS blood, and cytoarchitectural factors have

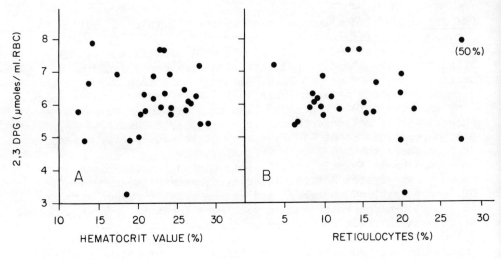

FIGURE 1A

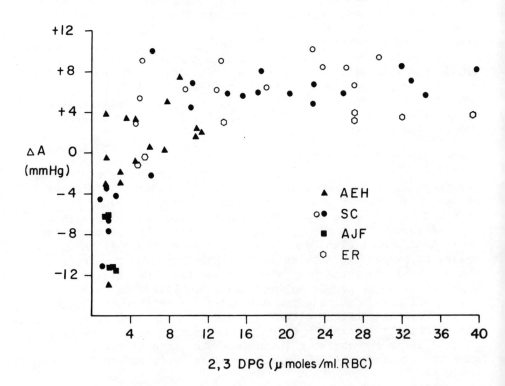

FIGURE 1B

been invoked as a cause of abnormal affinity of fetal red cells. It seems quite likely that a multiplicity of factors, in addition to the intracellular concentration of DPG, act in concert to govern oxygen affinity, not only in sickle cell anemia, but also in other pathophysiological states.

<u>Dr. Engel</u>: I think that we ought to maybe bring a little bit of order into the way we express our 2,3-diphosphoglycerate. I think that the many different ways of expressing it may add to the confusion. I would like to ask Dr. Charache whether he measured any difference in mean cell hemoglobin concentration? I mean if you express 2,3-DPG as 2,3-DPG in micromoles or in micromoles per milliliter packed cells, and you have a difference in your mean cell hemoglobin concentrations. Maybe you could interpret your data differently.

<u>Dr. Charache</u>: We are certainly aware of the points you have raised.

<u>Dr. Chanutin</u>: Dr. Hjelm, you're the expert in expressing concentrations of DPG by various manners. Would you comment on the question?

<u>Dr. Hjelm</u>: I think that it isn't time at present to decide what expression is the right one when one calculates intracellular components of erythrocytes. The point I would like to make here is that as has been stated by Dr. Engel, you may not include values from patients with varying concentrations of MCHC in your material, because then you also include a new variable among the other factors which can influence the content of 2,3-DPG.

<u>Dr. Chanutin</u>: I would like to ask Dr. Grisolia about how best to study this problem of determining oxygen dissociation curves, in terms of the ionic strength of the medium to be used. It seems to me that practically everyone has a different medium and there are large variations in pH; what in your opinion is the best medium to utilize?

<u>Dr. Grisolia</u>: I once asked my colleague, the Professor of Physiology, what he thought about that, and he hedged here and there and he said, "Well, maybe pH 7.2, and 0.1 M". I think that's probably just as close as you can be within the erythrocyte. On the other hand, if you want to do some comparative binding studies, I think one may be allowed to do so at concentrations far from physiological. I think this is a rather important point you are raising, because we have seen today, and probably we are going to see more, the necessity to bring together physiology and molecular events. To find out what really goes on inside <u>in vivo</u> systems is the hardest problem for modern biology!

Dr. Chanutin: But when you talk about physiologic conditions, with dilute hemoglobin solution, you've left the physiological world, haven't you?

Dr. Grisolia: Right, because right here you have in the case of the red cell the highest protein concentration known. Practically, there's not even room for water in there.

Dr. Chanutin: Dr. Hjelm, you're the expert in expressing concentrations of DPG by various manners. Would you comment on the question?

Dr. Hjelm: I think that it isn't time at present to decide what expression is the right one when calculating the intracellular components in human erythrocytes. The point I would like to make here is, that a further problem is introduced, when the content of intracellular components in the erythrocytes e g DPG, has to be compared in subjects with different values of MCHC.

REMARKS BY C.-H. deVERDIER, OPENING SESSION 2

Ladies and gentlemen,

This afternoon we are going to continue the discussion of the content of 2,3-diphosphoglycerate in red blood cells at different disorders.

Figure 1 summarizes the theoretically possible correlations between circulation, respiration and regulation of pH and intra-erythrocytic concentration of 2,3-diphosphoglycerate (DPG).

The delivery of oxygen per time unit to a tissue is the product of blood flow (Q) times hemoglobin concentration (C_{Hb}) times the difference in saturation between the arterial and venous blood ($Sat_a - Sat_v$). This product together with the oxygen consumption of the tissue determines the P_{O_2} of the tissue. The regulation of P_{O_2} through cardiac output and erythropoietin is well-known.

Changing the concentrations of DPG and hydronium ions creates possibilities to regulate the venous saturation (Sat_v) at a given P_{O_2}. The Bohr effect is familiar to all of us, but the magnitude of the effect of pH on DPG-binding to hemoglobin and on DPG-synthesis in the erythrocytes of the patient is not apparent at the present time. We hope to hear about these questions in the presentations by Dr. Rorth and Professor Astrup.

As DPG binds better to deoxygenated than oxygenated hemoglobin the time average degree of oxygenation of hemoglobin of the blood ought to regulate the total concentration of DPG, if one assumes that the enzyme systems of the erythrocyte tend to keep the free concentration of DPG at a fixed level.

I suppose the relative importance of these two regulation mechanisms - the pH mechanism and the mechanism through differential binding to oxygenated and deoxygenated hemoglobin - will be one main topic of the forthcoming discussion.

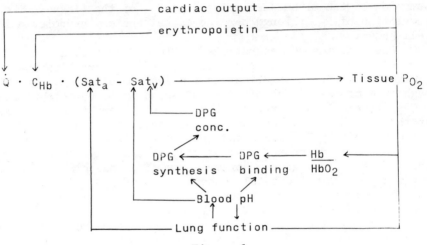

Figure 1.

DISCUSSION OF PAPER BY HJELM

<u>Unidentified Speaker</u>: If you explain your correlations to hemo-
globin level by means of the binding of DPG to reduced hemoglobin
and not oxygenated hemoglobin wouldn't you expect similar results
with all substances which preferentially bind to reduced hemoglobin? I notice that you find the ATP correlation in the opposite
direction.

<u>Dr. Hjelm</u>: ATP was inversely correlated with the hemoglobin con-
centration in whole blood only in subjects with hemoglobin values
within the normal range.

<u>Unidentified Speaker</u>: How do you explain the opposite direction of
the correlation?

<u>Dr. Hjelm</u>: We have tried to explain the inverse correlation
between the content of DPG and ATP in erythrocytes from subjects
with values for the hemoglobin concentration within the normal
range as a competition between the two compounds for binding sites
at the hemoglobin molecule, the concentrations of the free forms
of ATP and DPG being kept at a constant level. This hypothesis is
in accordance with the <u>in vitro</u> findings reported by deVerdier,
Garby, and Gerber (Eur. J. Biochem. 10, 110, 1969).

<u>Dr. Williamson</u>: Not very many people have measured the oxidized
and reduced form of glutathione, from which you can calculate the
redox potential of the TPN system for the erythrocytes, assuming
equilibrium with the glutathione reductase which is present in the
red cells in very large amounts. It would be very useful particularly
to correlate with the G-6-P, 6-phosphogluconate concentrations.
The equilibrium constant is very large since certainly most of it
is in the reduced form. I just wonder, do you remember what ratios
you get? To measure the oxidized form is an extremely difficult
technical problem. But it will be interesting to know what ratios
you get.

<u>Dr. Hjelm</u>: The ratio here was about 5% oxidized compared to
reduced, and I think that figure is too high. Thus I have used
the sum of the components to express the content of reduced
glutathione.

DISCUSSION OF PAPER BY BREWER ET AL.

Dr. Astrup: May I say a few words concerning oxyhemoglobin dissociation and carbon monoxide exposure. The effect of carbon monoxide on the oxyhemoglobin dissociation was discovered in 1896 by Haldane. It was later studied in 1912 by Smith and Haldane and studied again in 1933 by Roughton and subsequently by others. Now we have studied it too. The effect of the curve is due partly to the so-called Haldane-Smith effect, which is an immediate physical chemical effect on the hemoglobin molecule, so that the affinity for oxygen increases. The same occurs when hemoglobin is exposed to oxygen, and the affinity of the rest of hemoglobin increases and this causes the S shape of the curve. This is well known. There is a second effect of carbon monoxide according to our studies. The affinity of hemoglobin to oxygen is increased a bit more than can be explained by the Haldane-Smith effect on the curve. This we published three or four years ago. We didn't find the explanation of it until recently when we measured the 2,3-DPG values after exposure of human individuals to carbon monoxide for 24 hours. They had from 15 to 20% carboxyhemoglobin. We found a small reduction in 2,3-DPG varying from 5 to 10%, and we feel that this reduction is able to explain the increased affinity of hemoglobin for oxygen besides the Haldane-Smith effect of carbon monoxide. Now we come to the problem concerning oxygen tensions in arterial blood of smokers. May I just ask you how did you measure the arterial oxygen tensions?

Dr. Brewer: With radiometer electrodes.

Dr. Astrup: Did you measure 2,3-DPG values in smokers?

Dr. Brewer: Yes, we did. We found no difference between smokers and nonsmokers. Could I make one additional comment. I don't think that our data on carbon monoxide effects on DPG levels is in disagreement with Dr. Astrup's actually. We had to experiment for some time with rats in order to find appropriate carbon monoxide exposures which would cause the DPG to go up. We found that if we redosed the rats frequently with carbon monoxide and held them at high levels of carboxyhemoglobin (40-60%) we saw no change in DPG. Of course, the fact that it didn't go down is itself evidence that something besides hemoglobin binding effects on DPG is operating. We found the same thing with high levels of methemoglobin, which is a similar kind of experiment. We interpret these studies to mean that the two mechanisms are competing against each other, that is the hemoglobin binding mechanism tending to lower DPG, versus another mechanism which we call the hypoxia mechanism. The two mechanisms are working against each other. I would like to make our method clear in the rat studies to avoid confusion when people go back to their labs and try to reproduce these results. We dosed them to toxicity at 0 and 3 hours. The rat loses carboxy very rapidly. I think what we have is a hypoxia trigger which is there at 0 and 3 hours. The CO is blown off very rapidly and during the rest of the 3 hour period we don't have much of the DPG hemoglobin binding mechanism operating. Hypoxia during the first few minutes or so after CO exposure may be the trigger that makes the DPG go up. If you keep the carbon monoxide high constantly it doesn't work, at least in rats.

Dr. Duboff, University of Michigan: Did you note at what time of the menstrual cycle the samples from women were obtained? I take it all the subjects were in the child-bearing age?

Dr. Brewer: Yes, they were all young. No, we did not consider the menstrual cycle.

Dr. Duboff: Well, about 8 years ago I measured the lactate/ pyruvate ratio of the blood in young women in a study on the glycolytic metabolic blood changes throughout the menstrual cycle (Obst. & Gyn. 18,564, 1961) and found that there was a marked variation in the products of the Embden Meyerhof Pathway (EMP) versus hexose monophosphate pathway (HMP) relative to the cycle period with the EMP predominant during the follicular phase and declining with the onset of ovulation. There was a marked rise in the HMP over that of the EMP during the luleal phase with the EMP being restored and peaking at the fifth to sixth day of the cycle. Of course we were looking at the whole blood. Now I wonder to what extent RBC glycolytic changes would be influenced by the menstrual cycle.

Unidentified Speaker: Dr. Brewer, you have demonstrated differences between male and female red cells with respect to their glucose consumption. I wonder if you also found significant differences in their mean corpusle hemoglobin concentration (MCHC) because, if present, that can at least partly explain the difference, because of the way you have expressed the glucose consumption per gram of hemoglobin.

Dr. Brewer: We didn't look at the MCHC in this sample. This has been done in normal men versus normal women, and is about the same in the two sexes. So other than these being normal, healthy men and women, we don't know specifically what their MCHC was.

Unidentified Speaker: Because as you divide your glucose consumption in your sample by the hemoglobin, with even small differences in MCHC, say if you have 30 grams per 100 ml packed cells in man and 28 in females, that is already a difference of about 6 or 7%.

Dr. Brewer: Yes. I don't think that that is enough to account for the differences we are seeing here which are greater than 25%.

Further, even if we didn't correct the data, for differences in hemoglobin level and just expressed them per ml of whole blood, women still have a higher mean rate of glucose consumption.

Unidentified Speaker: Do you happen to have any control of red cell age such as red cell hexokinase activity? I know in our lab we don't even use our female personnel any more because they all have much younger blood cells. We have found that red cells in females are much younger and therefore might use more glucose.

Dr. Brewer: In general the red cell survival in women is about the same as that of men. Are you suggesting that the laboratory personnel in your lab are being bled so often that they have a young blood cell population?

Unidentified Speaker: No, but they're not pregnant. They're all menstruating.

Dr. Brewer: Yes, but this has only a slight effect on red cell survival.

Unidentified Speaker: I wonder about the possibility of hemoglobin polymorphism in the rats you studied. Is there any? How inbred is the strain?

Dr. Brewer: These are Hooded rats supplied to us as they come by the supplier. They are not specially inbred, although there is bound to be some inbreeding. We looked at the hemoglobins of some Hooded rats and didn't see any electrophoretic variation, but I am not positive about the ones I have shown you here.

Unidentified Speaker: Probably you realize, since you have gone about it in depth, that if there happened to be variation in the type of hemoglobin it would be possible to explain your results in your rat litters. This would involve, perhaps the relative ability of a variant hemoglobin to bind or not to bind 2,3-DPG.

Dr. Brewer: Yes. I think that that is a good point to look into. However, I am under the impression that there isn't much variation here with hemoglobin.

Dr. Filley: I am so delighted to find concordant results at this meeting. There are others who have reported a low arterial pO_2 in people with high carboxyhemoglobin. I would like to point out that Dr. Brodie in Philadelphia has actually found this out as well and has come up with an excellent explanation. However, that's what I am going to talk about tomorrow. It has to do with the uneven distribution of blood and gas in the lungs and if you think that this is a complicated meeting, you will find that if you're not familiar with pulmonary physiology, that that is also complicated. That's tomorrow.

GENERAL DISCUSSION

<u>Dr. Greenwalt</u>: It has now been established that fetal hemoglobin does not bind 2,3-diphosphoglycerate appreciably. In studies performed over a decade ago we observed low DPG in the red cells of rabbit pups. The level of DPG in the erythrocytes rose to adult rabbit erythrocyte levels during the first three weeks of life. Does anyone know whether rabbits have a different form of hemoglobin at birth? This might be a very suitable model for studying this phenomenon. These observations were published in the Journal of Cellular and Comparative Physiology 53, 307, 1959.

DISCUSSION OF PAPER BY WILLIAMSON

Dr. Loos: I should like to thank Dr. Williamson for his beautiful
explanation of some experiments we did. We were involved in the
problem of restoration of 2,3-diP-glycerate in DPG-poor bank blood.
We have incubated DPG-poor ACD-blood or red cell suspensions with
several additives but we never succeeded in generating more than
1 umole of DPG per ml of red cells. The only way we knew to
restore DPG-levels nearly to completion, was by incubation of red
cells in isotonic NaF solution with adenosine and pyruvate.
Recently we succeeded in generating 2,7 umole of DPG per ml of red
cells in 80 minutes by incubating DPG-poor ACD-blood with adenosine,
$MgCl_2$ and pyruvate at 37°C (details were presented in my paper).
So a crucial point in DPG-generation inside DPG-poor red cells is
the prevention of NAD-exhaustion by addition of pyruvate, as may
be derived from your presentation.

Dr. Grisolia: In addition to the regulatory effects so well
illustrated by the speaker I should like to make some comments on
the P-glycerate trident shunt. It should be of interest to the
audience the fact that acyl phosphatase controls chemotropic
effects particularly since certain reagents such as 1,3-diphospho-
glycerate are good chemotrophic effectors. It should be understood
that chemotrophic effects result in covalent bond formation, such
as for carbamyl phosphate and lysine to yield homocitrulline. It
is often a neglected consideration that reagents such as carbamyl-
phosphate or 1,3-diphosphoglycerate are made in large quantities
in the body, for example, it is self evident that each mole of
glucose yields 2 moles of 1,3-diphosphoglycerate during glycolysis
and that a normal diet may produce 2-4 moles of 1,3-diphosphoglycerate
per day. Again, a normal diet may yield nearly 1 mole of urea
(60 gm) and thus it will necessitate the formation of about 1 mole
of carbamyl phosphate which will be distributed during the day in
the liter of water or so contained in the human liver! It is then
no wonder that a high concentration of these reagents, and the fact
that they are highly reactive, may produce protein interaction
and modification. There are two points in this regard which I
would like to make. One is that, as shown in our laboratory, one
of the enzymes which is rapidly inactivated is triosephosphate
dehydrogenase, which produces 1,3-diphosphoglycerate. Second,
that as recently shown in our laboratory by Dr. Ramponi from the
University of Florence, histones can be readily carbamylated and/
or phosphorylated by carbamyl phosphate or 1,3-diphosphoglycerate
respectively. Therefore this is another level at which Diederich's
acyl phosphatase may have profound effect on regulation since it
acts both at enzyme and genetic regulatory sites!

Dr. Duboff, University of Michigan: As I sat here yesterday and
earlier today it has become apparent to me that I ought to go back
and relearn or review everything about phosphorous metabolism.

Essentially what you and others have presented here deals with phosphates as esters of carbohydrates. If the important thing is whether the carbohydrate as a glycerol is a monoester or a diester i.e., 2- or 3-phosphoglycerate, or 2,3-diphosphoglycerate and since you are dealing with equilibrium constants for these constituents in the sequence of events, should you not recognize the equilibrium constants for the two forms of the phosphate, namely the orthophosphate-pyrophosphate in any reaction, in which the direction of the reaction will go from left to right depending on the pH? If my memory serves me correctly the pyrophosphate has a very strong resonating bond between one of the oxygens and phosphorous, whereas this does not prevail for the other phosphate. It seems to me that anyone manipulating the glycerophates _in vitro_ must consider the chemistry and thermodynamics of the phosphate bonds.

Dr. Williamson: Yes, this is an interesting point. Most cells do contain extremely powerful pyrophosphatases. When people have tried to measure the content of pyrophosphate, it is extremely low, and so the species that one does need to take into account is actually inorganic phosphate. In the enzyme steps where pyrophosphate is formed, the pyrophosphate is probably snatched up and split, even perhaps using high energy phosphate. I haven't worked out the physical chemistry differences in the equilibrium you are talking about but I would just imagine that the pyrophosphate is always extremely low. Perhaps somebody else can comment.

Unidentified Speaker: Dr. Williamson, you have touched a lot of bases in an excellent review. I would just like to emphasize one point that may have slid by in all of the discussion. And that is the importance of ADP in controlling DPG concentration in the red cell. I think there will be quite a bit more said about it and I would just like to emphasize it briefly at this point. One of your sets of conditions showed a hangup in the triosephosphates and FDP which was relieved by increasing pyruvate. Under those conditions there was a decrease in ADP and I think the role of ADP in influencing phosphoglycerate kinase is going to come on strong. I also was pleased that you began to invoke the divalent cations in red cell metabolism because I think they have been neglected. Even calcium will become important in other connections, in relation to the membrane. Your concern about the Ki for DPG mutase, I think will remain because with a purified system it seems to be different than in intact cell or hemolysates. Actually Rapaport, who has shown nearly everything, has described the inhibition of the mutase with relatively decent concentration of 2,3-DPG, but much more than you would allow. We have done similarly with hemolysates.

Dr. Chanutin: There is one question I would like to ask you. You passed by the pentose phosphate shunt completely. Did you do that intentionally, or is it too complex?

<u>Dr. Williamson</u>: Well actually, I don't know what to say about it.
Maybe it should not be neglected.

<u>Unidentified Speaker</u>: There is another thing you did pass by and
that is the glucose-1,6-diphosphate.

<u>Dr. Williamson</u>: People better qualified than me can talk about
those points.

DISCUSSION OF PAPER BY ROSE

<u>Dr. deVerdier</u>: I want to congratulate you for this interesting
work. From my own experiences I know the difficulties involved in
work with DPG phosphatase as the activity of this enzyme in the red
blood cell is very low.

I would like to make a comment about the strong ability of
DPG phosphatase to exchange phosphate groups between monophosphoglycerate (PG) and 2,3-DPG. DPG phosphatase was purified according
to an earlier publication (Fol. Haematol. <u>90</u>, 215, 1968). At a
final purification step electrofocusing was introduced. Fig. 1
shows the clear-cut separation between DPG phosphatase (tested as
liberation of i P^{32} from $DP^{32}G$) on PG mutase (tested photometrically
by coupling with enolase, pyruvate kinase and lactate dehydrogenase)
although the mutase still contains phosphatase activity. Material
from the phosphatase and mutase peak was tested in the systems
outlined in Table I. The transfer of radioactivity from PG to DPG
was measured in 0.1 M tris-maleate buffer at pH 0.5 and the result
was obtained by paper chromatographic separation of DPG and PG
through a solvent system (n-propanol/NH_3/water 20/10/3).

Comparing the ability of the phosphatase and the PG mutase to
exchange phosphate groups one finds that the activity of the former
is remarkably higher. Preliminary results with differently labelled
PG and DPG indicate that the mechanism for the two exchange reactions
differs.

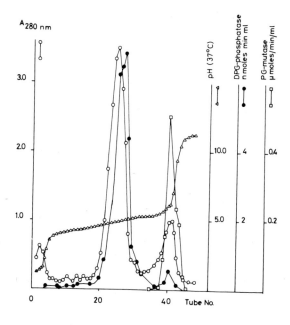

Figure 1.

TABLE 1

Activities of a DPG phosphatase and a PG mutase preparation investigated indifferent test systems

	DPG phosphatase preparation (EE 15)	PG mutase preparation (EE 15)
DPG $\longrightarrow$ PG + P' (DPG phosphatase)	348	22
3-PG $\xrightarrow{\text{DPG}}$ 2-PG (PG mutase)	< 300	10.200
PG + DPG $\rightleftharpoons$ PG + DPG	402.000	2.560

Activities expressed as nmoles/hr/ml enzyme preparation.

Dr. Grisolia: I would like to ask Dr. Rose if she knows whether the glycolate 2-P activates the phosphatase activity of the mutase.

Dr. Rose: Yes, glycolate 2-P is a very good activator of the phosphatase activity of the mutase. We have submitted a paper using this reaction for the quantitative determination of DPG.

Dr. Grisolia: Well I think that this is very important because some of the people in the audience may not be as well aware of the mutase as also having phosphatase activity. This is also linked to the question of Dr. deVerdier. I think this is a very exciting finding of Dr. deVerdier, since this change between the monophosphoglycerate and the 2,3-DPG is terribly dependent upon the ionic strength of the media. Indeed this was the point raised yesterday about the enormous change in kinetic constants with the ionic strength. It seems to me that it is self-evident that one of the first things to try is to find out whether ionic strength affects, as we discussed yesterday, the phosphatase or the exchange reaction of your phosphatase. The other question which I would like to know is, does anyone know if the KCl also affects the phosphatase activity of the mutase?

Dr. Rose: KCl inhibits the phosphatase activity of the mutase.

Unidentified Speaker: It seems to me, Dr. Rose, that even if you believe that the regulation is mostly at the DPG mutase, somehow, if there are such marked changes in the concentration of 2,3-DPG in the rabbit cell, there must be a mechanism whereby you can get rid of it also rather quickly. Therefore, phosphatase activity must play an important role at certain times.

Dr. Rose: Yes, I agree with that. It can be increased by an increase in the concentration of phosphate in the physiological range, because the Ka for phosphate was 0.7 millimole. The concentration of phosphate in the red cell normally is about 0.4 millimolar. I would think that any kind of increase in that range would affect the rate of the enzyme. One can account in this way for rates in the range of 0.5 umcles/hr/ml of cells.

Dr. Grisolia: I should like to make a point clear for the record. That is that Dr. Towne, in our laboratory, showed for the first time 15 years ago that 2,3-diphosphoglycerate is the product of diphosphoglyceromutase. In other words, Rapoport's evidence for the reaction was entirely indirect, he showed an increase of utilization of fructose 1-6 diphosphate on addition of red cell mutase, while Towne and Rodwell first and then Joyce demonstrated by unequivocal and classical methods the identity of the product. In addition they showed that contrary to the early reports of

Rapoport, who claimed that diphosphoglycerate mutase is present only in red cells, many tissues contain the enzyme and one of the best sources is muscle.

Dr. Bartlett: We looked for phosphoglycolate many years ago very carefully, and had no evidence for any down to a level of at least 1/10 that which had been originally reported. If it is present in the red cell, it must be in extremely small amounts.

I think some results that Gerlach has, and which I have, indicate that the labeling of DPG after incubating human red cells with p^{32} inorganic phosphate under conditions where there was no change in the concentration of 2,3-DPG, suggest that all of the DPG present in the cell is freely available to the MPG mutase. This was under conditions where we would expect, from the reports presented here at the conference, that there would be a considerable degree of binding of the DPG to hemoglobin. This is of special interest with respect to the mechanism of the synthesis of extra 2,3-DPG in hypoxia, since complete inhibition of the DPG mutase by 2,3-DPG would be expected in any case.

Unidentified Speaker: I would like to shift the area of the discussion a little bit from biochemistry to physiology. It seems to me that there are two apparent discrepancies here. The first one is that it is very difficult to reconcile the fact that DPG is in fact synthesized in the red cells with the Ki values. The second one is that increasing levels of inorganic phosphate should, in the intact cell, decrease the level of DPG whereas in fact, as we saw yesterday in Astrup's paper, the relationship is the other way around. One approach to find out about these apparent discrepancies might be to study the enzymes in the presence of high concentrations of hemoglobin. I wonder if you have done that.

Dr. Rose: Yes we have done that with both enzymes. We passed concentrated hemolysates through a sephadex column and assayed in as high concentration as we could. The rates were consistent with what we get for dilute hemolysates.

Dr. Grisolia: I should like to ask from the experts in 2,3-diphosphoglycerate phosphatase what regulates this enzyme, since as reported here by many the level of 2,3-DPGA increases and decreases rapidly within the red cell. This will necessitate a much larger activity than reported by Rose (in the absence of an activator). Moreover, there will be inhibition of activity once certain levels of product have been reached. These briefly outlined considerations indicate that there is a very close control in this enormously high protein medium which is the interior of the red cell.

DISCUSSION OF PAPER BY GERLACH ET AL.

Dr. Harkness: These are very provocative, interesting data. The decomposition of 2,3-DPG in oxygenated and deoxygenated cells is rather puzzling. I was worried about the intracellular pH. Did you have any chance to measure it or calculate it? Would the intracellular pH be much different in the deoxygenated and oxygenated cells?

Dr. Gerlach: We have neither measured nor calculated the intracellular pH in oxygenated or deoxygenated cells. As to my knowledge it has not yet been clarified whether the intracellular pH changes in deoxygenated cells. In our experiments the extracellular pH was kept constant at pH 7.35 both under aerobic and anaerobic conditions.

Dr. Brewer: I think Asakura et al. (J. Biochem. (Tokyo) 59, 524, 1966) have found the decay of 2,3-DPG to be different under aerobic and anaerobic conditions. Do you have any explanation for the difference in results?

Dr. Gerlach: In our experiments the RBC were incubated without glucose. Under these conditions there was no difference in the rate of decrease of 2,3-DPG in oxygenated and deoxygenated cells. Asakura's paper deals with the decrease of 2,3-DPG in RBC incubated in the presence of glucose. Under these conditions the metabolism of 2,3-DPG is different in RBC incubated aerobically and anaerobically. This could also be seen from the last table of my paper.

Dr. Astrup: I would just like to congratulate you on your nice findings. I think they are very close to the findings we presented and I feel that your results also indicate that it is the pH of the cells which is very important indeed for regulating the 2,3-DPG concentration.

Dr. Filley: Again it is nice to find some concordant results between your findings and Dr. Astrup's interesting scheme. You raised the question, however, as to what is primary here. I suspect that the pH is a means to an end. What may be primary is the pCO_2 damage caused by hyperventilation. Reason: The intracellular pH is affected by the pCO_2 outside extremely rapidly because this is the one species that we have been discussing that moves most rapidly between the inside and the outside of the cells.

Dr. Gerlach: I would agree that the initial changes in 2,3-DPG are brought about by pH. But there must be some other factors controlling the maintenance of high DPG levels after a long period of hypoxia, as for instance the diminution of the saturation of hemoglobin with oxygen. It is known that the pH changes in acute hypoxia are almost completely reversed during chronic hypoxia.

Unidentified Speaker: With respect to your last remark I would like to point out that it is not certain that people at high altitudes have a normal pH. If they stay there for a long period of time the pH is still elevated. For instance, at sea level we have a pH of 7.4, and if we go to a higher altitude our pH would go up to 7.45 or 7.48. But being not a high altitude native, after a long period of time we would find ourselves with a pH of probably 7.42. A native of a particular altitude would have a normal pH of 7.4.

Dr. Gerlach: Over which period of time does the pH remain elevated:

Unidentified Speaker: As far as I know, from some of the work that has been published it stays for four months actually. We did some measurements in lowlanders who had been at altitude for months and there was always a pH which was consistently higher than that in the natives of this area. These were people who were from this country, from Europe, and from wherever else.

Dr. Astrup: One further comment concerning the acid-base status of dwellers at high altitudes. I haven't seen many data here, and it might be that there are small differences between the pH levels in arterial blood at sea level and at high altitude. Perhaps only 0.02 pH units would be sufficient to explain the increase in 2,3-DPG.

Dr. Lenfant: It is true that there are very few intracellular pH measurements available. However, I would like to say that pH may be one thing but bicarbonate may be another. I am not certain that there is a pH difference between a sea level dweller and a high altitude dweller, but we know that there is a difference in bicarbonate. That may be something which should be introduced into this picture. Since the altitude dwellers have a higher pCO_2 they must have a higher bicarbonate. This is a significant difference of, I am sure, several milli-equivalents.

Dr. Lionetti: Your finding about sulfate is very interesting, since it is a normal blood constituent and may exercise a role in the regulation of 2,3-DPG content of RBC. Relative to ADP, several years ago we discussed a situation in hemolysates of fresh cells previously depleted of 2,3-DPG. If the hemolysates were incubated with extracts of stored cells, the synthesis of DPG was inhibited. We followed this up and found that it was ADP and AMP, which inhibited DPG synthesis. We speculated that the phospho-glycerate kinase competes with the DPG mutase for 1,3-DPG. ADP accumulated in the red cells during storage has a tendency to pull the carbon toward lactate instead of allowing synthesis of 2,3-

DPG. So our point was that the synthesis was inhibited. The phosphatase which we attempted to study was not activated under those conditions.

Dr. Kitchen: Dithionite is quite a reducing agent. This could result in deoxygenation of your hemoglobin and might ultimately explain your results, rather than a direct effect of the agent.

Dr. Gerlach: We have not measured the oxygen tension in presence of the different sulfur compounds. But the concentration of dithionite was smaller than those necessary for deoxygenation of hemoglobin in our RBC suspensions.

Unidentified Speaker: Coming back to the DPG utilization, I wonder if the phosphatase experts would like to comment on two points. One is that I have been impressed by the similarities shown here in your data and the data of other authors with respect to 2,3-DPG phosphatase activity in hemolysates. There seems to be an autocatalytic type of effect. As the time increases, you get more activity and I wondered what the explanation for this is. And the second point concerns a report of Gomperts a few years ago that the 2,3-DPG phosphatase is bound to the membrane and has vectorial aspects (Fol. Haematol. (Leipzig) 90, 196, 1968).

Dr. Gerlach: We did some experiments to find out whether the 2,3-DPG phosphatase actually has directional properties. Our results not yet published demonstrate, however, that the 2,3-DPG phosphatase liberates the inorganic phosphate primarily inside the cell. Therefore the 2,3-DPG phosphatase seems not to be a vectorial enzyme of the red cell membrane liberating inorganic phosphate outside the cell into the medium as Gomperts concluded from his experiments. With respect to your first question it might be speculated that the slower decrease of 2,3-DPG in hemolysates in the beginning of incubation is due to some synthesis of 2,3-DPG from triosephosphates or fructose diphosphate which could be present in hemolysates in the initial phase of incubation.

Dr. Rose· According to my experiments 2,3-DPG phosphatase is a soluble enzyme. The activity is the same in stroma-free and in whole hemolysates. - I was interested in the chloride concentration in your experiments, because I think that you are activating the phosphatase. I haven't tried all those sulfur compounds you used, but I found that sulfite is an activator and sulfate is a very potent inhibitor of the phosphatase. Under my conditions I would require chloride to show effects of either sulfite or sulfate. Do you have chloride in your system?

Dr. Gerlach: Yes, we incubate red cells in plasma or in Locke-solution containing normal amounts of chloride. Only in the hemolysates chloride content was reduced to one third.

Dr. Greenwalt: Dr. Gerlach, I was interested to hear that you found 2,3-diphosphoglycerate more rapidly and extensively labeled by $^{32}PO_4$ in the presence of reduced hemoglobin than when the hemoglobin was oxygenated. I am not certain of the significance of the more rapid and extensive labeling of DPG in the erythrocytes of adults than in cord blood which we observed (Blood 19, 468, 1962). It appears to parallel your findings for fetal hemoglobin has much less affinity for DPG than even the oxyhemoglobin A in the cells we were studying.

DISCUSSION OF PAPER BY FILLEY

<u>Dr. Garby</u>: Dr. Filley, would you please repeat the last hypothesis, slowly?

<u>Dr. Filley</u>: Every time the oxyhemoglobin dissociation curve is moved the CO_2 dissociation curve is also moved. These are linked processes. Now the fact that they are linked means that we have to consider the mechanism for the linkage, and so far as I know, the most potent mechanism for this effect is the exchange of protons between the two systems. It is this exchange of protons which makes the CO_2 curve move because hemoglobin is a stronger acid when it's oxygenated in the lung and therefore delivers protons to the CO_2 system, driving out the CO_2 from the lung.

<u>Dr. Garby</u>: I'm very confused, because I thought this has been known for a long time.

<u>Dr. Filley</u>: So it has; there's nothing really new about this. All I'm doing is quoting from the past, and I hope I'm making some kind of a point.

<u>Dr. Garby</u>: Then I'm not so confused any more. How about the DPG then? You had some thoughts on how it might be affecting the dissociation curve.

<u>Dr. Filley</u>: All I can say about this is the following: My ideas are based on the work of Henderson, who in 1908 laid the foundation of acid base physiology by considering a system which consisted of CO_2, bicarbonate, and phosphate, and who proved that the bicarbonate must be the most important buffer because it's part of an open system, whereas the phosphate is in a closed system. Now if phosphate, as we've certainly known all these years, has been functioning and was used by most of the chemists to show how buffering processes occur, it strikes me as not purely coincidental that a particular phosphate, located in exactly the right place, namely inside the cell in high concentration, might be acting as a buffer, either directly or by affecting the pKs on the hemoglobin molecule, therefore helping to facilitate proton exchange...So the hypothesis is that 2,3-DPG contributes, in a particularly powerful way, by virtue of its chemical structure and in particular its location on the hemoglobin molecule, (to the extent that it is on it, which I'm afraid I'm not clear about) simply facilitates the process of proton exchange between the bicarbonate and hemoglobin systems.

<u>Dr. Brewer</u>: If this is a buffering effect only, how can you account for the specificity of DPG versus other phosphates?

Dr. Filley: Well, I understand, as a matter of fact, that it is not so terribly specific; one can move this curve around with other materials simply by changing the concentration enough; is it not true that NaCl can push the curve around?

Dr. Brewer: I'm still a little bothered by the fact that you can't move the curve to anywhere near the extent with inorganic phosphate, say, as you can with 2,3-DPG. This suggests to me that there's more than a buffering effect on the system, such as a conformational change of the hemoglobin molecule resulting from DPG binding.

Dr. Filley· There certainly could be. I certainly don't want to make this hypothesis an all or none proposition.

Dr. Bartels: I think we should admit that in the heavy working muscle and in the placenta, the Bohr effect is very important, but not in the lung, where it is normally explained, even in very good textbooks of physiology.

Dr. Filley: Thank you very much, Dr. Bartels.

DISCUSSION OF PAPER BY GROVER

<u>Dr. H. Bartels</u>: Your values of arterial oxygen content at sea
level indicate that your llamas had lower hemoglobin concentrations than have been reported previously. Can you explain
this?

<u>Dr. R. Grover</u>: Hemoglobin values published by others, and by
ourselves, are as follows:

Hemoglobin gm/100 ml	Hematocrit %	Altitude Meters	Number of Animals	References
18.8	41	s.l.	1	Bartels et al (1)
17.5	-	s.l.	4	Hall et al (2)
12.8	-	2810	1	Hall et al (2)
12.1	-	4710	1	Hall et al (2)
11.1	-	5340	1	Hall et al (2)
15.1	38	4200	12	Reynafarje et al (3)
9.9	-	4540	1	Meschia et al (4)
10.6	-	s.l.	3	Banchero et al (5)
11.8	-	3400	3	Banchero et al (5)
12.3	26	1600	4	Banchero et al (5)

(1) Bartels, H., Hilpert, P., Barbey, K., Betke, K., Riegel, K.,
     Lang, E.M. and Metcalfe, J.: Am. J. Physiol. 205:331, 1963.

(2) Hall, F.G., Dill, D.B., and Guzman Barron, E.S.: J. Cell.
     Comp. Physiol. 8:301, 1936.

(3) Reynafarje, C., Faura, J., Paredes, A., and Villavicencio,D.:
     J. Appl. Physiol. 24:93, 1968.

(4) Meschia, G., Prystowsky, H., Hellegers, A., Huckabee, W.,
     Metcalfe, J., and Barron, D.H.: Quart. J. Exp. Physiol.
     45:284, 1960.

(5) Banchero, N., Will, J.A., and Grover, R.F.: Physiologist
     12:166, 1969.

The obviously lower values we obtained may reflect the fact
that our animals were quiet and undisturbed by the blood
sampling procedure; the blood was drawn through a small
catheter inserted percutaneously earlier. Higher values
in some published reports may have resulted from excitement
and contraction of the spleen, which in sheep can increase
the hematocrit as much as 10-20% (Turner, A.W. and
Hodgetts, V.E.: Australian J. Exptl. Biol. Med. Sci.
37:399, 1959).

Dr. H. Bartels: I would like to point out that the llama, like
the white mouse and the golden hamster, has a relatively
large amount of hemoglobin in each red cell. The mean corpuscular hemoglobin concentration in the llama we studied
was 46%, and in your llamas it was 47%, whereas in man it is
only 35%. This enables the llama to have a relatively high
oxygen carrying capacity at a comparatively low hematocrit.
Thereby, he enjoys the advantages of maintaining a low blood
viscosity which facilitates blood flow and oxygen transport.
         As you mentioned, the position of the dissocia-
tion curve is not necessarily an advantage or a disadvantage.
Sheep and llamas graze together in the high Andes. Both
species thrive and reproduce well at high altitude in spite
of their very great differences in the affinity of hemoglobin
for oxygen. The camel, a relative of the llama, also has
hemoglobin with a high affinity for oxygen. Thus, it is
apparent that a dissociation curve unusually far to the left
functions equally well in the camel at sea level and the
llama at high altitude. Therefore the position of the
dissociation curve does not correlate with successful
adaptation of various animal species to high or low altitude.

Dr. R. Grover: I certainly agree with you that the affinity of
hemoglobin for oxygen is only one of several important
factors which determine oxygen transport, tissue oxygenation,
and ultimately survival.

Dr. G. Brewer: One could say that each species is adapted to
its own particular dissociation curve. Would it not be fair
to say that while the position of the dissociation curve
may be relatively unimportant between species, it may be of
greater importance within a given species?

Dr. R. Grover: That is probably ture. In species with a rightward dissociation curve, venous PO_2 tends to be relatively
high. This would minimize the need for tissue adaptations
(e.g. short diffusion pathway, increased myoglobin concentration) to preserve tissue PO_2. Within such an individual,
shifting the dissociation curve to the left could produce
tissue hypoxia (unless oxygen transport were greatly increased).

Dr. Astrup: Within a given species, the position of the
dissociation may be very important. I am thinking of work
done at Colorado State University in Fort Collins north
of Denver (S. Cueva and D.H. Will: Blood oxygen transport
in cattle "susceptible" and "resistant" to high mountain
disease. In Current Research in Chronic Respiratory Disease;
Eleventh Aspen Emphysema Conference held June 1968.
U.S. Public Health Service Publication No. 1879, pp. 81-86).
Cattle native to low altitude are prone to develop "high
mountain disease" when taken to altitudes above 3000 m.
Chronic atmospheric hypoxia causes severe pulmonary

hypertension. When right heart failure eventually develops, the associated edema fluid tends to accumulate in the dependent portions of the neck and thorax. Because this edematous swelling is often prominent in the pre-sternal region, cattlemen coined the term "brisket disease", since the parasternal muscles constitute the brisket of beef ("corned beef" is brisket).

Cueva and Will compared two groups of female Hereford cattle obtained at 3000 m. altitude. One group was "susceptible" (S) to "high mountain disease", having developed heart failure while at altitude. When they were moved to low altitude, they recovered. The other group was considered "resistant" (R) because they had developed no evidence of "high mountain disease" at 3000 m. Both groups were in good health when these studies were conducted at low altitude.

The oxygen-hemoglobin dissociation curves were determined in vitro. Group R had a curve significantly to the right of Group S. Expressed as the PO_2 at 50% saturation (T50), R = 35.17 mm Hg and S = 29.65 mm Hg (pH 7.4 at 37°C).

Dr. R. Grover: That is a very interesting observation with the general implication that in animals with hemoglobin with a lower affinity for oxygen (Group R), the unloading of oxygen at the tissue level is facilitated, thereby preserving tissue oxygenation. Conversely, "susceptible" animals may have greater tissue hypoxia. In more specific terms, there is the suggestion that animals with a lower T50 (Group S) may have a lower PO_2 in pulmonary arterial blood, which, in turn, may contribute to pulmonary arterial constriction and hence more severe pulmonary hypertension.

I have talked with Dr. Will who tells me that the story is now more complicated. He has studied dissociation curves in calves born to the females in the original two groups. These calves have never been to high altitude. Consequently, unlike their mothers, none has ever been in heart failure. Calves of R have a lower T50 than calves of S, which is the converse of the original groups (R higher than S). This raises questions not only regarding genetic differences between R and S in determining T50, but also between the possible role of the position of the dissociation curve in the pathogenesis of "high mountain disease".

Dr. H. Kitchen: As you know, two types of hemoglobin occur in sheep: type A with a high affinity for oxygen, and type B with a low affinity for oxygen. Whitlock has reported that at the same low altitude, sheep with hemoglobin A have consistently higher hematocrits than sheep with hemoglobin B. (Evans, J.V. and Whitlock, J.H.: Genetic Relationship Between Maximum Hematocrit Values and Hemoglobin Type in

Sheep. Science 145:1318, 1964).

Dr. R. Grover: This fits very nicely with our concept of oxygen transport regulating red cell mass. With a given oxygen transport and a consistant quantity of oxygen extracted from the blood, the venous PO_2 will be lower when the hemoglobin affinity for oxygen is higher (type A). This implies a lower tissue PO_2, greater stimulation of red cell production, and ultimately a higher hematocrit. At equilibrium, the greater oxygen carrying capacity of the blood will increase oxygen transport, and extraction of the same quantity of oxygen will be achieved with less reduction in PO_2, i.e. a higher tissue PO_2.

Dr. H. Kitchen: Do you have data on the hemoglobin type of the sheep you reported here?

Dr. R. Grover: No, these sheep were not hemoglobin-typed.

DISCUSSION OF PAPER BY LENFANT ET AL.

Unidentified Speaker: Dr. Lenfant, the people that you tested with
Diamox - did they tolerate the change in altitude as well as those
not treated?

Dr. Lenfant: Oh, yes, much better. These people were in fine
shape when they got up there. All the rest of us were not in such
fine shape. It's amazing to see the differences between the two
groups. Those people (who took Diamox) were active and unconcerned
and we were tired and just wanted to rest.

Dr. Miller: I'm delighted that we're talking about the physiological
significance of these conditions. It may be that within the broad
range there is little in the way of physiological significances.
In light of what Dr. Grover said, in his talk, could either of you
gentlemen tell me what a critical PO_2 is for man, and what evidence
there is for this?

Dr. Lenfant: I am not quite certain there can be such a simple
question. It depends on the circumstances. Obviously, when you
are at altitude but resting, you are not hypoxic in the generic
sense which we would like to keep for this expression. However
one is going to become hypoxic if he starts doing things and moving
around, because then he won't be able to supply enough oxygen to
his tissues for an increased demand. This is where a shift of the
oxygen dissociation curve, I feel, becomes important. In fact,
we have done some calculations to show the importance of that shift.
They show that if one goes to altitude and does not increase his
hemoglobin, nor shifts his dissociation curve, his working ability
will be decreased by about 50%. Now if one has a shift of his
curve, his working ability will be up to about 75% of what he can
do at sea level. The last 25% will be gained if he has also a
hemoglobin increase.

Unidentified Speaker: In your people who got up to altitude and
didn't shift their curve to the right, we may make an analogy between an individual who starts with a normal position, and then
shifts it to the left. Now if we shifted a normal person far
enough to the left, perhaps Dr. Grover might comment on whether
we would reach a point at which the mixed venous PO_2 would become
critical for organ function. Is that known?

Dr. Grover: I don't think it's known.

Dr. Lenfant: This is an interesting question that I can illustrate
with an example. In our hospital some people were doing work with
diabetic patients.   These patients were deprived of their
insulin and therefore became severely acidotic. When we measured

P_{50} and DPG in these patients we found very significant changes. The P_{50} fell by 3 to 5 mm Hg, and the DPG decreased by 25%. At that time pH was about 7.15 or 7.2. I assume that if these people were given a massive dose of bicarbonate they would become relatively hypoxic by suddenly shifting their in vivo curve to the left because of alkalosis and DPG depletion. However, if they would correct their pH slowly, there would be no great problem.

Dr. Grover: Dr. Faulkner says that the critical PO_2 is known.

Dr. Faulkner: Wendell, University of Florida, studied the critical PO_2, not in humans but in dogs. It is about 10-15 mm of mercury in mixed venous blood.

Dr. Grover: What's the criterion for critical?

Dr. Faulkner: Well, critical PO_2 is simply where you keep decreasing the partial pressure of oxygen til the metabolism is affected; so the critical PO_2 is defined as that point at which metabolism is impaired.

Unidentified Speaker: I know data on men which are, I think, 15 years old. In young healthy people as we have seen them, you lose consciousness at around 15 mm of oxygen tension in mixed venous blood, plus or minus 2 mm.

Dr. Metcalfe: It seems to me that this is a situation in which mixed venous values can be terribly misleading, because of organ function. I think we would all agree that unconsciousness is a sign of organismic function, the function of the total organism, but not that of perfused hind limb, for instance, which has a very rich capillary supply. Oxygen consumption doesn't fall until venous blood from that limb gets down to about 5 mm of mercury. So mixed venous blood reflects, unfortunately, changes in the distribution of blood flow, and if you suddenly send most of your blood up to your cerebral circulation, you may mask the effect of the decrease in PO_2. So I think that mixed venous PO_2's are very insecure measurements.

Dr. Filley: I'd like to underline what's just been said, and put in one more plug for CO_2; namely, the critical PO_2 is an almost impossible thing to define unless you want to talk about death or consciousness, or something; you have to define what it means. Now, if you say that it's unconsciousness, then the unconsciousness depends on the CO_2 much more than the PO_2 because that determines how much blood goes to the brain. Because the vessels of the brain are sensitive to PCO_2 and probably via pH again; these two are always coupled. So I think the critical PO_2 in whole man really needs definition before you put some kind of number down and say now I know what critical PO_2 is.

Unidentified Speaker: I think you have to talk about individual organs too.

Unidentified Speaker: We have heard quite a lot about the metabolic regulation of DPG levels but I think it is unclear until now why ATP increases, taking into account that the pH maximum for ATP concentration is about 7.2.

Dr. Lenfant· I am not certain that I can answer this particular question; perhaps Dr. Torrance can. But I can tell you that in all of these conditions that we have discussed we found an increase in ATP, although always to a much lesser extent than for DPG.

Dr. Loos: In 1959 Henderson and LePage (J. Biol. Chem. 234, 3219, 1959) published experiments of perfusing livers of mice with blood. The mice had been preinjected with adenine-8-C^{14}, so the livers were loaded with adenine-8-C^{14} labelled nucleotides; when these livers were perfused with blood, adenine-8-C^{14} could be isolated from the erythrocytic ATP-pool of this blood. They found also that when a non-labelled mouse liver was perfused with blood with a labelled erythrocytic ATP-pool, adenine-8-C^{14} could be isolated from the liver nucleotides. From these experiments they concluded that the total adeninenucleotide pool in red cells is in a dynamic state; somewhere in the circulation adenine is taken from extra-erythrocytic pools and elsewhere it is given to extraerythrocytic pools. Recently Syllm-Rapoport et al. (Blood, 33, 617, 1969) confirmed this postulation for the human circulation.

Dr. Garby: This problem, I think might be very interesting to study. What is the correction to be used with respect to pH and temperature for cells that do not have a normal DPG content? You are using the correction factors, I suppose by Severinghaus and coworkers for temperature and for pH. You are using them also for red cells which are deficient in DPG.

Dr. Lenfant: Well, for pH we use ours. The way our oxygen dissociation curve determination is set up we get the Bohr effect and therefore we use our own corrections. Now for temperature, I'm a bit concerned, here, which temperature you are talking about. I mean I don't see where the temperature change you are concerned with fits.

Dr. Garby: I'm sorry; in your experiments it doesn't matter, but there are other experiments where you might encounter temperature differences.

DISCUSSION OF PAPER BY FAULKNER ET AL.

Unidentified Speaker: What happens to DPG after exercise? How long is it before the DPG returns to resting levels?

Unidentified Speaker: At the University of Pennsylvania we have studied a number of patients at various work loads. The lactate level stays elevated but the DPG level returns to normal. Is this not contradictory to your data?

Dr. Faulkner: I do not recognize any cause and effect relationship between the lactate concentration and the DPG concentration. At different time periods in submaximum work we have also seen them vary independently.

Dr. Garby: Are you certain that your DPG method is independent of the lactate concentration?

Dr. Brewer: Yes, the DPG method is independent of lactate.

Unidentified Speaker: What was the physical condition of these subjects?

Dr. Faulkner: In the 50 min tests we had 5 trained and 5 untrained subjects. Because the trained subjects appeared to have a more stereotyped DPG response in exercise we used 4 highly trained subjects in the 10 min tests.

Unidentified Speaker: You mentioned the measurement of pH in Mitchell's study. Did you measure pH?

Dr. Faulkner: We measured the pH in the blood of the antecubital vein before and during the 50 min ride on the bicycle ergometer. The very slight decrease was not significant. We did not measure the pH during the 10 min tests.

Unidentified Speaker: In the maximum exercise tests of Mitchell there was a very dramatic drop in pH, wasn't there?

Dr. Faulkner: Yes, the pH in the brachial artery was 7.4 and the pH in the femoral vein was 7.12.

Unidentified Speaker: Right. Now do you have any idea what could be called the mean red cell pH in exercise compared to that at rest? This would be important in terms of what Dr. Astrup discussed earlier. This would have to do with the pH of all the red blood cells in the system and would also involve the possibility that there is a different condition of blood in the arterial system compared to the venous system when one exercises. Have you any information on that?

Dr. Faulkner: The pH, oxygen tension, and carbon dioxide tension are very different in the venous blood compared to the arterial blood in maximum exercise. There is also a change in the amount of blood in different parts of the system. In exercise, there is constriction of the capacity vessels and an opening up of capillaries in the contracting muscle.

Unidentified Speaker: Right. I have always imagined that the blood that was sitting around in the veins loafing at rest would be brought into the picture. Would Dr. Astrup have any comments on this because it does not fit his pH theory?

Dr. Astrup: As far as I can see the pH changes cannot explain the changes in DPG you have found. I would also say that during very short periods of maximal exercise the pH of the blood does not change very much because lactic acid is released into the blood and this stimulates respiration. The enormous increase in ventilation keeps the pH within quite normal limits. We have measured this.

Dr. Faulkner: Our subjects had minute ventilations of over 100 liters/min during the maximum oxygen uptake test.

Dr. Astrup: So the pH did not change very much and neither did the pH in the red cells.

Dr. Lenfant: I just would like to mention here two experiments we have done in the area of what you are talking about. One day we took a blood sample from a subject who had been running on a treadmill for an hour or so. After about $1\frac{1}{2}$ hour we found an increase in DPG which was quite significant, about 40%, and a shift in the oxygen dissociation curve giving a P_{50} of 31 mm Hg. (In our lab the normal is about 26.6 mm Hg.). The other experiment might bring more confusion than anything else. Dr. Shappel in our hospital has been collecting some samples from the coronary sinus in subjects who were paced to the point of angina; in these people he found an increase in lactic acid, no change in DPG, but a shift in the oxygen dissociation curve. In this case there is some kind of discrepancy between all these parameters.

Dr. Rørth: I have a slide. These are patients from a coronary unit being trained after hospital care. We have measured the venous oxygen saturation in the pulmonary artery before and after 20 minutes submaximum work, and we found no consistent change in DPG. Perhaps you could find a significant increase in P_{50}?

Dr. Lenfant: I've got to say in respect to the changes in P_{50}

that they are very small. But we have 8 subjects and all have increased their P_{50} during pacing. We feel that it is a significant change.

Dr. Faulkner: Dr. Rorth, what was the intensity of exercise?

Dr. Rørth: Oh, I cannot remember that for sure; these were coronary patients with different exercise tolerances.

Dr. Faulkner: Could you give me any idea was it on a bicycle ergometer?

Dr. Rørth: Yes.

Dr. Faulkner: You don't know what the work load was? Because this would be crucial; that is, if you work people at very low work loads, the DPG does not change at all, even if you work them for hours.

Dr. Rørth: But what I would like to point out is the lack of correlation between venous oxygen saturation and the DPG levels because it seems to me that one has been looking at the DPG level as being regulated by the venous oxygen saturation, and that cannot be the case.

Unidentified Speaker: Did you measure the pH?

Dr. Rørth: Yes, pH and standard bicarbonate also were measured and there was no constant changes.

Dr. Horejsi: I would like to ask a question. Is there any information about the distribution pattern of lactate dehydrogenase isoenzymes in these white and red muscles? And my second question: Is there any change of isoenzymes of lactate dehydrogenase pattern after severe exercise and in trained people?

Dr. Faulkner: In answer to your first question, yes, there are different LDH isozymes in red and white muscle. The LDH-1 isozyme predominates in red muscle cells and LDH-5 predominates in white muscle cells. I don't know of any data on changes in isozymes with acute exposures to exercise. Goluch and his associates (1961) have shown an increase in LDH activity in heart muscle with training and Moger and his associates (1968) have observed a decrease in H-subunit and an increase in M-subunit during adaptation to hypoxia.

DISCUSSION OF PAPER BY METCALFE AND DHINDSA

<u>Dr. Harkness</u>: We have been partly responsible for the notion that caprine erythrocytes contain no 2,3-DPG. We were unable to demonstrate this compound in the red cells of the goat using the column and chemical methods of Bartlett. Using the enzymatic methods of Grisolia and coworkers, we have subsequently found a range of 0.06-0.15 umoles 2,3-DPG per ml of cells. Furthermore, the activities of both the enzyme responsible for its synthesis, diphosphoglyceric acid mutase, and the specific 2,3-DPG phosphatase are only 1-2% of the levels in human red cells.

This amount of 2,3-DPG is nevertheless several-fold greater than the K_m of the purified caprine erythrocytic PGA mutase for this cofactor. The PGA mutases of human and caprine erythrocytes are, in fact, similar in every respect studied.

<u>Dr. Metcalfe</u>: I think the only comment that I should make is that apparently goat hemoglobin is sensitive to 2,3-DPG; that is, if you add DPG, the dissociation curve of goat hemoglobin shifts, and you have to use it in the same amount as in the human to cause the same amount of shift.

<u>Unidentified Speaker</u>: What kind of dogs were you using?

<u>Dr. Metcalfe</u>: These were mongrels. The new ones are all Labradors and I hope that we'll either get a pure population or at least a definable one, and then we can see if it's breed related. That's certainly one of the things that occurred to us.

<u>Unidentified Speaker</u>: This suggests again a genetic regulation of DPG, perhaps.

<u>Dr. Metcalfe</u>: Yes, that's a possibility.

<u>Dr. Filley</u>: Dr. Metcalfe, I was particularly impressed when you said that the purpose of oxygen transport was to deliver oxygen at a rate <u>just great enough</u>. Now the implication would be in part, that it's uneconomical to deliver it at any higher rate because it is energy-expensive. What about the very practical problem that is now arising in clinical medicine with regard to the other reason why you don't want it any more than just great enough, namely oxygen toxicity from too high a PO_2? I mention this because if the answer is ever going to come it's not going to come from the pathologists looking at the possible thickenings of the lung, but from the biochemist who is going to tell us under what chemical conditions too much oxygen is bad. The clinicians are not getting very far with this problem of oxygen toxicity. So I put this out as a point for discussion, because in addition to wasting oxygen transport economy in this parsimonious way that you speak of, also

maybe it's bad to have more than a certain amount.

Dr. Metcalfe: Yes, in fact I meant to imply that it's bad. It seems to me clearly demonstrable that any increase in environmental oxygen pressure is resisted by the organism just as decreases in environmental oxygen are. Bartels in his lecture in the Lancet (2,599-604, 19 Sept., 1964) pointed out that we have really all evolved, perhaps with the exception of the llama and a few others, in an atmosphere which requires about the same kind of transport mechanism to the tissue capillaries so that cells are supplied at a pO_2 of 3 or so. They don't want any more; they don't want any less, but they also don't want any more. As clinicians we all seem to act as though if a little oxygen's good a lot of oxygen's better, and I think that's something we mustn't fall into.

Dr. Lenfant: We have an interesting observation in fish in regard to what you just said about adaptation for survival. The bottom feeding sharks have a low hematocrit and a curve which is very much shifted to the left as shown by a P_{50} of 10 mm Hg. But on the other hand, the Bonito shark which is a very fast swimmer (as a matter of fact if you keep it from swimming it dies from asphyxia) has a hemoglobin concentration of about 18 and a P_{50} of about 25 mm Hg which is extremely high for a fish. I believe that it is indeed related to their survival; they need such adapted blood properties because of their feeding habits. They feed from tuna fish, and therefore they have to swim very fast.

EDITOR'S NOTE: The recording of the discussions of the following
session was particularly incomplete. Thus, the shortness or
absence of these discussions is due to technical problems and not
due to a lack of interesting and enthusiastic interchange.

DISCUSSION OF PAPER BY BARTLETT

Dr. Harkness: We have published similar data on the organic
phosphates of the erythrocytes of several of these same species
and others. We also observed that feline erythrocytes contain very
little 2,3-DPG. Rapaport and Guest in 1941 using acid stable
phosphate as a measure of 2,3-DPG content also reported low 2,3-
DPG in the domestic cat.

Dr. Bartlett: Why do you think this is so?

Dr. Harkness: I assume that as is the case in the goat and the
sheep that animals with low 2,3-DPG in the erythrocyte have a
hemoglobin with a low enough affinity for oxygen that a cofactor
for deoxygenation is not required to adequately oxygenate the
tissues. I don't specifically have information about the oxygen
dissociation curve of feline hemoglobin.

Dr Kitchen: The cat has two hemoglobins as demonstrated by
electrophoresis and there is a quantitative difference in the two
electrophoretically distinguishable components.

Dr. Harkness: Yes, but what about the oxygen dissociation curves
of these hemoglobins?

Dr. Kitchen: I don't know, but I believe it is published in
Biochim. Biophys. Res. Comm. by B. Sullivan.

Unidentified Speaker: The P_{50} for oxygen of cat hemoglobin is 36.

DISCUSSION OF PAPER BY DERN

Dr. Shafer: Did red cell survival correlate as well with the fall
in ATP during storage as with the final ATP levels

Dr. Dern: No. While there was a good correlation between final
ATP and red cell survival, there was a poor correlation between
poststorage survival and both initial ATP and, as expected from
this, with the rate of fall of ATP. It now appears that poststorage ATP levels may be determined by two separate hereditary
mechanisms. A man's prestorage or inherent ATP level appears to
be controlled by a hereditary mechanism, as shown by Brewer some
time ago, and it also appears that there may be a secondary
mechanism, also inherited, which determines how fast an individual's
ATP level will fall during storage. The final ATP, therefore, is
a function of an individual's initial ATP level and his rate of
ATP decay. Our attempts to develop a test to permit prediction
of the rate of fall in advance have been unsuccessful. Because
of the variability we've encountered, we have just about given up
on this problem.

Dr. Bartlett: Has anyone ever done a survival study like this?
Incubate fresh blood without substrate, that is without glucose,
to run down the level of ATP. Actually, there are two different
types of things that one could do. One could run down the ATP
level fairly rapidly, or one could run down total adenine nucleotides. If the ATP level falls to less than 1/3 of the original,
the survival of these cells when transfused should give a better
idea if it is only ATP level that is critical. It's beginning
to look as if stored cells require a certain size pool of ATP
in order for it to survive a few circulations until it can
rejuvenate itself.

Dr. Dern: I do not know of any studies of this kind that have
been done. We have started making estimates of how fast the ATP
runs down on incubation without glucose, but have proceeded no
further.

Dr. Brewer: I was rather impressed by your differences in
survival with mixing and nonmixing. At least in one set of
experiments, storage seemed quite superior when mixed. Was the
mean ATP level different with the mixed compared to the unmixed
samples?

Dr. Dern: May I make one point clear. The survival is actually
not superior in the mixed, but rather very poor in unmixed
samples. I think that this point is critical. It does not appear to be a blood banking problem. Apparently, the occasional
mixing that occurs in routine blood banking situations is almost

as good as continuously mixing throughout the storage period. To
answer your question, the ATP level in mixed samples was
invariably higher when compared to the unmixed samples. In fact,
with respect to the individual data, the ATP and cell survival
data for both mixed and nonmixed samples fit the regression curve
that was shown.

DISCUSSION OF PAPER BY LOOS AND PRINS

<u>Dr. Bartlett</u>: An interesting question which has already been men-
tioned concerns whether a hemoglobin complex of DPG enzymatically is
active within the red cell and in the analytical procedure described
here which uses hemolysates. How much of the DPG is complexed to
hemoglobin in these hemolysates?

<u>Dr. Loos</u>: I have no idea about the rate of splitting of the DPG-
hemoglobin complex but I guess that in a 27,000-fold dilution it
would be split completely; moreover it should be noticed that the
dilution is made with 1 mM NH_4OH, especially with the intention to
split the DPG-hemoglobin complex, as at alkaline pH the dissociation
of the complex is promoted.

<u>Dr. Loos</u>: Dr. Bartlett, I have a delayed comment on your paper if it
is allowed. You told us that the compound glucose-1,6-diP is a
characteristic feature of red cells. We found about 0.08 umole
glucose-1,6-diP per 10^{10} human lymphocytes.

<u>Dr. Bartlett</u>: That's a pretty good amount. I think that is very
interesting because we looked at quite a number of rabbit tissues -
liver, kidney, brain, lung, heart, and up and down the intestinal
tract - and we were unable to find any glucose or mannose diphosphate
in any where near these amounts. There was a small amount in the
skeletal muscle. That was the only place we could find it. A
colleague in our laboratory has been working for the past few years
on granulocytes and he has found glucose and mannose diphosphate in
these cells. We have also found some DPG in granulocytes apparently
not due to red cell contamination. In our rabbit tissue experiments
we have not seen any DPG in any tissue except that which could be
accounted for by the contamination with red cells. I think you
have told me that you have also found some DPG in lymphocytes?

<u>Dr. Loos</u>: Yes, I found also about 0.16 umole 2,3-DPG per 10^{10}
human lymphocytes.

<u>Dr. Loos</u>: (In response to a further question about the effects of
various diluents on results.) I should have mentioned this before
but I did all the work together with Dr. Prins and actually he was
the one who suggested the use of lysates instead of extracts. In
our first experiments we diluted the blood with water instead of
1 mM NH_4OH; we found some indications that a relation occurred between the oxygenation of the blood and the amount of DPG which was
found in the lysates. To avoid any influence of the blood oxygenation on the DPG-level in our assay system we decided to dilute with
1 mM ammonia instead of using water.

<u>Dr. Harkness</u>: In the experiments on regeneration of 2,3-DPG in
depleted defibrinated blood using Mg^{++}, pyruvate, and adenosine

was it necessary to add the Mg^{++}? In other words is there enough Mg^{++} in the cell for maximal rates of reaccumulation?

Dr. Loos: I don't know. We should have done that control. We only did this experiment the past week!

DISCUSSION OF PAPER BY VALERI

Dr. Miller: This is certainly a very pressing problem for transfusion in general and in particular in the transfusion of the individual in an acute hypoxic emergency who requires a lot of blood. It seems to me that when you need a lot of blood the time change is extremely important, because you need to get that oxygen to the tissue in seconds. Is the DPG content critical, and how rapidly does the rise come in DPG? So any kind of data that we can get on this is extremely important and we need much more.

Dr. Brewer: The correlations you report between DPG and red cell mass deficit seems to me to be a more sensitive way of studying the correlation Eaton and I reported some time back between hemoglobin and DPG (Proc. Nat. Acad. Sci. 61, 756, 1968).
    I wonder if it would be appropriate to consider recommending to blood banks that we use certain kinds of blood for certain kinds of patients: fresh blood for the more acutely ill patients, and older blood, for example, for the chronic anemia type patient who is well stabilized and has plenty of time to build up his DPG?

Dr. Valeri: That is a very pertinent suggestion. A blood bank certainly has to consider these things. These are really the problems that we will eventually have to face.

Dr. deVerdier: I would like to comment a little about the resynthesis of DPG. In collaboration with Drs. O. Akerblom, L. Garby and C. Hogman at the University Hospital, Uppsala the resynthesis of DPG was studied in ACD-adenine stored erythrocytes after reentry into the circulation. The results obtained so far indicate that the synthesis of DPG is slower in cells stored for 35 days than in cells stored for 12 days. The storage dependency on the rate of resynthesis ought to be further investigated.

Unidentified Speaker: How much actual difference is it going to make in the transfer of oxygen from hemoglobin to the tissue, if you have no DPG, or practically no DPG, as compared to the normal level.

Unidentified Speaker: I think that from calculations from the shift of the curve the change expected theoretically is comparable to the results that have been found.

Dr. Brewer: I was quite interested in your creatine results. Do you have any further information about that? Does creatine have any effect on the dissociation curve?

Dr. Valeri: We are very excited about red cell creatine. We have observed that creatine has no effect on the oxyhemoglobin dissociation curve in vitro. Altschule has discussed an earlier observation that patients with cardiac decompensation usually have creatinuria and that the creatinuria regresses with clinical improvement. We tend to think that red cell creatine is a very sensitive indicator of tissue hypoxia because in all conditions where we see elevated red cell 2,3-DPG creatine is also increased. The mechanism for the elevated creatine may be increased permeability of red cells to creatine released from hypoxic tissue. Our speculation is that creatine may be related to the red cell membrane function. I would appreciate further comments concerning the elevated creatine observed in red cells.

Dr. Garby: Do you know of the paper, I think 2 years ago, in which somebody reported that there was an extremely good correlation between creatine and age of red cells? In most of the patients that you reported here I think that there was no question that the mean red cell age was lower, so that I was not so very excited about your creatine findings.

Dr. Valeri: We are aware of the paper of Griffiths and Fitzpatrick. These investigators reported very high reticulocyte counts. In our patients only slight increases in reticulocyte counts were observed and it is our opinion that the reticulocytosis cannot account for elevated red cell creatine levels.

DISCUSSION OF PAPER BY DAWSON

<u>Dr. Bartlett</u>:   Do some of you hemoglobin specialists have a comment
on this?

<u>Dr. Garby</u>:   Did you say that the right-hand shift induced after
sodium chloride persisted <u>in vivo</u>?

<u>Dr. Dawson</u>:   This is what Valtis & Kennedy said, I haven't done
this. This was only produced <u>in vitro</u> in my studies. Valtis &
Kennedy did theirs <u>in vivo</u>. They transfused the blood and saw
that the effect persisted.

<u>Dr. Garby</u>:   Do you have an explanation for that because the salt
should diffuse out, shouldn't it?

<u>Dr. Dawson</u>:   We have no explanation .

<u>Dr. Dawson</u>:   (in response to a question regarding availability of
products with a high salt content) I was asking someone in a
discussion last night whether saline solutions with concentrations
higher than physiologic are available and approved for intravenous
use. And I think there are some, or at least one. I'd like to
know what they are. It could be that this effect, a shift to the
right of the oxygen dissociation curve, may result from a decrease
in the intracellular pH. I have not yet measured the intracellular pH in the salt studies. A large part of my understanding
of this phenomenon has come from discussions with Dr. Norman
Fortier. I suspect that the pH is lower, at least he explained
to me that with each of these salts the pH could be lower. I was
looking for this kind of explanation because the chloride concentration in the red cell increases only with the chloride solutions
and large increases in MCHC occur only with the sodium-potassium
salts. Also, data which I didn't present, on the chloride salts
of lithium, cesium, and choline, show the same effect as sodium
chloride.

<u>Dr. Loos</u>:   With respect to the pH changes which might occur after
addition to the cells, the ammonium chloride addition certainly
would do this. I am using ammonium chloride as a lysing agent
for my red cells in the preparation of lymphocytes, and I did
some experiments to find the optimal conditions for that. In your
experiments how much lysis occurred with the ammonium chloride?

<u>Dr. Dawson</u>:   There is a small amount or increase in the plasma
hemoglobin and it is the only increase that was obtained with the
salts used. The plasma hemoglobin of control blood was 24-25 mg %
and this increased from 33.3 to 33.9 with ammonium chloride.
The sodium chloride, potassium chloride, and sodium acetate did not

cause an increase in plasma hemoglobin.

Unidentified Speaker: So you added the ammonium chloride in addition to the plasma, so you made it hypertonic?

Dr. Dawson: I'm not sure it's that hypertonic. The MCHC values with ammonium chloride decreased only very slightly; I'm not sure it's significant, from control of 30.8 to 28.2.

Unidentified Speaker: How soon after addition of the salts is the effect seen?

Dr. Dawson: This occurs certainly in all the experiments within 2 hours because we usually complete the experiments within an hour and certainly within 2 hours.

Dr. deVerdier: During this Symposium we have only been discussing the effect of DPG and ATP on the oxygen-hemoglobin dissociation curve. Under artificial conditions as blood storage other phosphocompounds may reach molar concentrations equivalent to that of hemoglobin and may thus exert an effect on the affinity of hemoglobin to oxygen. A study of the effect of inosine on stored red blood cells (C.-H. deVerdier, O. Akerblom, L. Garby and C. Hogman: Int. Symp. Modern Problems of Blood Preservation. March 17th - 18th, 1969 Frankfurt) was extended by the same investigators to include also freshly drawn erythrocytes. In these the concentration of DPG increased only slightly whereas fructose 1,6-diphosphate (FDP) went up to about the same molar level as DPG (Fig. 1). Addition of FDP and DPG to stripped hemoglobin revealed a shift of the oxygen dissociation curve to the right for both substances. According to these preliminary results DPG had a somewhat more pronounced effect on the oxygen affinity than FDP.

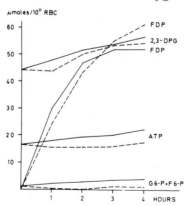

Figure 1.